£6.00

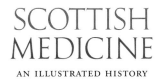

SCOTTISH MEDICINE

AN ILLUSTRATED HISTORY

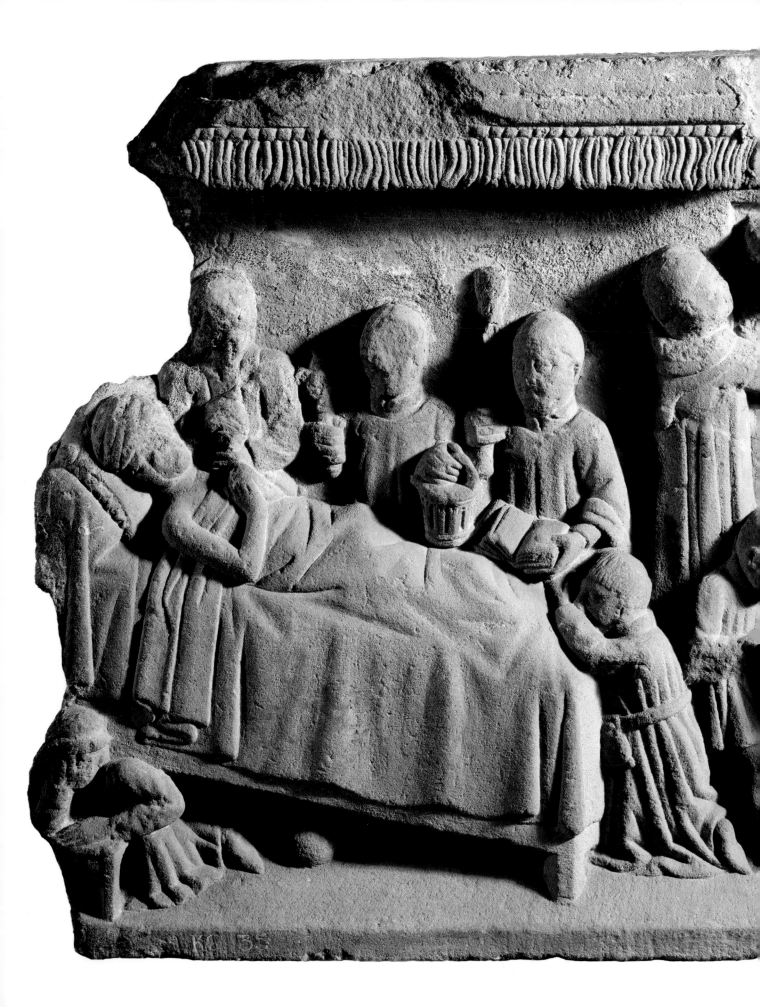

SCOTTISH MEDICINE

AN ILLUSTRATED HISTORY

Helen Dingwall,

David Hamilton,

Iain Macintyre,

Morrice McCrae

and

David Wright

BIRLINN

First published in 2011 by
BIRLINN LIMITED
West Newington House
10 Newington Road
Edinburgh
EH9 1QS

www.birlinn.co.uk

ISBN: 978 1 78027 018 0

British Library Cataloguing-in-Publication Data
A catalogue record for this book is available from the British Library

Designed and typeset by Mark Blackadder

Printed and bound in Malta by Gutenberg Press Ltd.

CONTENTS

———

ABBREVIATIONS

ASH	Action on Smoking and Health
BMA	British Medical Association
EMS	Emergency Medical Scheme
EUL	Edinburgh University Library
FPSG	Faculty of Physicians and Surgeons of Glasgow
GCS	Glasgow Coma Scale
GUL	Glasgow University Library
HIMS	Highlands and Islands Medical Service
IMR	Infant Mortality Rate
LHSA	Lothian Health Services Archive
MOH	Medical Officer of Health
NHS	National Health Service
RCPE	Royal College of Physicians of Edinburgh
RCSEd	Royal College of Surgeons of Edinburgh
RCPSG	Royal College of Physicians and Surgeons of Glasgow
RMS	Royal Medical Society
SSHM	Scottish Society of the History of Medicine
SWH	Scottish Women's Hospitals

FOREWORD

Scotland has made a remarkable, rich contribution to medicine, health care and medical education, both within its borders and further afield. At the start of the twenty-first century it is appropriate that this wealth of experience and expertise should be reassessed and updated. Medicine in Scotland has not remained isolated but has drawn on the developments and discoveries in other places, and learned from these, while at the same time exerting a major influence on health care across the world.

One aspect of medical history which has always fascinated me is the way in which the focus of experience and expertise has moved around the world. Western medicine provides a good example. Beginning in Salerno in the twelfth century, then moving to Bologna, Padua, Montpellier, Paris, Leiden, Edinburgh, Paris, Berlin, and Glasgow by the late nineteenth century and thence to the USA and beyond, the centres of excellence have travelled across the continents. These 'medical magnets' have been the places to go to learn the newest techniques and developments and work with the world's best. Edinburgh was the key 'medical magnet' in the late eighteenth century. It was an exciting place, full of remarkable people and ideas, in philosophy and in the arts as well as the sciences and medicine, which drew people from all over the world to learn. The Edinburgh Medical School had been built on the experience of medical education in Leiden, and Edinburgh itself was then overtaken by Paris. Why? What factors caused this rise and fall, and can we learn from them? What are the characteristics of 'medical magnets'?

The outstanding medical teachers in these centres were usually innovators. They took a different path and made others think differently. This change in direction could be related to a new discovery, technique, or procedure, diagnostic test, research programme or a new way of presenting knowledge. They also had connections, often a world-wide network of contacts, which allowed them to correspond with like minds wherever they happened to be in the world. Many travelled widely and knew other leading figures personally.

They were also passionate about their subject and enjoyed passing on their learning. They enthused and inspired, and were interested in their students, in whose development they would take a personal interest. As a result they had many disciples and acolytes who would travel across the world carrying the messages and knowledge of each master, enhancing his reputation and strengthening the bonds between centres. The stories of those from Scotland are presented and highlighted in this book.

In more recent times those involved in health care have tended to work in teams, a process begun by societies that were formed to bring people together to share experiences. Teams were often formed by colleagues of equal distinction who created an environment which was conducive to new thinking, a milieu which encouraged different ways of approaching a problem. In some instances the external environment was especially favourable, as in the case of the Hunter brothers in London, who were able to fill the vacuum resulting from the small number of medical graduates from Oxford and Cambridge at the time.

Yet it is the more recent history of medicine in Scotland which now, more than ever, deserves to be recorded and reviewed. From the inception of the National Health

Service in 1948, the medical, nursing and allied professions have been part of a huge experiment in how best to deliver medical care and health services to a national population. It has been a remarkable success, but over the last 60 years there have been successive changes, which continue. Two additional factors make the position even more complex. The first is the enormous advances which have occurred in clinical practice. These, in the lifetime of those writing this book, have transformed the possibilities of care and treatment available to patients. The second factor is the advent of devolution in Scotland and the creation of a Scottish Parliament in 1998. This has meant that the National Health Service in Scotland (always slightly different from that in England) has been able to develop further its own particular characteristics, and has moved progressively away from the style of the NHS in England.

Throughout this long and distinguished history of medicine in Scotland, the health of the public has provided the focus of attention. Currently health in Scotland is poorer than that in England in almost all indices. This is especially true in some parts of west central Scotland. Why should this be the case when Scotland has produced so much in medical terms? There are many factors which determine health: the environment, social and economic factors, lifestyle, genetic and biological influences and health services. Yet it is the last which may well be least important in improving public health. Scotland's poor health record will hopefully be rescued, but it will take a considerable effort, not all of it by the medical profession.

Books like this are invaluable, not only because they chronicle and illustrate events, but because they provide the basis on which to interpret the reasons for change and to learn from the outcome. History then provides a framework for creating policy. The future of medical care, as in other walks of life, depends to a large extent on our understanding of the past, making this book all the more relevant.

SIR KENNETH CALMAN
Chairman, National Trust for Scotland
Chancellor, University of Glasgow
2011

INTRODUCTION

Over the centuries Scotland has played an outstanding role in world medicine. While histories of Scottish medicine have been produced in the last three decades, it is now more than 75 years since the last fully *illustrated* history was published. J. D. Comrie's *History of Scottish Medicine* (1932) is a masterly book, but it is very much a product of its time, emphasising the history of great doctors and great institutions while paying relatively little attention to their political, social and cultural context. Since then, there have been remarkable advances in medical science and healthcare, with techniques of investigation and treatment advancing beyond what could have been imagined in the 1930s. These advances have been accompanied by a great increase in public interest in matters relating to health and a new blossoming in the study and scholarship of the history of medicine. For all these reasons a new book seems well justified.

Why a history of Scottish rather than British medicine? Medicine in Scotland has an ethos and traditions of its own. History has shaped the development of medicine in ways that are distinctive from those of her European and British neighbours. The emphasis on education became apparent in Scotland in pre-Reformation times, when four universities served a tiny nation, an emphasis that was later enhanced by the Reformers' aim to have a school in every parish. From the beginning medical education was made open to members of almost every section of Scottish society. Scottish medicine has never been elitist, and Scottish medical schools have always sought to pay due attention not only to the health of the individual patient but also the health of the community. As a result of the breadth of the curriculum offered, students were attracted from every part of the English-speaking world. For many generations Scottish-trained doctors have chosen to make their careers in every part of Britain, her Empire and beyond, often in some form of public service. One of the aims of this book is to illustrate the ways in which Scottish medicine, wherever practised, has been and remains distinctive.

By making illustrations a core feature of the book, we hope to make the history of medicine attractive to a public accustomed, now more than ever, to receiving information supported by images that enhance and elucidate the message. Wherever possible we have made use of the work of Scottish artists and photographers, and Scottish subjects, using not only images from collections in Scotland but also relevant works from elsewhere. We have aimed to make effective use of captions by including, where relevant, some interpretation of the meaning and symbolism of the images. In this way we hope that, wherever possible, each image can tell a story in its own right and be able to stand independently from the text, while remaining integral to the overall narrative.

As the book is intended primarily for a general readership, we have avoided technical terms and medical jargon as far as possible. And rather than providing detailed footnotes or references, we have compiled a comprehensive, thematic bibliography to allow further study of the plentiful written sources which are now available. Relevant sources are now increasingly accessible through the internet and we have therefore included a list of websites where further information and more illustrations can be studied.

We have tried throughout to portray the history of

medicine in the social and political context in which it took place. To facilitate this we have included a timeline which places events in world and Scottish history and world and Scottish medicine in their chronological context. Before the mid-twentieth century, the focus of medical history was largely concerned with great doctors, institutions and discoveries. Since then, as medical history has developed, there has been an increasing emphasis on portraying medicine from the patient's perspective, and we have tried to describe Scottish medicine as it has affected the patient or consumer.

Each of the five main chapters has been written by a different author, but we have attempted to ensure that core themes are covered in all chapters. Each author covers a chronological period, but the boundaries between chapters are flexible in order to allow aspects of some major themes to be discussed in the most appropriate places in the book.

This is not a comprehensive history of Scottish medicine and does not claim to be. It does not, for example, cover dentistry, nursing, and the paramedical professions. We hope, nonetheless, that it offers new information, new insights and new perspectives on medical history in a small, complex, fascinating country, where the importance of medicine was, and remains, out of all proportion to its size.

ACKNOWLEDGEMENTS

———

This book was made possible by generous financial support from the Royal College of Surgeons of Edinburgh, the Royal College of Physicians of Edinburgh, the Royal College of Physicians and Surgeons of Glasgow, the Scottish Society of the History of Medicine, the Carnegie Trust for the Universities of Scotland and the Russell Trust.

The Royal College of Surgeons of Edinburgh also provided rooms, allowing the authors to meet regularly over the two-year period when the book was being planned and written. We are grateful to Siabhan Doughty of the College's finance department who looked after the finances of the project.

We received help from many librarians and archivists, too numerous to list here, but we would like to thank in particular the following, all of whom provided material and images from their organisations at no cost to the project: Iain Milne and Estela Dukan at RCPE; Marianne Smith and Steve Kerr at RCSEd; Carol Parry at RCPSG; Anna Smith and Venita Paul at Wellcome Library, London.

Malcolm MacCallum, the Partnership Manager of the Scotland & Medicine partnership, contacted the partners on our behalf and, as a result of this approach, many of the partners provided images at no cost or reduced cost. It is a pleasure to acknowledge their generosity.

We are grateful for the advice and help from John Burnett, Caroline Wickham-Jones and Mary Kemp Clarke. Malcolm Nicolson took on the onerous task of reading the manuscript and provided a wealth of constructive comments and suggestions.

High quality illustration is a core feature of the book and we were keen to commission new art work from young artists. Our thanks to Susie Wright and Dave Morrow, who provided reconstructions of historical scenes, and to Allan Shedlock for photography.

At Birlinn Tom Johnstone cheerfully and patiently took on the unenviable task of dealing with five authors. He guided the project from its inception, and was always available for help and advice. We gratefully acknowledge too the input of Neville Moir, of the book designers Jim Hutcheson and Mark Blackadder, and of Jan Rutherford, Kenny Redpath and Sarah Morrison who arranged the publicity.

Finally it is a pleasure to acknowledge the many other organisations that provided images at no cost or reduced cost, who are acknowledged in full in the list of picture credits.

WORLD HISTORY

Alexander the Great, (356–323BC), invaded Asia

Foundation of Christianity (33AD)

Main Roman invasion of Britain started (43AD)

Rise of Mayan Civilisation (c300AD)

Anglo-Saxons invade Britain (450AD)

WORLD MEDICINE

Doctrine of humours expounded by Empedocles

Hippocrates (460–377BC)

Greek physicians came to Rome

Sophisticated surgical techniques described
in India (Susruta Samhita)

De Medicina by Celsus

Dioscorides (c40–c90AD) (His De Materia Medica
provided detailed descriptions of medicinal plants)

Galen (129–c216AD) Left a major body of work and ideas
which influenced western medicine for many centuries

Plague in Rome kills 5000 (c250–265AD)

WORLD HISTORY

Early domestication of plants and animals (9000BC)

First towns and cities developing in the
Middle East (c4000BC)

Civilisation in China (1600BC)

Foundation of Rome (763BC)

Alexandrian School (mid-second century AD)

WORLD MEDICINE

Codex Hammurabi created in Babylon (c1790BC)

Traditional Chinese medicine established

Edwin Smith and Ebers papyri created describing medical and
surgical procedures in Egypt (c1600–1550BC)

Medicine described as the 'noble' art by Homer

WORLD HISTORY

Byzantine conquest of North Africa (535)

Birth of prophet Mohammed (570)

Muslim invasion of Spain (711)

WORLD MEDICINE

Spread of Greek Medicine into Arabic world

Plague in Europe (669)

Al-Razi (Rhazes) (865–925)

Ibn Sina (Avicenna) (980–1037)

10000BC–500BC | 500BC–500AD | 500–1000

SCOTTISH HISTORY

Colonisation of Scotland after the last Ice Age (c9000)

Hunter gatherers (roasted hazelnuts, shell middens) (c6000)

Neolithic village at Skara Brae in Orkney (c3000)

Bronze Age settlement (c2200)

Climate deteriorated following eruption
of Hekla in Iceland (c1159)

Iron Age farmers (c700)

SCOTTISH MEDICINE

Archaeological evidence of trepanning.
(Bronze Age skull, Bute) (c2000)

SCOTTISH HISTORY

Roman victory at Battle of Mons Graupius (c84AD)

Building of Antonine Wall (c143AD)

St Ninian's Christian mission at Whithorn (c397AD)

SCOTTISH MEDICINE

Druidic and Pictish medicine used
plants in conjunction with ritual.

Evidence of Roman medicine,
surgery and surgical instruments

Healing wells and objects used,
including charms, stones and amulets

SCOTTISH HISTORY

St Columba's monastery founded at Iona (563)

St Cuthbert (c684–687)

Battle of Dunnichen (685)

Town of St Andrews founded by 747

Iona burned by Vikings (802)

Death of Kenneth McAlpine, union of
Scots and Picts (858)

SCOTTISH MEDICINE

Early Christian medicine including bloodletting

Holy wells visited by pilgrims seeking healing

Saintly relics used for cures

Leech Book of Bald (early 10th century)

TIMELINE

This timeline is intended to provide a more
general, global background context to the
detailed coverage of Scottish medicine within
the main text of the book. It is selective,
and arranged by time period in four main
sections – World History, World Medicine,
Scottish History and Scottish Medicine.

1000–1200

WORLD HISTORY
Norman Conquest of Britain (1066)

Crusades (1095–1291)

Domesday book compiled in England (1086)

WORLD MEDICINE
Foundation of Medical School at Montpelier (c1137)

Medical School at Salerno in Italy (1050)

Arabic and Greek medical texts translated into Latin

Edict of Pope Innocent III limiting the involvement of the clergy in medical practice (1163) *Ecclesia abhorret a sanguine*

SCOTTISH HISTORY
David I introduces feudal system (1124)

Somerled defeated by Scottish king in Battle of Renfrew (1164)

SCOTTISH MEDICINE
Flourishing of monastic medicine and medieval hospitals

Gaelic medical manuscripts with translations of Hippocrates and Galen

Michael Scot, churchman and physician (1175–1232)

1200–1400

WORLD HISTORY
Inca dynasty founded (1200)

Signing of Magna Carta in England (1215)

Genghis Khan invades Russia (1223)

Marco Polo reaches China (1275)

Kublai Khan invades Japan (1281)

Ming dynasty founded in China (1368)

WORLD MEDICINE
University of Padua founded (1222)

Mansuri Hospital founded in Cairo (1284)

Europe devastated by Great Plague (1346–7)

SCOTTISH HISTORY
Southern border of Scotland established by Treaty (1237)

Western Isles ceded to Scotland by Norway in Treaty of Perth (1266)

Battle of Stirling Bridge (1297)

Defeat of English at Bannockburn (1314)

Declaration of Arbroath (1320)

Robert II becomes second Stewart king (1371)

SCOTTISH MEDICINE
Edward I treated at Torphichen Priory after the battle of Falkirk (1298)

Arrival of Black Death in Scotland (1350)

1400–1600

WORLD HISTORY
Johan Gutenberg used type for printing (1440–55)

Fall of Constantinople (1453)

New World discovered by Columbus (1492)

Reformation in Northern Europe (from 1517)

Copernicus described rotation of earth around the sun (1543)

Circumnavigation of world by Francis Drake (1577–80)

WORLD MEDICINE
Syphilis epidemic in Europe (1496–1500)

Influenza pandemic in Europe (1510)

Founding charter of Royal College of Physicians given to London physicians by Henry VIII (1518)

Paracelsus burns works of Galen (1527)

Publication of Andreas Vesalius' *De Fabrica Humani Corporis* (1543)

Ambroise Paré published treatise on surgery including treatment of wounds (1580s)

Invention of microscope by Jansen (1590)

SCOTTISH HISTORY
Foundation of St Andrews University (1412)

Foundation of Glasgow University (1451)

Orkney and Shetland annexed to Scotland (1472)

Archbishopric of St Andrews erected (1472)

Foundation of Aberdeen University (1495)

First printed book in Scotland (1508)

George Wishart burnt at the stake for heresy (1546)

Reformation in Scotland (from 1560)

Death of George Buchanan, humanist (1581)

Foundation of Edinburgh University (1583)

Execution of Mary, Queen of Scots (1587)

SCOTTISH MEDICINE
James IV (1473–1513) patronised science and medicine

Act for isolation of syphilis (grandgore) patients (1497)

Seal of Cause founding Incorporation of Surgeons and Barbers of Edinburgh (1505) (ratified by James IV in 1506)

Edict for treatment of lepers in Edinburgh (1528)

Surgeons exempted from bearing arms in battle (1567)

Publication of Gilbert Skeyne's *Ane Breve Descriptioun of the Pest* (1568)

Faculty of Physicians and Surgeons of Glasgow founded (1599)

WORLD HISTORY

Gunpowder Plot in English Parliament (1605)

First English settlement in America (1607)

Bacon publishes *Novum Organum* describing scientific method (1620)

Newton explains gravity (1687)

WORLD MEDICINE

William Harvey describes circulation of blood (1616)

Society of Apothecaries of London founded (1617)

Publication of Harvey's *De Motu Cordis* (1628)

Royal Society of London founded (1660)

Publication of Robert Hooke's *Micrographia* (1665)

Thomas Sydenham attempts to classify diseases (1670s)

Royal College of Physicians of Ireland founded (1667)

Observation of bacteria by Leeuwenhoek (1683)

WORLD HISTORY

Robert Walpole appointed first British Prime Minister (1721)

Steam engine developed from Newcomen model by James Watt (1765)

James Cook lands in Australia (1770)

Slavery declared illegal in Britain (1772)

American Revolution (1776)

French Revolution (1789)

WORLD MEDICINE

Hermann Boerhaave appointed Professor of Medicine at University of Leiden (1714) and establishes clinical teaching there.

First appendicectomy performed by Claudius Aymand (1736)

First hospital in United States founded (1752)

Linnaeus' classification of diseases (1763)

John Hunter's *Treatise on the Blood, Inflammation, and Gunshot Wounds* (1794).

Edward Jenner develops vaccination for smallpox (1796)

WORLD HISTORY

First national census in Britain (1801)

Start of Napoleonic Wars (1803)

Potato famine in Europe (1840s)

Revolutions in Europe (1848)

WORLD MEDICINE

Foundation of Royal College of Surgeons of England (Company of Surgeons from 1745) (1800)

Ephraim McDowall performs first elective abdominal operation (1809)

Stethoscope invented by Laennec (1816)

Isolation of alkaloids from plants (1817)

First issue of *The Lancet* (1823)

Foundation of British Medical Association (1832)

Anatomy Act in Britain (1832)

Public demonstration of ether as an anaesthetic in Boston (1846)

Ignaz Semmelweiss publishes on principles of asepsis (1849)

Elizabeth Blackwell gains first MD by female, in America (1849)

1600–1700   1700–1800   1800–1850

SCOTTISH HISTORY

Union of crowns of Scotland and England (1603) under James VI and I (1567-1625)

National Covenant (1638)

Execution of Charles I (1649)

Cromwell becomes Lord Protector (1654)

Restoration of monarchy (1660)

Publication of first Scottish newspaper, Mercurius Caledonius (1661)

First Glasgow to Edinburgh coach service (1678)

Order of Thistle founded by James VII (1687)

Crown offered to William and Mary (1689)

Presbyterian church settlement, making Presbyterianism the state church in Scotland (1690)

Foundation of Bank of Scotland (1695)

SCOTTISH MEDICINE

Incorporation of Surgeons and Barbers founded in Glasgow (1656)

Foundation of Royal College of Physicians of Edinburgh (1681)

Publication of first edition of *Edinburgh Pharmacopoeia* (1699)

SCOTTISH HISTORY

Union of parliaments of Scotland and England (1707)

Jacobite Rebellion (1715)

David Hume's *Treatise on Human Nature* (1739)

Jacobite Rebellion (1745)

Battle of Culloden (1746)

Discovery of 'fixed air' (carbon dioxide) by Joseph Black (1754)

Birth of Robert Burns (1759)

Adam Smith's *Wealth of Nations* (1776)

First *Statistical Account* of Scotland (1791–8)

SCOTTISH MEDICINE

First Chair of Medicine at Glasgow University (1714)

Separation of barbers and surgeons in Edinburgh and Glasgow (1722)

Foundation of Medical School at Edinburgh University (1726)

Opening of first infirmary in Edinburgh (1729)

Opening of Royal Infirmary in Edinburgh (1741)

Opening of infirmary in Aberdeen (1742)

Lind experiments on treatment of scurvy (1747)

Start of clinical teaching in Edinburgh by John Rutherford (1748)

Incorporation of Surgeons of Edinburgh becomes Royal College (1778)

Foundation of Montrose Royal Asylum (first such institution) (1781)

Andrew Duncan launches appeal for Lunatic Asylum (1790)

Foundation of Glasgow Royal Infirmary (1774)

SCOTTISH HISTORY

Highland Clearances

First edition of *Scotsman* newspaper (1817)

First commercial railway from Edinburgh to Dalkeith (1826)

Burke and Hare Trial (1828)

Disruption of Church of Scotland (1843)

Poor Law (Scotland) Amendment Act (1845)

Potato famine in highlands and islands (1846–9)

Tay Bridge disaster (1879)

SCOTTISH MEDICINE

Foundation of Anderson's Institution (later College) in Glasgow (1800)

Birth of James Young Simpson (1811)

Act to Regulate Madhouses in Scotland (1815)

Cholera epidemic (1832)

Outbreaks of typhoid and typhus (1842)

Poor Law (Scotland) Amendment Act (1845)

Robert Liston performs first operation in Britain under ether (1846)

David Livingstone's African travels (1840s/50s)

First use of chloroform as anaesthetic by James Young Simpson (1847)

Royal Commission on Lunatic Asylums (1855)

Nuisance Removal Acts (1850s)

Great Exhibition in London (1851)

Crimean War (1853–6)

American Civil War (1861)

Discovery of wireless telegraphy by Marconi (1895)

Boer War (1899–1902)

● WORLD MEDICINE
Medical Act and foundation of General Medical
Council in Britain (1858)

Louis Pasteur proves that putrefaction caused by germs (1861)

International Red Cross founded (1864)

Sophia Jex-Blake enters Edinburgh University as
first British female medical student (1869)

Isolation of tubercle bacillus by Koch (1882)

Immunisation for anthrax, cholera and rabies (1880s)

Discovery of X-Rays by Röentgen (1895)

● WORLD HISTORY
Death of Queen Victoria (1901)

First powered flight by Wright brothers (1903)
Suffragette movement founded in Britain (1903)

Sinking of Titanic (1912)

Easter Rising in Dublin (1916)

World War I (1914–18)

Theory of Relativity published by Albert Einstein (1916)

● WORLD MEDICINE
Blood transfusion enabled after elucidation
of blood groups (1901)

First ECG recording made by Eindhoven (1902)

Introduction of barbiturates (1903)
Marie Curie publishes on radioactive substances (1903),
becomes first female Nobel Laureate

Harold Gillies establishes unit for facial
surgery during World War I

Influenza pandemic kills an estimated 50 million people (1918–20)

1850–1900

1900–1920

● SCOTTISH HISTORY
Nuisance Removal Acts (1850s)

Tay Bridge disaster (1879)

Crofters Act (1886)

Opening of Forth Rail Bridge (1890)

● SCOTTISH MEDICINE
Act for Regulation of Care of Lunatics (1857)

Joseph Lister appointed Professor of Surgery at Glasgow (1861)

Henry Littlejohn appointed Medical Officer of
Health in Edinburgh (1862)

Public Health (Scotland) Act (1867)
Lister publishes first papers on antiseptic surgery (1867)

Dentists Act (1878)

Foundation of Edinburgh Hospital for Women and Children (1885)

First medical research laboratory established by Royal
College of Physicians of Edinburgh (1887)
Treatment for tuberculosis by Sir Robert Philip (1887)
Opening of Edinburgh School of Medicine for Women (1887)

Foundation of School of Medicine of the
Royal Colleges in Edinburgh (1895)

First clinical X-Ray Department in the
world in Glasgow Royal Infirmary (1896)

Public Health (Scotland) Act (1897)

● SCOTTISH HISTORY
First Ibrox disaster (1902)

Royal Commission on the Poor (1905)

National Insurance Act (1911)

Glasgow rent strikes (1915)

'Bloody Friday' riot in Glasgow (1919)

First television pictures transmitted by Logie Baird (1926)

● SCOTTISH MEDICINE
Milk Depots set up (1902)

Royal Commission on Physical Training (1902)

Foundation of Glasgow Hospital for Women (1903)

Dewar Committee established (1912)

Highlands and Islands Medical Service (1913)

Mental Deficiency and Lunacy Act (Scotland) (1913)

Operation of Scottish Women's hospitals (WWI)

WORLD HISTORY

Soviet Union established (1922)

General strike in Britain (1926)

Wall Street Crash (1929)

Adolf Hitler takes power in Germany (1933)

Mao Tse Tung long march (1935)

Spanish Civil war (1936–38)

World War II (1939–45)

WORLD MEDICINE

Family Planning Clinic opened by Marie Stopes (1921)
Discovery of insulin (1921)

Discovery of Vitamin D (1922)

Discovery of penicillin by Fleming (1929)

BCG vaccination for tuberculosis introduced (1924)

Anti-malarial drugs introduced (1932)

ECT used to treat depression

Sulphonamides introduced (1935)
First leucotomy performed by Muniz (1935)

First kidney dialysis machine invented (1938)

WORLD HISTORY

Atomic bombs dropped on Hiroshima and Nagasaki (1945)

Start of Korean War (1950)

Treaty of Rome, founding the European
Economic Community (EEC) (1957)
Sputnik 1 satellite launched by Soviet Union (1957)

WORLD MEDICINE

Clinical use of penicillin (1941)

Contraceptive pill developed by Pincus (1951)

Heart-lung pump used for open cardiac surgery (1953)
Structure of DNA elucidated by Wilkins, Crick and Watson (1953)

Psychotropic drugs given for mental illness

Salk develops polio vaccine (1955)

DDT used for treatment of malaria

Polio and diphtheria vaccinations introduced in UK (1958)

1920–1940

1940–1960

SCOTTISH HISTORY
Paisley cinema fire (1929)

Evacuation of St Kilda (1930)

Foundation of Scottish National Party (SNP) (1934)

Empire Exhibition (1938)

Sinking of Royal Oak in Scapa Flow (1939)

SCOTTISH MEDICINE
Macleod and Banting awarded Nobel Prize for
Medicine for their work on insulin (1923)

Morbidity Statistics Scheme (1930)

Cathcart Report (1936)

Emergency Hospital Service established (1939)

SCOTTISH HISTORY
Blitz on Clydebank (1941)

SNP first victory in Motherwell by-election (1945)

First Edinburgh International Festival (1947)

Last hanging in Scotland (1953)

Dounreay nuclear power station opened (1957)

SCOTTISH MEDICINE
Construction of Emergency Medical Scheme Hospitals (1940s)

Polish School of Medicine opened at Edinburgh University (1941)

Beveridge Report (1942)
Clyde Basin Experiment (1942)

National Health Service (1948)
First randomised controlled trial published by
Crofton on use of Streptomycin in TB (1948)

Opening of Sighthill Health Centre, Edinburgh (1953)

Triple therapy for tuberculosis introduced (1950s)

Alexander Todd awarded Nobel Prize for work on Vitamin B12 (1957)
Publication of key paper on ultrasound by Ian Donald (1957)

WORLD HISTORY
Cultural Revolution in China (1966–76)

Cuban missile crisis (1962)

First man on moon (1967)

Britain joined EEC (1972)

Yom Kippur war and oil crisis (1973)

WORLD MEDICINE
Dame Cicely Saunders pioneers hospice movement (1967)
First heart transplant performed by Christiaan Barnard (1967)
Introduction of beta blockers (1960s)

Abortion Act (1970)

CAT scanners developed (1970s)

Louise Brown, first test-tube baby born (1978)
Last cases of smallpox in Britain (1978)

Royal Commission on NHS reports (1979)

Revived popularity of herbal medicines in the West

Eradication of smallpox worldwide (1980)

WORLD HISTORY
Personal computers introduced (1981)

Falklands War (1982)

Fall of Berlin Wall (1989)

First Gulf War (1990)

Break-up of Soviet Union (1991)
Liberation of Kuwait (1991)

Bosnian conflict (1992)

Treaty of Maastricht renamed EEC as
European Community (EC) (1993)

Invasion of Iraq (2003)

WORLD MEDICINE
Magnetic Resonance Imaging (MRI scans) developed (1977)

First clinical account of AIDS (1981)

Development of minimal access (keyhole) surgery (1980s)

MMR immunisation introduced in UK (1988)

Introduction of new drug classes, including statins
and H2 receptor antagonists

Anti-retrovirals introduced to combat HIV/AIDS (from mid-1980s)

1960–1980

1980–PRESENT

SCOTTISH HISTORY
Discovery of North Sea Oil (1965)

Ordination of women allowed by
Church of Scotland (1968)

Second Ibrox Park disaster (1971)

Local Government (Scotland) Act (1974)

Devolution Referendum fails to meet
required majority (1979)

SCOTTISH MEDICINE
First Chair of General Practice in the world
established at Edinburgh University (1963)

R D Laing begins therapeutic
community psychiatry (1964)
Aberdeen typhoid epidemic (1964)

Establishment of Scottish Health
Education Unit (1968)

Foundation of Scottish Council for
Postgraduate Medical Education (1970)

Glasgow Coma Scale (1974)

SCOTTISH HISTORY
Lockerbie disaster (1988)

Stone of Destiny returned to Scotland (1996)

Second devolution Referendum, majority in favour (1997)

Scottish parliament reconvened (1999)

Closure of last Scottish deep coal mine (2002)

Opening of New Scottish Parliament Building (2004)

Scottish National Party forms minority government (2007)

Calman report on devolution (2009)

SCOTTISH MEDICINE
Black Report on Social inequality (1980)
SHAPE Report on mental health/care of elderly (1980)

Vaccine against Hepatitis B developed by Murray (1982)

Forrest report recommends screening for breast cancer (1986)

Sir James Black awarded Nobel Prize for Physiology or Medicine (1988)

Start of care in the community for mental health (1990s)

Establishment of Scottish Intercollegiate Guidelines Network (1993)
Clean Air Act (1993)
Calman report on training of Hospital doctors (1993)

Cloning of Dolly the sheep. Team led by Ian Wilmutt (1996)
E-Coli outbreak in Wishaw (1996)
Opening of first Maggie's Centre in Edinburgh (1996)

European Working Time Directive (2004)
Establishment of NHS24 (2004)

Ban on public smoking (2005)

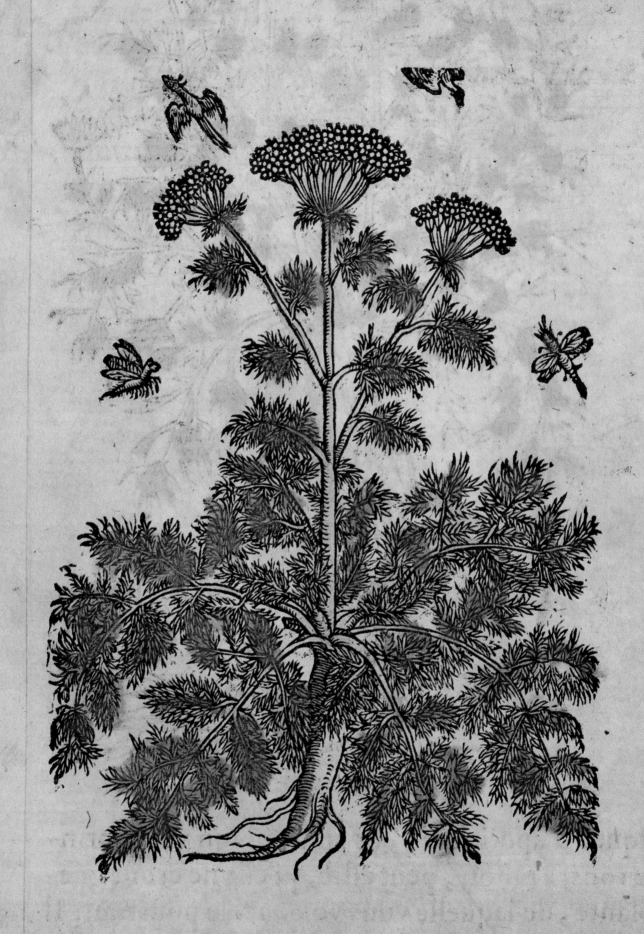

CHAPTER ONE

NOMAD TO NATION, NATION TO REFORMATION

David Wright

————

In the year 1350, there was in the kingdom of Scotland,
so great a pestilence and plague among men, (which also
prevailed for a great many years before and after, in divers
parts of the world – nay, all over the whole earth) as, from the
beginning of the world even unto modern times, had never
been heard by man, nor is found in books, for the enlightenment of those who come after. For, to such a pitch did that
plague wreck its cruel spite, that nearly a third of mankind
were thereby made to pay the debt of nature.

JOHN OF FORDUN
(before 1360–*c*1384), *Chronicle of the Scottish Nation*
(p 358 in the 1871 translation by WS Skene)

————

O Lord! that is to mankynd hail succure,
Preserve us fra this perrelus pestilens.

[O Lord, who is mankind's entire and only help,
Preserve us from this perilous pestilence.]

ROBERT HENRYSON
(*c*1450–1505), *Ane Prayer for the Pest*

INTRODUCTION

This chapter spans more than ten thousand years, from the Ice Age to the Reformation, and it traces the beginnings of medicine from the accumulated knowledge of scattered small family groups. It has been possible to identify challenges to health and ideas about the causation of disease and to describe the healers and remedies available to those who were unwell. The country now known as Scotland did not exist at the beginning of this period. Its development involved battles and power struggles and its boundaries changed considerably. By the end of the period its future structure was becoming clearer.

Henry Home (Lord Kames, 1696–1782), the eighteenth-century Scottish philosopher, described four stages in man's development, from hunter-gatherers to herders of domesticated animals, then through organised agriculture with villages and farms to the final stage of urban development with towns. This is a helpful concept, though there may be variation in different places and under different conditions.

As communities formed and grew, they realised the advantages of working together efficiently and discovered the benefits of mutual protection. However, larger populations led to pests, such as rats, and to the increasing presence of animal-derived micro-organisms. With these factors came an increased risk of epidemic disease, although exposure to disease also provided the potential to develop resistance.

The period is considered in two parts, because of its great length. The first starts when settlers began to colonise the land as the ice receded, and finishes around the end of the first millennium. The second part looks at the next five hundred years or so, as increasing pressures, particularly in towns, led to the development of strategies and structures that are recognisable today. The boundary between this chapter and the next is not clearly cut, as it is better to deal with some subjects in one chapter rather than in the other.

FROM NOMAD TO NATION

In the period to the end of the first millennium, a number of themes will be explored. These include the progression of man from survival on the move to life in a farming community, the introduction of metal for tools for agriculture and warfare, the consequences of the arrival of the Romans, the coming of Christianity, and the influences of the various peoples who contributed to the development of the country of Scotland.

In the earliest times there was no direct written record and much of the evidence comes from materials that have survived for centuries because of their ability to resist destruction. Stone in buildings and some metals, for example bronze, silver or gold, particularly when used in tools, can remain unchanged for thousands of years, particularly when under the soil or the sea. In general, animal and plant materials tend to deteriorate and leave little to be examined. Bones are more likely to be preserved than soft tissues, while seeds and nuts, if protected, may remain intact enough for identification. Pollen, particularly in samples of peat taken from bogs, may have survived unchanged for thousands of years.

Making the best use of such evidence includes knowing where to search, obtaining material without damaging it or its environment, and applying a wide range of modern investigative procedures, including carbon dating, microscopic analysis, DNA studies, pollen identification and sophisticated scanning techniques. New information continues to emerge as developing technology sheds more light. Buildings provide information about living conditions, skeletal remains about posture, trauma and disease, while the examination of traces of food and the analysis of pollen give clues to diet and lifestyle of hunter-gatherer or farmer.

The greatest threats to health during this period were warfare or famine, while at times epidemics of infectious disease had devastating effects. Knowing which plants were poisonous and which had a therapeutic effect may have made the difference between life and death. Fire brought benefits as well as hazards. It deterred predators, but it also made burns more likely. Heat from fire increased chances of surviving the cold and light allowed better visibility for man in the darkness. Cooking food shortened the time needed to eat it, allowing time for other activities by all members of the family, as well as making food safer to eat, more palatable and more easily absorbed. Preservation of food with salt or smoke may have made a critical difference between staying alive or starving to death.

Hunter-gatherers

Scotland began to be populated when conditions were free enough from ice to permit survival. Although the earliest evidence of human activity so far comes from a site at Biggar, between the Clyde and Tweed valleys, where stone tools have been found that have been dated to about 12,000 BC, many of the early dwelling sites that have been investigated archaeologically have been coastal.

Scotland's mainly acidic soils do not provide sufficiently good conditions to allow the preservation of much organic material, but, in sites near the sea, piles of shells, collected by the early inhabitants and known as shell middens, have provided conditions alkaline enough to preserve tools made of bone or antler. Most of the shells are limpets, and there is evidence that they were cooked, which would have helped to preserve them, as well as making them easier to eat. Apart from shellfish, bones from fish and from birds suggest other animal protein sources. Most plant food remnants have not survived, but investigation of an archaeological site on Colonsay has shown large numbers of hazelnut shells, which had been burned in order to cook and preserve the nuts. Also found were lesser celandine tubers, known to have been used by indigenous North American peoples.

Survival for early settlers would have been helped by their wide knowledge of the environment, of plants and animals and of the implications of seasonal changes. The people were hunter-gatherers. Movement from place to place was necessary to find food and to lessen the likelihood of local over-exploitation. Travel also provided access to a wider range of edible berries and nuts, leaves and roots. Birch and hazel trees gave wood and bark for a variety of uses, including shelters, baskets and weapons, as well as for fuel. Animals, which included deer and elk, gave food, skins and antlers, which could be used to make

tools. Other tools such as arrowheads, cutting edges and scrapers, were made from stone, particularly flint. Some of the stone artefacts came originally from other sites, illustrating the exchange of ideas and materials and the ability to travel overland and by sea.

Little is known about risks that existed and diseases that were present, because of the absence of human skeletal remains. Accidents, attacks by animals or exposure to cold and wind are likely to have been factors in shortening life expectation. While men may have had more involvement in hunting, women may have played a greater role in cooking and in identifying and gathering plants that were edible or useful, for such things as dyeing or drying for preservation. Familiarity with the use of plants to treat illness would have developed knowledge and skills which could be passed on orally from mother to daughter, increasing the importance of the role of women in the health of a community.

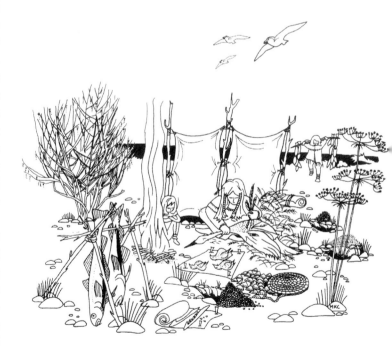

1.1 Reconstruction of a hunter-gatherer site at Crail, Fife. The sea is close, providing fish and shellfish. With the year well advanced, food, including birds, berries and seeds, is being prepared for cooking and preservation. The use of flint and bone for tools, of wood and hide for shelter and of wood for fire can also be seen (*Illustration by Mary Kemp Clarke*).

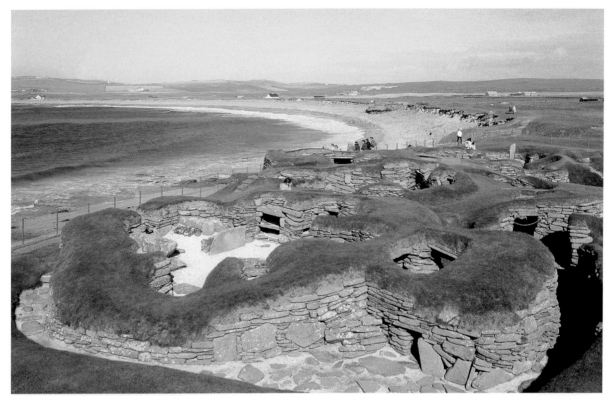

1.2 Skara Brae in Orkney. A storm in 1850 exposed ancient stone buildings, and subsequent excavations have shown eight houses separated by passages. Each house had beds, a fireplace and dressers, all made of stone, and an entrance which could be closed from inside. The beds on the right of each entrance were larger than those on the left, suggesting that the right side of the house was for the men and the left for the women. The houses were built into, and surrounded by, the midden, which acted as a shelter from the wind and provided insulation against the cold (© *Historic Scotland*).

Early Farmers

From around 4000 BC, nomadic hunter-gatherers in Scotland began to settle in communities. Trees were chopped down with stone axes and wood was burnt, with ash helping to make the ground more fertile. As time went on, the range of what was eaten decreased. While food came from a variety of sources, including wild plants, hunted animals and the sea, there was increasing reliance on crops such as early forms of wheat and barley, and domesticated animals such as sheep, goats and cattle. This required less travelling, but also meant that safe storage became necessary and therefore secure constructions began to appear. Where trees were not available, particularly on the islands in the north and west, stone was used for buildings.

Some of these stone buildings have survived, buried underground by blown sand, preserving artefacts and human remains, and these tell us something of the life at that time. Orkney has many such archaeological sites, dating from the period 3200–2200 BC, including the wonderfully preserved houses at Skara Brae and the cham-

bered cairn at Isbister. At Isbister, where extensive human remains have been found, the bones of 43 people reveal that most of them had been in their twenties, with only a few males reaching the age of 50. Their stature was very similar to late twentieth-century Orcadians, with an average height of 170cm (5 ft 7 in) for males and 162 cm (5 ft 4 in) for females. Though perhaps surprising, it is unclear to what extent these heights relate to diet or to genes. Some of the female skulls show forehead deformities, which suggest that they used head bands to help carry heavy weights.

Eggs of *Trichuris trichiura*, whipworm, a roundworm parasite of the bowel, have been found in material taken from the Skara Brae midden. Severe infestation with whipworm would have produced diarrhoea and anaemia. Two plant remains found in Skara Brae may have had medicinal uses. Fragments were discovered of the rhizome, or rootstalk, of yellow iris, which has been used, until recent times, in many civilizations as a purgative, or alternatively to stop diarrhoea, to stop bleeding, to relieve the

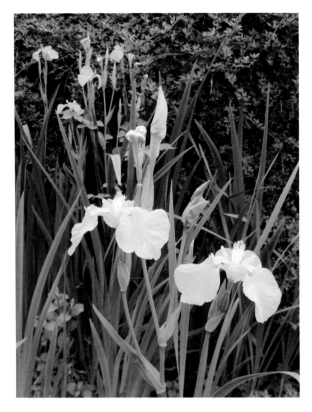

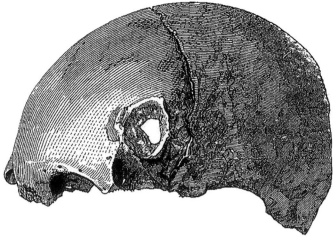

1.3 *Left*. Yellow Iris (also called Yellow Flag). This plant is found in wet meadows and ditches. In addition to the many medical uses of the rhizome described above, the leaves were used for thatching and for making a green dye (*Bron Wright*).

1.4 *Above*. Drawing of a Bronze Age skull. This shows a hole probably made by scraping with flint, in the procedure known as trepanning. The bone shows evidence of healing, indicating that there was survival, for some months at least, after the procedure. There is also a ridge around the hole, showing that there had been chronic infection (*From T.H. Bryce*, Proc. of Soc of Antiquaries of Scotland, *1903, 38 (14 December), p. 67*).

pain of toothache or a sore throat, as a constituent of poultices applied to wounds and, powdered and taken as snuff, to clear the blocked nose of a cold. Mature puffballs were also found, the fine powder from which has been used for centuries to stop bleeding from cuts, such as those inflicted by sharp surfaces.

The Use of Bronze and Iron
Around 2000 BC, objects made of metal began to appear. Bronze, an alloy of copper and tin, was hard and durable and could be cast into shapes to make tools, weapons and armour. Its introduction was associated with a change in burial practice, with communal burial chambers being replaced by single tombs or cists.

The incomplete skull in Fig. 1.4 is from the remains of a woman found in a cist on the island of Bute, showing what may be evidence of trepanning, where a hole has been made through the bone, probably with a flint tool. Trepanning has been found in many different parts of the world and may have been carried out in various circum-

stances, for example following unconsciousness due to a head injury or brain haemorrhage, after an epileptic fit, as a treatment for mental illness, or perhaps for superstitious reasons unrelated to ill-health.

The skeletal remains of a man in his sixties, found in another cist, at Boarhills in Fife, show a number of features which have medical significance. The teeth were very worn from eating food which was gritty and abrasive. The left hip shows evidence of chronic infection and signs of previous injury. There are signs of two wounds which had probably been fatal, one a crushing blow to the head, and the other a heavy stroke, probably from an axe, which had damaged the vertebrae in the neck, exposing and perhaps dividing the spinal cord.

Findings from a cave, occupied during this period, which was excavated in the 1930s, at Covesea, near Lossiemouth, Morayshire, included a number of skeletons of children who appeared to have been decapitated, but whether these were sacrificial victims, or they represented a ritual which occurred after death, is unclear.

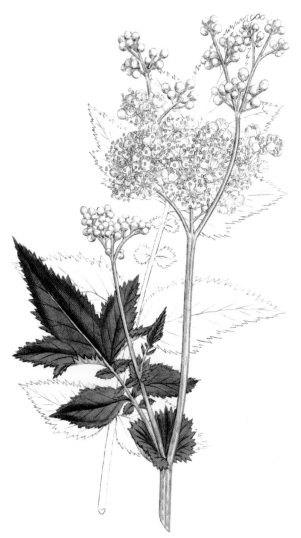

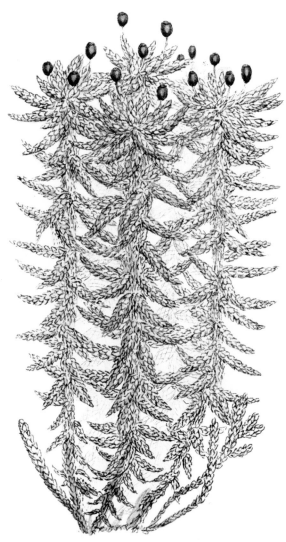

1.5 Illustration of Meadowsweet by James Sowerby (1757–1822). This plant grows in damp places and is likely to have been more common in the past than in modern times, when drainage for agriculture has led to a marked loss of wet grassland. In addition to its use in the making of mead, it has been used in the brewing of beer and for dyeing (© *Royal Botanic Garden, Edinburgh*).

1.6 Illustration of Sphagnum Moss by James Sowerby (1757–1822). This plant grows in very damp places, particularly in bogs, where it is a major constituent of peat. Mosses help to retain water in bogs by their great ability to absorb fluid, and this property has led to their being used by man in many circumstances, such as for wound dressings or in place of towels for drying or mopping up (© *Royal Botanic Garden, Edinburgh*).

A report on Bronze Age skeletons retrieved from 70 Scottish short cists over a period of many years showed a mean height of 171 cm (5 ft 7 in), (ranging from 157 cm to 178 cm), for men and 160 cm (5 ft 3 in), (ranging from 156 cm to 166 cm), for women, again similar to twentieth-century heights, although these remains may represent a group of privileged individuals with better nutrition and living conditions than were usual at the time.

The realisation, around 700 BC, that iron could be used to produce weapons and tools which were harder and more durable, brought further changes to the way that people lived. It became increasingly necessary to protect communities from sudden attacks. The tops of isolated hills developed into hill forts, protected by ditches and ridges. Brochs, massive stone towers, and crannogs, artificial islands in lochs providing a base for fortified towers on wooden stilts, were built for protection.

Health and Healing

Remains from Bronze Age burials have shown pollen grains of meadowsweet, heather and small leaved lime. One possible explanation for this is that they were in honey or in mead, an alcoholic drink made from fermented honey, which had been placed in the graves.

Pliny's Account of the Medicine of the Druids

Pliny's *Natural History* gave very detailed instructions on how the Druids gathered their medicinal herbs, showing how important the observation of ritual was to them.

> Care is taken to gather it [selago] without the use of iron, the right hand being passed for the purpose through the left sleeve of the tunic, as though the gatherer were in the act of committing a theft. The clothing too must be white, the feet bare and washed clean, and a sacrifice of bread and wine must be made before gathering it: it is carried also in a new napkin. The Druids of Gaul have pretended that this plant should be carried about the person as a preservative against accidents of all kinds, and that the smoke of it is extremely good for all maladies of the eyes.
> Pliny, *Natural History*, Book XXIV, section 6.

> The Druids, also, have given the name of 'samolus' to a certain plant which grows in humid localities. This too, they say, must be gathered fasting with the left hand, as a preservative against the maladies to which swine and cattle are subject. The person, too, who gathers it must be careful not to look behind him, nor must it be laid anywhere but in the troughs from which the cattle drink.
> Pliny, *Natural History*, Book XXIV, section 63.

Selago and samolus are thought to be the plants known now as *Selago huperzia* (Fir Clubmoss) and *Samolus valerandi* (Brookweed). Although their Latin names are suggestive, these were actually given by Linnaeus in the eighteenth century and were derived from traditional usage rather than the certainty that they were the plants described by Pliny.

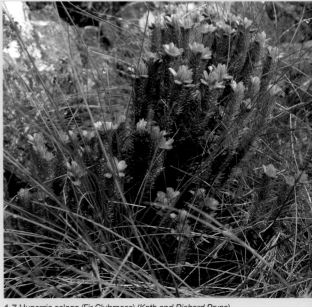

1.7 Huperzia selago (Fir Clubmoss) (*Kath and Richard Pryce*).

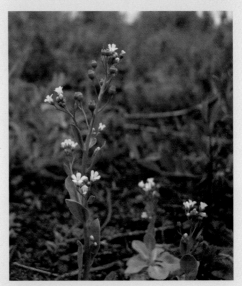

1.8 Samolus valerandi (Brookweed) (*Kath and Richard Pryce*).

Meadowsweet, whose name may relate to mead, was used to flavour drinks and also to relieve pain and reduce fevers. It contains salicylic acid derivatives, and the drug aspirin derives its name in part from *Spiraea ulmaria*, the original Latin name for meadowsweet. Sphagnum has also been found in burial cists. When dried, this moss was used for tinder, but another common use from ancient times has been in the dressing of wounds, and this has persisted, with collection on a national scale taking place in Scotland during the First and Second World Wars.

A stone storage compartment in an Iron Age broch, at Howe in Orkney, has yielded a charred seed from each

of three plants with medicinal properties, skull-cap, dead-nettle and sheep's sorrel. Skull-cap has anti-inflammatory properties, an infusion of dead-nettle has been used to treat burns and sheep's sorrel has been used to increase the flow of urine in urinary disease.

Burns and violent injuries would have been common. Skills in the dressing of wounds and in the treatment of illness, from minor problems such as colds, headaches and toothache, to major life-threatening disease, would have been passed on within family groups. Knowledge of plants and their use evolved over generations. Lack of improvement in the patient or dangerous side effects might lead

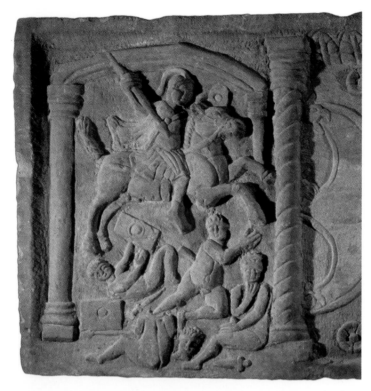

1.9 A carved Roman stone from the Antonine Wall found at Bridgeness, West Lothian. It shows an armoured Roman cavalryman attacking four less well-protected enemies, naked but with shields. One has a spear in his back, another has been beheaded and the other two look as though they will offer no resistance. Such images may have been used to demoralise those who might have considered opposing the might of Rome (© *National Museums Scotland*).

to rejection of the plant altogether, reduction of the amount used or use of a different part of the plant. Success could reinforce confidence in the plant, encourage further use and form the basis of what was, in essence, medical treatment.

The Romans in Britain

From the time of the Romans, there are written accounts of life in Britain (strictly, the geographical area that was to become Britain). However their accuracy is open to doubt, as some may have been based on hearsay and some may have sought to tell one side of a story for political purposes. In the years 83–84 AD, the Roman general Agricola fought against the Caledonian tribes under their leader Galgacus. Agricola's son-in-law, Tacitus, wrote a detailed account of Agricola's activities, which included a description of the battle of Mons Graupius, said by Tacitus to be north of the firths of Forth and Tay. According to Tacitus, before the battle the Caledonians had formed an alliance of tribes and commemorated this with rites and human sacrifices. Such human sacrifices were also described by Pliny, another Roman writer, who, in his *Natural History*, noted that these were carried out by the Druids, who he called *genus vatum medicorumque* [seers and healers]. Pliny also wrote that the Druids used various herbs such as selago and samolus. Selago (clubmoss) was used to protect against various sorts of accidents and, in

the form of smoke, for the treatment of eye complaints. Samolus (brookweed) was used to treat illness in cattle.

Although, by Tacitus's account, the Romans were successful against the Caledonians at the battle of Mons Graupius, over the next two centuries there were defeats as well as victories, and the frontier of the Roman Empire changed regularly. Hadrian's stone wall, built around 120 AD between the Tyne and the Solway, and the largely turf-built Antonine Wall of around 140 AD, between the Forth and the Clyde, still have enough of a presence to remind us tellingly of the power of Rome. However, their effects on the people to the north of the walls were relatively limited. By 163 AD there were only isolated camps north of Hadrian's Wall. There was another campaign in 208 by Septimius Severus, but this too became a lost cause after his death at Eboracum (York), in 211 AD.

The Roman author Herodian, who recorded Severus's campaign, has left us a vivid description of the land and its people.

Most of the regions of Britain are marshy, since they are flooded continually by the tides of the ocean; the barbarians are accustomed to swimming or wading through these waist-deep marsh pools; since they go about naked, they are unconcerned about muddying their bodies.

Strangers to clothing, the Britons wear

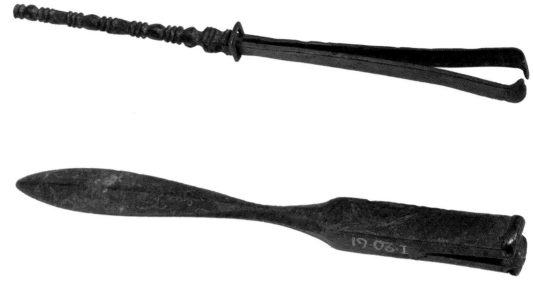

1.10 Bronze forceps, dating from between 140 and 210 AD, found at Cramond, near Edinburgh. The two opposing surfaces at the left end were pushed together, allowing objects, even small ones, to be firmly grasped (© *National Museums Scotland*).

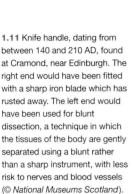

1.11 Knife handle, dating from between 140 and 210 AD, found at Cramond, near Edinburgh. The right end would have been fitted with a sharp iron blade which has rusted away. The left end would have been used for blunt dissection, a technique in which the tissues of the body are gently separated using a blunt rather than a sharp instrument, with less risk to nerves and blood vessels (© *National Museums Scotland*).

ornaments of iron at their waists and throats; considering iron a symbol of wealth, they value this metal as other barbarians value gold. They tattoo their bodies with coloured designs and drawings of all kinds of animals; for this reason they do not wear clothes, which would conceal the decorations on their bodies.

Extremely savage and warlike, they are armed only with a spear and a narrow shield, plus a sword that hangs suspended by a belt from their otherwise naked bodies. They do not use breast-plates or helmets, considering them encumbrances in crossing the marshes.

Herodian, *History of the Roman Empire since the Death of Marcus Aurelius*, Book 3, Section 14

Roman Medical Care

As well as the advantages of superior arms and communications, the Romans had a well organised system of health care, with sanitation in their living quarters and an efficient medical service, providing support in the field and transport to the hospital areas which were in the forts and fortresses. The fortress and temporary camp at Inchtuthil in Perthshire, probably constructed in the first

century AD, but never completed and only briefly occupied, demonstrates how sophisticated this could be. The hospital had two main wings, on either side of a central courtyard. Each wing had a central corridor, from either side of which there was access to patients' accommodation, which consisted of many small rooms. The design is remarkably similar to that of a modern hospital, in which cubicles have replaced open wards, in an effort to reduce cross infection.

Text books, such as those of Celsus, describe sophisticated surgery for wounds, and there have been several finds of surgical instruments, including a collection at Cramond, which dates from between 140 and 210 AD. Such instruments could have been used in a variety of circumstances. A forceps might have been used cosmetically, to grasp and remove eyelashes, or for medical reasons, to lessen damage to the eye if an eyelash was growing inwards.

Another interesting find, from Tranent in East Lothian, gives an insight into the relative sophistication of the organisation of Roman medicine. It is an inscribed stone stamp for Roman prescriptions. A different reversed inscription was carved on each side, to be used for pressing out the name of a treatment for eye problems, identifying a particular liquid or ointment whose details would have been known to the person making it up. Such eye salves were frequently described, for example in the writings of Marcellus and Scribonius Largus. One recipe, from the latter, contained pompholyx (an ash from smelting metal), myrrh, burnt copper, saffron, hematite (iron ore), opium and other ingredients, rubbed together and made up in Chian wine. Spikenard, a fragrant herb, was added to make it smell pleasant.

The fact that several of the Roman artefacts which have survived relate to conditions affecting the eyes may be significant, showing the importance of the eyes in many aspects of life.

Archaeological excavations of a Roman building at Bearsden, Glasgow, have shown various plant remains, such as common mallow, opium poppy and linseed, which may have had medicinal use. A fragment of an amphora, marked with an inscription denoting the medicinal plant horehound, was found at Carpow, a fort on the south of the Firth of Tay. This suggests that the amphora had been used for the storage of wine which contained horehound. Such preparations were used for the treatment of coughs and chest problems, and were recommended by the Greek author Dioscorides (author of the best known early pharmacopoeia, *De Materia Medica*, dating from 50–90 AD).

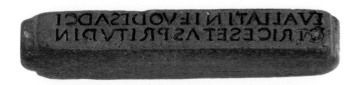

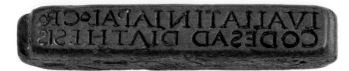

1.12 L VALLATINI APALOCROCODES AD DIATHESIS
[The mild crocodes of Lucius Vallatinus, for affections of the eyes] (An eye salve which was based on crocuses)

1.13 L VALLATINI EVODES AD CICATRICES ET ASPRITUDINES
[The evodes of Lucius Vallatinus for cicatrices and granulations] (An aromatic application used to reduce or prevent scarring of the eyelids)

1.12 and **1.13** Two sides of a steatite Roman prescription stamp, found at Tranent, East Lothian. Note that the writing is reversed, as the stamps were used to make impressions on wax or clay. The stamps named two different eye salves. Directions for making these up would have been widely known, so that they could be made locally if the ingredients were available (© *National Museums Scotland*).

Analysis of excavated material from a sewage-filled ditch at the Bearsden site has given insights into Roman diet, bowel parasites and hygiene. Remains of food included fragments of lentils, field beans and the cereal crops, emmer and spelt, together with seeds from raspberry, bramble, bilberry and wild strawberry. Eggs of the whipworm, *Trichuris trichiura*, and the roundworm, *Ascaris lumbricoides*, were found. The Romans usually used marine sponges for cleanliness in latrines, but these would have been difficult to obtain locally, and the finding of mossy material in the ditch suggests that this may very well have been used instead.

The End of Roman Influence

After the death of Severus, the Romans fought no more major campaigns in Scotland, though there are frequent records of incursions into areas they controlled from the northern tribes, particularly the Picts in 297 AD and the Picts and Scots in 367. By 411 the Romans had left Britain for good. Their influence in Scotland was mixed. Their presence had been intermittent and was mainly as an army of occupation, although during 400 years there must at times have been significant interaction with the local population. The Romans left behind knowledge of medicinal plants and the plants themselves, which may have persisted for many centuries, adding to the eclectic mixture of influences which has over the centuries, contributed to 'Scottish' medicine.

William Camden, writing in the sixteenth century about Hadrian's Wall in Cumberland, noted:

There continueth a settled perswasion among a great part of the people there about, and the same received by tradition, that the Roman souldiers of the marches did plant heere every where in old time for their use certaine medicinable herbes for to cure wounds, whence it is that some Empiricke practitioners of Chirurgery in Scotland flocke hither every yeere in the beginning of summer to gather such Simples and wound herbes, the vertue whereof they highly commend as found by long experience, and to be of singular efficacie.

The Life of the Picts

The Picts have left no written record of their history and there is some debate among historians as to who they were, where they came from and where they were located. Some of the knowledge that we have of them comes from encounters described by Romans or later by Anglo-Saxons such as Bede. Living in the area to the north of the Forth and Clyde, they have left striking carved stones which give insight into the way they lived. Images of sheep and goats show that the Picts were agricultural, that they hunted bear, deer and boar and that they fished for salmon. They must also have spent much time fighting, as images of men on horseback, in armour and protected with shields and helmets, show. Weapons included spears, swords and bows and arrows; and injuries, such as fractures and perforating wounds of the chest and abdomen, would have been common.

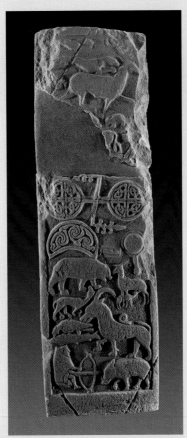

1.14 The Drosten Stone, St Vigeans, Angus. This is a Pictish carved stone, dating from the ninth century, which shows sheep, goat, bear, a raven and a salmon and an archer about to shoot a boar with bow and arrow. The stone is displayed in the recently refurbished museum in the village of St Vigeans in Angus (© RCAHMS).

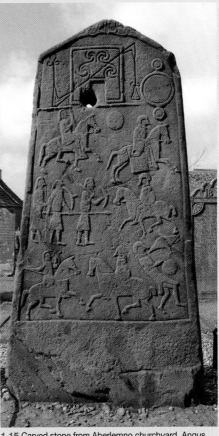

1.15 Carved stone from Aberlemno churchyard, Angus. The stone probably dates from the eighth or ninth centuries, and may commemorate the battle of Dun Nechtain, or Nechtansmere, when the Picts defeated the Northumbrians in 685 AD. It shows soldiers on foot and on horseback, protected by helmets and round shields with sharp bosses and armed with spears and swords (© RCAHMS).

From the Fifth to the Tenth Centuries

The peoples of the north of Britain, in the centuries after the Romans left, came from a number of origins. They were partly the descendants of the tribes that existed before the Romans arrived, and partly invaders from the west and the south east. Initially, the Picts occupied the area north of the Forth and Clyde and the Britons were in the south. By the fifth century, a kingdom of Gaels from the north of Ireland had been established in Argyll, and from the seventh to the tenth centuries, the Angles moved up from the south east. In the Western and Northern Isles and on the east coast, from the ninth century onwards, there were Norse influences, which in some parts lasted for centuries. Information about health, disease, medicines or healers in this period comes partly from written evidence, particularly from Bede and Adamnan, and partly from archaeological evidence, from sites which can be identified with the different cultures.

Early Christian Saints

Christianity had been adopted by the Romans during the fourth century and, according to tradition, existed in south west Scotland from the fifth century, associated with St Ninian and Whithorn, in Galloway. Bede's *Ecclesiastical History of the English People*, admittedly written several hundred years later, recorded brief details of St Ninian,

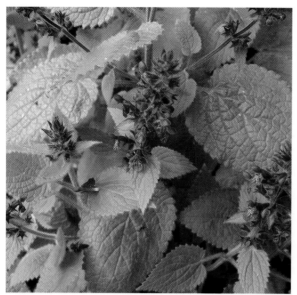

1.16 Marsh woundwort. The leaves were used to make poultices which were applied to wounds to help healing. Some of the compounds obtained from the plant have antiseptic properties. The plant has a distinctive unpleasant smell when a leaf is rubbed between the fingers, and this may have helped in its easy identification (*David Wright*).

who brought Christianity to the southern Picts. Archaeological investigation of the early monastery at Whithorn that existed from the fifth century showed seeds of coriander, dill, black mustard, bramble, nettle, woundwort, elder and hemlock. Apart from the use of these plants in either cooking or dyeing, they also had medicinal uses. Although they may have been collected in the wild, their presence may indicate that some or all were grown deliberately.

Bede also wrote of the life of St Columba, who came from Ireland and founded a monastery on Iona in 563. Adamnan, the ninth Abbot of Iona, who wrote a *Life of St Columba*, gave more details of the work and health of the community. The settlement on Iona had a hospitium, where travellers and pilgrims could be accommodated and those who were ill could be looked after. The monks had a gardener, Laisran Mocumoie, and grew herbs which were presumably used in the making of medicines. Adamnan records that problems such as nosebleeds and fractures were dealt with very practically, though Columba and his followers probably considered illness as resulting from failure to behave in a Christian way. Bede's *Life of St Cuthbert* (635–687) records the existence of healers (called leches, see text box), who treated the sick. However, Bede emphasised that St Cuthbert was able to cure cases that the leches and their medicine were unable to help. The implication of this was that he was an agent of God. This

view of disease, that it was due to divine displeasure and that divine intervention was necessary for restoring health, persisted for hundreds of years. It had the effect of lessening the influence of earlier, more rational ideas about causation and treatment and it inhibited the development of new ways of thinking about health and illness.

Another notable feature of the early centuries of Christianity was that sources of water, which for thousands of years had had a special significance, became associated with Christian saints rather than with non-Christian gods. This adoption by the Church, incorporating familiar things and adapting them, may have helped to lessen the reliance on pagan beliefs, while it reinforced the idea that the new Christian religion had healing powers. In addition it may have made a positive contribution to the health of communities by emphasising the advantages of water in the maintenance of cleanliness and hygiene. These pools and wells were widespread and many have retained a hold on public imagination until recent times, with some still regularly visited for their supposed curative powers. Many bear the names of Christian saints, but some do not, and this may reflect their pre-Christian origins.

The most important threats to health during these centuries were violence and famine. The low density of population, and the absence of easy communication, meant that travelling long distances was not common and the spread of epidemic disease was less likely.

Bede described the occurrence of a major epidemic in 664, while St Cuthbert was at Melrose, in the Scottish borders, which was at that time part of the kingdom of Northumbria. The Northumbrian King Oswald had, with St Aidan, founded the monastery at Melrose, just before this. Outbreaks of the disease had started in the south of England earlier that year and had spread north into Northumbria.

Bede wrote that St Cuthbert:

was seized with a pestilential disease, of which many inhabitants of Britain were at that time sick. The brethren of the monastery passed the whole night in prayer for his life and health . . . They did this without his knowing it; and when they told him of it in the morning, he exclaimed, 'Then

The Middle English word Leche comes from the Old English *læce*, which meant a healer or physician. Læce comes, in turn, from a much older word and suggested the actions of collecting, gathering and choosing. Other variations from the same roots are the old Irish *liaig* (physician) and the modern Swedish *läkare* (doctor).

However, the word leech has also been used for a blood sucking creature. Although its origins may be similar, from a word suggesting getting and holding, it conveyed a different concept from that of a healer. The deliberate use of leeches to suck blood as a treatment for disease goes back at least to Ancient Egyptian times, but in early medicine it did not occupy a major role.

In Bede's time, in the eighth century, the word leche indicated a healer, and two centuries later, the Saxon healer Bald gave his name to the *Leech Book of Bald*, a manuscript with recipes, charms and other suggestions for improving health.

In fourteenth-century Scotland the word still signified a learned healer, someone held in high regard. In 1386, King Robert II of Scotland gave, in heritage, a number of islands, including Jura, Calwa and Sanda, to 'Ferchard Leche', Farquhar the physician.

As the training of physicians in later centuries became more organised, the word continued to be used for healers, often including those without formal training.

One of the traditional ways of treating illness from early times was taking blood from a patient to restore what was perceived to be an imbalance of the four humours, blood, phlegm, black bile and yellow bile. Often, blood was removed by opening a vein with a small knife or lancet. Increasingly in the eighteenth and nineteenth centuries, the blood-sucking medicinal leech, *Hirudo medicinalis*, was employed for this purpose, as it was easier to use than the lancet. At the peak of their use, millions were being used each year.

The two meanings of leech became synonymous. The leech was the blood-sucking creature which inspired horror and was associated with illness, but the word also came to signify the doctor himself, as a bloodthirsty and grasping creature. The high regard in which a *leche* had been held in the past had gone.

With the development of modern medicine, bleeding became less frequently used and, as the blood-sucking leech fell out of favour, it became less common to refer to doctors as leeches. A word which replaced it, still implying disrespect, is a term which also has a venerable history, quack.

In the twentieth century, use of the medicinal leech, *Hirudo medicinalis*, underwent a revival. Carefully bred and prepared in a sterile way, leeches are now used to improve wound healing, by facilitating blood flow in skin grafts after plastic and reconstructive surgery.

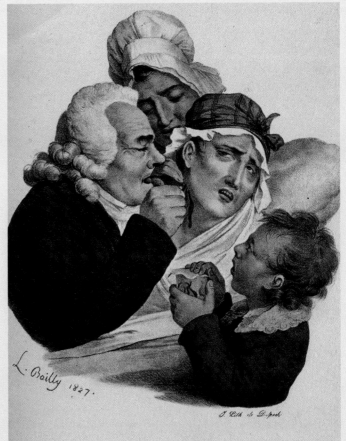

1.17 A physician administers leeches to a patient. Colour reproduction of a lithograph by F-S. Delpech after L. Boilly, 1827. The illustration, from the period when the use of leeches was at its peak, shows the anxiety on the face of the patient and the woman accompanying her, the detailed concentration of the physician who is applying the leech and trying to get it to attach to the neck, the size of the leech and the open mouthed awe of the small child holding the other leeches. This may possibly be a case of tonsillitis or a quinsy, a tonsillar abscess, for which leeches were used up to the twentieth century (*Wellcome Library, London*).

St Cuthbert's Healing Miracles

Bede's life of St Cuthbert was written around 720 AD. It provided the inspiration for the twelfth century illuminated manuscript which is in the Bodleian Library, (University College MS 1650). Bede's text and the illustrations describe what were seen at the time as miracles.

The first image (Fig. 1.18), illustrates an occasion when Cuthbert's knee became so swollen and painful that he was unable to walk. A man passing by on horseback told him: 'Boil some wheaten flour in milk, and apply the poultice warm to the swelling, and you will be well.' Having said this, he again mounted his horse and departed. Cuthbert did as he was told, and after a few days was well. He at once perceived that it was an angel who had given him the advice. (Bede's *Life of St Cuthbert*, Chapter 2.)

The second image (Fig. 1.19) shows St Cuthbert healing a young man with plague. St Cuthbert prayed, 'and bestowing his blessing, expelled the fever, which all the care and medicines of the physicians had not been able to cure. The young man rose up the same hour, and having refreshed himself with food, and given thanks to God, walked back to the women who had brought him.' (Bede's *Life of St Cuthbert*. Chapter 32.)

The third image (Fig. 1.20) shows another cure by St Cuthbert, this time of a young child dying of plague. St Cuthbert 'blessing the boy, kissed him and said to his mother, "Do not fear nor be sorrowful; for your child shall be healed and live, and no one else of your household shall die of this pestilence." To the truth of which prophecy the mother and son, who lived a long time after that, bore witness. (Bede's *Life of St Cuthbert*, Chapter 33.)

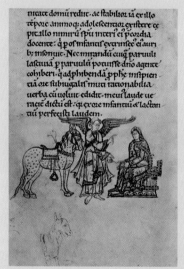

1.18 St Cuthbert's knee being healed by a stranger (*Wellcome Library, London*).

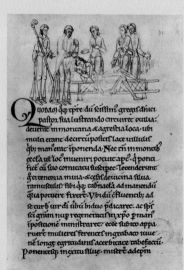

1.19 St Cuthbert healing a young man with plague (*Wellcome Library, London*).

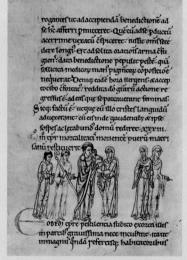

1.20 St Cuthbert healing a child dying of plague (*Wellcome Library, London*).

why am I lying here? I did not think it possible that God should have neglected your prayers: give me my stick and shoes.' Accordingly, he got out of bed, and tried to walk, leaning on his stick; and finding his strength gradually return, he was speedily restored to health: but because the swelling on his thigh, though it died away to all outward appearances, struck into his inwards, he felt a little pain in his inside all his life afterwards.

The effects of this plague in Scotland seem to have been less than in England or in Ireland, where some sources record that a third of the population died. Bede recorded a high mortality at the monastery at Jarrow, where only two of those who could read or preach survived. It is unclear what the cause of this plague was, although it was described by the Irish as a *buide connail* [yellow plague]. Some have suggested that it was related to the plague of Justinian that had spread from Constantinople in 541–2.

The Holy Pool of St Fillan

Water has had a special significance in healing for many centuries. The early Christian saints encouraged belief in the curative powers of water and, in Britain, particularly in Celtic areas, many sites such as wells or pools have retained their hold on popular belief until recent times. The following quotation, which includes comments from the late eighteenth century, describes St Fillan's pool on the River Fillan, near Tyndrum in Perthshire. It mentions, as do many of the old charms for disease, the cure of animals as well as people.

On the 9th August 1798, he rode from Tyndrum to the holy pool of Strathfillan, which towards the end of the first quarter of the moon, was resorted to by crowds of the surrounding peasantry, who expect to be cured of their diseases . . . A rocky point projects into the pool, on the one side of which the men bathed and on the other the women. Each person gathered up nine stones from the pool, and after bathing walked up to a hill near the water where there are three cairns, round each of which he performed three turns, at each turn depositing a stone. 'If it be,' he says, 'for any bodily pain or sore that they are bathing, they throw upon one of these cairns that part of their clothing that covered the part affected; and if they have at home any beast that is diseased, they bring some of the meal that it feeds upon and make it into paste with the water of the pool, and afterwards give it to the beast to eat, which is an infallible cure, but they must likewise throw upon the cairn the rope or halter with which the beast is led. Consequently the cairns are covered with old halters, gloves, shoes, bonnets, nightcaps, rags of all sorts, kilts, petticoats, garters and smocks.'

When mad people are bathed, they throw them in with a rope tied around the middle, after which they are taken to St Fillan's church, where there is a large stone, with a niche in it, just large enough to receive them. In this stone trough, which lies in the open churchyard, they are fastened down to a wooden framework and there left for a whole night with a covering of hay over them and St Fillan's bell is put on their head. If in the morning the unhappy patient is found to be loose, the saint is supposed to be propitious [and recovery is likely to take place].

Joseph Anderson,
Scotland in Early Christian Times,
The Rhind Lectures in Archaeology.
Edinburgh, David Douglas, 1881, p.192.

Below is a photograph of St Fillans pool as it is now (Fig. 1.21), paired with a reconstruction of a scene described above (Fig. 1.22). The rocky outcrop descending into the river, which makes two separate pools, can be seen. This allowed a degree of privacy for the men, bathing in the foreground, and the women in the background. The hill on the left, at the top of the outcrop, with three cairns, was where articles of clothing and animal halters were left in the hope of a cure for various problems. One of the men in the reconstruction has a rope around his body and is being immersed by the two men on either side, who have brought him here because he has trouble with his mind. After bathing, he will be taken afterwards to the chapel of St Fillan, seen on the horizon, in the centre, where he will be left tied up overnight, in an attempt to bring about recovery.

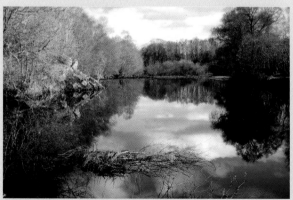

1.21 The River Fillan, near Tyndrum in 2010 (*Peter Wright*).

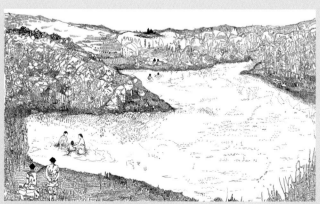

1.22 Reconstruction of a scene at the Holy Pool of St Fillan, Strathfillan, Perthshire (*Illustration by Susie Wright*).

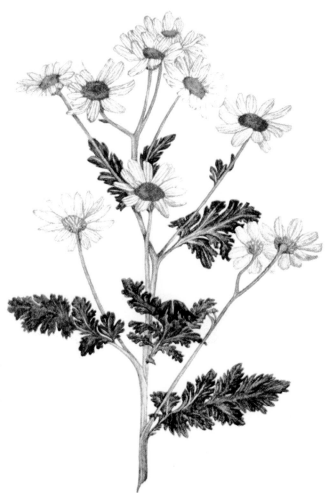

1.23 Feverfew (*fefer-fuge* in Anglo-Saxon, *febrefugia* in Latin). Another easily recognised plant with a distinctive smell. Remedy XXXIa in the *Lacnunga* contains feverfew as one of many ingredients in a '*salve that is good for headache*'. In the twenty-first century, feverfew still retains a reputation for the treatment of headaches and is available from Napiers, the herbalists of Edinburgh, in tincture or capsule form (*Kathryn Ball/Wellcome Images*).

Identifying the cause of particular epidemics that have occurred in the past is not easy. Even though contemporary descriptions might be careful and accurate, it was not until the nineteenth century, when specific organisms began to be identified, that distinction between many diseases could be made with certainty.

Eleventh and Twelfth Centuries

During this period, times of peace continued to alternate with conflict as national boundaries were contested. Although in the west and north there was considerable Norse influence, in the southern part of Scotland attitudes to health and healing owed much to Anglo-Saxon ideas and beliefs. Malcolm III of Scotland, known as Malcolm Canmore, who reigned from 1058 to 1093, spent part of his life in Anglo-Saxon England, before the Norman Conquest. His wife, Margaret, was the grand-daughter of the Anglo-Saxon King Edmund II. Sources of information about this period include *Lacnunga*, an Anglo-Saxon magico-medical commonplace book, and the *Leech Book of Bald*. Their origins are a mixture of Greek and Roman sources, and of Celtic and northern European traditions. Although Christianity had been the accepted religion for centuries, much of the material in the books is pagan. There are charms which call specifically on the Apostles, others which invoke Woden, and some seeking both pagan and Christian help. Some recipes are based on plants, such as fennel, sage and feverfew, and some are based on animals, such as gall of boar.

While only limited conclusions can be drawn from these few sources, it is clear that many different conditions and illnesses were recognised. Well over a hundred different plant species were listed. For these to be available, they would have had to have been collected from a range of different habitats, at varying seasons of the year. As well as stems, roots, leaves, flowers and berries, substances derived from animals were used, such as fats, which were used to facilitate the absorption of plant materials through the skin. Treatments and charms were recorded for animal as well as human diseases, emphasising the importance of animals for the economy and for survival. While much would have been learned by memory, there was considerable advantage in recording recipes in a more permanent way. Although this meant that the body of knowledge could spread beyond a limited number of practitioners, in practice the number of people who had access to what was written and who could read it must also have been limited.

Summary

Two general themes have emerged from this review of several thousand years. The first is at an individual level, with the gradual collection, over many generations, of a body of practical ideas about health and its management, particularly in the treatment of wounds and other injuries and the use of plant and animal materials for certain conditions. As this evolved, certain people within families,

Anglo-Saxon Leech Books

Only a few Anglo-Saxon manuscripts relating to medicine survive. In 1865 the Rev T. O. Cockayne published a translation of one of these, the *Leech Book of Bald*. Bald was a leech or physician and the remedies were written down for him by Cild, a monastic scribe. The book contains many recipes used for a variety of conditions or diseases, some serious and some slight. A number of recipes are likely to have been based on known effects, one for example noting that a poppy, rubbed down with oil and applied to the skin, would moderate a person's wakefulness. Many included, or consisted solely of, charms. In the example below, the word *aernem*, which occurs five times, is thought to be from the old Irish *ar neim* [against poison]. Neat is a word for cattle. These charms emphasise the importance of animals to man, whose survival may have depended on them for food, transport and work.

> For flying venom and every venomous swelling, on a Friday churn butter, which has been milked from a neat or hind all of one colour: and let it not be mingled with water, sing over it nine times a litany, and nine times the Paternoster, and nine times this incantation.
>
> Acrae, aercrae, aernem, nadre, aercuna hel, aernem, nithaerb, aer, asan, buithine, adcrice, aernem, meodre, aernem, aethern, aernem, allu, honor, ucus, idar, adcert, cunolari, ratcamo, helae, icas xpita, haele, tobaert, tera, fueli, cui, rabater, plana, uili.
>
> That is valid for every, even deep wounds.

Another leechdom, or charm, used Scottish beeswax for an animal that was 'elf shot', a term used for an illness that was thought to have a supernatural cause.

If a horse or other neat be elf shot, take sorrel seed and Scottish wax, let a man sing twelve masses over it, and put holy water on the horse, or on whatsoever neat it be, have the worts always with thee.

> T. O. Cockayne, *Saxon Leechdoms*, Vol II, Book 1, XLV, no 5, *Leech Book of Bald*.

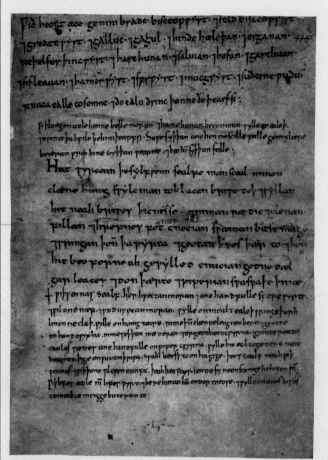

1.24 Collection of recipes for treating heartache, lung disease, 'wenns' and tumours and liver disease. The manuscript was written by three different hands in the eleventh century, in Anglo-Saxon, and was probably originally in a monastery (*Wellcome Library, London*).

or within larger groups as they came together, developed considerable skills and knowledge, which could be made available to the community. The second, more complex, theme, is at the level of society, which varied at different times in different places. For centuries, any development of settlements that occurred was on a small scale and scattered. The arrival of Roman civilisation brought, to at least part of the country, a sophisticated approach to structure and organisation, surgery and medicine, hospitals and hygiene. As the Romans withdrew, the influence of the Roman Church began to make itself felt, producing widespread effects on the way that people thought and lived, in ways which could be both supporting and inhibiting.

FROM NATION TO REFORMATION

The second part of this chapter looks at events from Anglo-Saxon times to the Reformation. Themes include the further development of the role of the Roman Church, the increasing size of towns, Scotland's relationships with other countries in Europe, and factors relating to communication, including the introduction of printing. Perhaps most important of all was the ebb and flow of events during these four or five centuries, with wars, famines and epidemics and intermittent periods of stability, prosperity and growth.

The Church was important in several ways. At their peak, the monasteries were major landowners, and their wealth, though often turned inwards and upwards, could provide support for the local community as well as for pilgrims and other travellers in times of need and ill-health. They were centres of learning, passing on knowledge through practice and experience, by the growing and use of herbs and by their creation and care of manuscripts. Religion had a significant influence on how people thought about disease, both in its cause and its outcome. The Church was also involved in many of the medieval hospitals that came into existence. In time, where the

charitable sentiments that led to the foundation of these institutions became lost, their exploitation by the church was one of the factors fuelling the unrest that led to the Reformation.

The increasing size of the centres of population had a number of implications. Conditions developed which favoured epidemics, such as problems with clean water supply and the disposal of rubbish, the presence of vermin and shortages of food. However, with bigger towns came better organisation, and this led to Burgh regulations and the appointment of officers, such as cleansers and physicians. Towards the end of the period, Edinburgh was big enough to allow the setting up of guilds or incorporations, in which areas of practice could be delineated and standards set, effectively excluding non-members.

Scotland was orientated much more towards Europe than to England in the south, and relationships with Europe were vital in maintaining and developing a country situated at the edge of the continent. Trade with France and the countries of the Baltic was to remain important to Scotland for centuries. Education, for those who could afford it, was available at universities in France

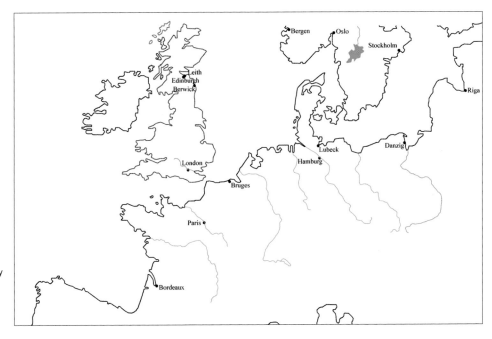

1.25 Trade between Scotland and Northern Europe in the period 1000–1600 AD. The main Scottish port was Leith, but there were many other East coast ports, including Anstruther, Berwick, Bo'ness, Crail, Culross, Dunbar, Dysart, Kirkcaldy, Montrose and Prestonpans. Exports included coal, fish, grain, hides, malt, salt and wool. The main ports in Europe with which Scotland traded included Bergen, Bordeaux, Bruges, Danzig, Hamburg, Lubeck, Oslo, Riga and Stockholm. Goods imported included apothecaries' drugs, glass and pottery from the Low Countries, brandy and wine from France, and iron ore and timber from the Scandinavian and Baltic countries (*Illustration by Susie Wright*).

and Italy and, later, in the Low Countries. Traffic was in both directions, with knowledge and skill being exchanged as well as food and other materials.

Communication was of great importance. Contact was maintained by word of mouth, with important messages being written. Rumour and myth could be easily spread and were difficult to stop. Charlatans could prosper and magic be believed. Movement between towns was by foot, or by horse, and towns themselves were surrounded by walls and could usually only be entered through a limited number of gates. Ports developed to facilitate movement of ships. Latin continued to be important as the language of the universities. The printing of books in Scotland began in 1507, but it was not until 1568 that the first medical book in Scots appeared. In Gaelic speaking areas, particularly in the Islands, manuscripts in Gaelic provided an alternative to the oral transmission of ideas and information.

The strength of the ebb and flow of events over the centuries was significant. Periods of war with England, particularly in the period between 1296 and 1547, brought defeat and victory, death and injuries, famine and destruction. Even in times of peace, famines could occur after years of plenty. Politically, at national and local levels, periods of stability alternated with instability, with progress suddenly replaced by disorder.

The major challenges to health, apart from famine and warfare, were the epidemic diseases such as plague and typhus. Syphilis and leprosy were widespread. The records of the Burghs give many examples of local regulations passed to deal with these challenges to the health of the community, such as restricting movement into towns and defining those who could offer accommodation to visitors.

Treatment

People could seek help in the treatment of their illnesses from a wide range of those who might be called healers. At the beginning of the period this included those in religious orders, but as time went on the clergy were less likely to be involved. In 1163, an edict of Pope Innocent III, containing the words *Ecclesia abhorret a sanguine,* forbade those in the church from taking blood and restricted their involvement in medical practice.

Patients with fractures or similar injuries might have sought help from those with experience in setting bones. In most communities there were women whose knowledge and skills would have been needed for such things as assistance with labour, the management of childhood disease and the care of the dying. A few towns with a large enough population had surgeons and physicians and some would have had apothecaries, with less formal training but with experience of the use of a variety of treatments.

Many people went on pilgrimages to religious sites. It was widely believed that the commitment shown in making the journey would be rewarded.

Pilgrimage in Medieval Scotland

Pilgrimage for medical reasons was undertaken to seek a cure (for the pilgrim or others), or to give thanks for a life saved. Non-medical reasons included the seeking of indulgence (a reduction in the time to be spent in Purgatory). Journeys were made to specific sites which were associated with saints, usually because the saint had lived and died there or had carried out miraculous cures. Thus Whithorn was associated with St Ninian, Iona with St Columba and Glasgow with St Kentigern (St Mungo). Occasionally, as at St Andrews, pilgrims came because of the presence of holy relics associated with the saint which had been acquired from abroad.

The longer and more arduous the journey to the point of pilgrimage, the greater the benefit that might be expected. With many sites away from the main centres of population, pilgrim routes developed, along which were monasteries and hospitals to provide accommodation and care for those needing rest, support or treatment.

The pilgrims provided a reason for existence and a welcome source of income for these places of care along the route, and pilgrims' donations provided a major source of income for the church which lay at the end point of their journey, allowing for the construction of larger and more impressive surroundings of the shrine. At the most popular sites, pilgrims would have been directed carefully from the entrance of the church to the shrine where the body of the saint or the relics were situated. Prayers would have been said, and offerings made in hope of cure, or thanks given for an alleviation of suffering. Models of

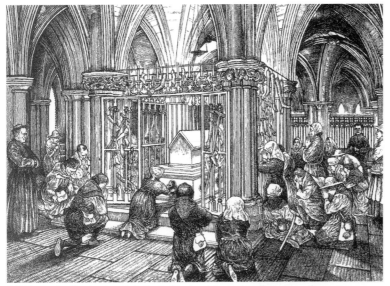

1.26 Reconstruction drawing of pilgrims in Glasgow at the tomb of St Kentigern. The scene depicted is of a feast day, with the gates around the tomb opened to allow direct contact with the sepulchre. Hanging on the metal gates are crutches and models of arms and legs, which have been left by those who are seeking cures or by those who have been healed (*from Peter Yeoman's Pilgrimage in Medieval Scotland (Historic Scotland), illustration by David Simon*).

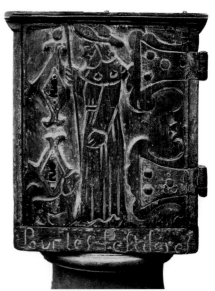

1.27 Wooden Plague box. The box, used for collecting money for those suffering from plague, is carved with an image of St Roch dressed as a pilgrim. Pilgrims were recognised by their simple robes and broad-brimmed hats, and often carried a long staff (*Wellcome Library, London*).

parts of body which were diseased, such as an arm or a leg, (and known as *ex voto* offerings), were brought, and might be displayed thereafter around the shrine as a tribute to its power.

In early times Iona, St Andrews and Whithorn were the most important places for pilgrims to travel to, with St Kentigern's tomb in Glasgow becoming popular after a *Life of Kentigern* appeared in about 1180, not long after the martyrdom of Thomas Becket in 1174.

James IV made many pilgrimages during his reign from 1488 to 1513, and his journeys give an idea of the sites that were being visited during these years. He regularly made a southern pilgrimage to Whithorn from 1491 onwards, and to the shrine of St Duthac, at Tain in Easter Ross, from 1493 onwards. While many of his pilgrimages seem to have been as penance for the guilt he felt about the death of his father, a pilgrimage made to Whithorn in 1507 was because of concern about the health of his wife, Margaret Tudor, and his new-born son.

Several saints were associated with specific problems of health. St Roch was particularly associated with plague or pest. A chapel dedicated to his memory, perhaps with the hope of protecting the town from plague, existed on the Burgh Muir in Edinburgh and was another of the sites visited by James IV in his 1507 pilgrimages. A church

named after St Roch was built at Garngad in the north east of Glasgow, in 1506, in the area subsequently known as St Rollox.

St Triduana's chapel at Restalrig, a few miles from the centre of Edinburgh, was a place of pilgrimage for the blind and those with other eye complaints. According to tradition, St Triduana, a Christian saint, had beautiful eyes which attracted the attention of Nechtan, king of the Picts. Her response was to pluck them out and sent them to him, impaled on a thorn. She thereafter lived as a recluse at Restalrig, and after her death her shrine became a place of pilgrimage for those who wished to be cured of eye disease. Sir David Lindsay (1486–1555), the Scottish poet, wrote of those who went 'To Sanct Tredwell to mend their eine'. St Triduana's chapel in Restalrig can still be visited. In addition there is a well in Holyrood Park a mile or so away, known variously as St Margaret's or St Triduana's Well. St Margaret's Well had existed near the Restalrig site, but was removed in 1860 to make way for railway developments. It was reconstructed in Holyrood Park on the site of another well, St David's, and details of the old building can still be seen through a grille placed in front of the well.

In summary, while many pilgrims during medieval times travelled for personal or social reasons, many went

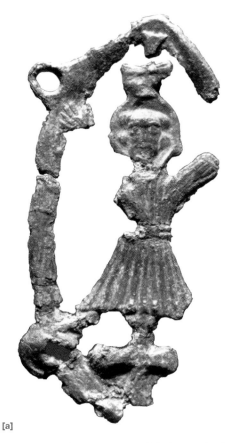

[a]

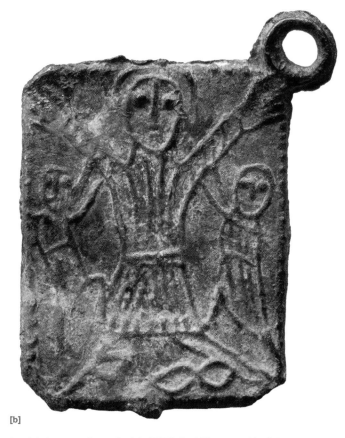

[b]

1.28a and b Two fourteenth-century pilgrim badges, showing images of St Andrew. Both badges show traces of corner rings. Badges such as these had a ring at each of the four corners, which were used for pinning to the traveller's coat so as to identify them as pilgrims. The one on the left was found during excavations at Perth in 1977 (© *Perth Museum and Art Gallery, Perth & Kinross Council*). The one on the right was found during excavations at St Andrews in 1989 (© *Fife Council Museums: St Andrews*).

for reasons associated with the preservation or restoration of health. Such journeys continue today, as the popularity of pilgrimages to Lourdes and Santiago de Compostela shows.

Major Epidemics of Disease

During this period, Scotland, in common with other European countries, endured major outbreaks of disease, including plague, leprosy and syphilis. Although we can now attribute these diseases to specific organisms, as has already been noted, this precision cannot be applied to medieval concepts of illness, so that the terms plague or pestilence may refer to several epidemic diseases, and those said to be suffering from leprosy or syphilis (grand gore or the great pox) may instead have had manifestations of non-contagious skin disease.

Plague was often associated with famine, leading to considerable loss of life. Creighton, in *A History of Epidemics in Britain*, estimates the frequency of what he

called famine pestilences as occurring, on average, about once a generation. The fourteenth-century writer, John of Fordun, mentions several of these in his *Chronicle of the Scottish Nation*. These include famines in 1196, 1321 and this, in 1344:

> In the year 1344, there was so great a pestilence amongst the fowls, that men utterly shrank from eating, or even looking on a cock or a hen, as though unclean and smitten from leprosy, and . . . nearly the whole of that species was destroyed.
>
> John of Fordun, *Chronicle of the Scottish Nation*
> (p 358 in the 1871 translation by W. S. Skene)

An epidemic like this among livestock had serious consequences for humans, making it impossible for some to maintain the precarious balance between survival and starvation. However, the next plague, which arrived in Britain in 1348 and spread to Scotland by 1350, was unprecedented. John of Fordun, writing of events which happened in his lifetime, gave details of its affects.

> By God's will, this evil led to a strange and unwonted kind of death, insomuch that the flesh of the sick was somehow puffed out and swollen, and they dragged out their earthly life for barely two days. Now this everywhere attacked especially the meaner sort and common people; seldom the magnates. Men shrank from it so much, that, through fear of contagion, sons, fleeing as from the face of leprosy or an adder, durst not go to see their parents in the throes of death.
>
> John of Fordun, *Chronicle of the Scottish Nation* (p 358 in the 1871 translation by W. S. Skene)

This epidemic, known as the Black Death, occurred at this time because of a combination of circumstances. It probably started in China, spreading steadily westwards from 1346. In Europe the population had risen, towns were bigger and more crowded and transport between them was becoming easier and faster. The disease was almost certainly bubonic plague (caused by the bacterium *Yersinia pestis*), communicated to humans by the bites of infected fleas carried on rats, commonly present in the houses of the poor, whose resistance was often lowered by poor nutrition. Those affected developed swellings (buboes) in the groin and fever, and became severely ill. When the lungs were infected (pneumonic plague), infected droplets could be spread by coughing and sneezing and subsequent inhalation, and this led to very rapid spread from person to person.

The overall mortality in Scotland from this epidemic may have been less than in some other parts of Europe, because the population was small and widely distributed, but in later outbreaks, when communications had improved, the epidemics may have spread more rapidly and further. An immediate consequence of the reduction in population was that there were fewer people to deal with harvests, and this, coupled with any adverse effects from cold winters and wet summers, meant that famine was more likely. Later, however, for the survivors, the drop in numbers meant that more food was available, land

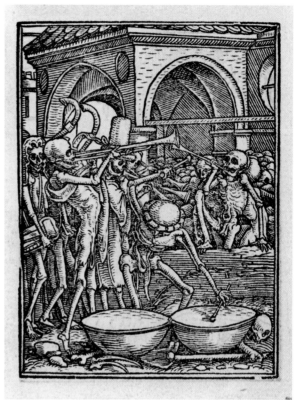

1.29 An illustration of the type known as the Dance of Death, by Hans Holbein (1497–1593), printed by woodblock. Such images were typical of a time when death from famine, war or epidemics of disease was common. It shows a band made up of skeletons playing drums and various brass instruments. Most images of this type show skeletons dancing, often leading the living towards death. The image is one from a Dance of Death library collected in the nineteenth century by William Gemmell (1859–1919), a Glasgow doctor, which was bequeathed to Glasgow University on his death. The original collection of 76 items has been increased to some 150 items covering several hundred years of the dance of death tradition (*University of Glasgow Library*).

became cheaper and those who were fit and able to work commanded higher wages.

Over the next few centuries, there were regular epidemics of plague or typhus (another epidemic disease, caused by an organism called *Rickettsia prowasekii* and associated with lice), and this led to more organised attempts to limit the spread of disease. These included restricting travel from areas that might have been affected. In the smaller towns in the Borders, the risk was mainly from the south (from England) or from the north (from towns such as Edinburgh). In 1468, the burgh of Peebles adopted local regulations by which the four ports of the town were closed, the walls of the town were to be repaired and movement to and from Edinburgh was forbidden.

For the towns that were ports on the East coast, a

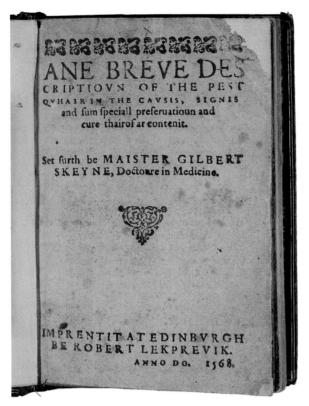

1.30 Title page of Gilbert Skeyne's *Ane Breve Descriptioun of the Pest Quhairin the special causis, signes and some speciall preservatioun and cure thairof ar contenit.* [Wherein, the special causes, signs and some special preservation and cure thereof are contained] Published in Edinburgh in 1568 by Robert Lekprevik (*National Library of Scotland*).

serious risk was from trade with Europe, particularly with the Baltic ports, such as Danzig. Quarantine became common. In Leith, ships which were thought to be a risk were kept for 40 days on one of the islands in the Forth, Inchcolm, Inchkeith or the Isle of May, and restrictions were imposed on the importation of their cargoes.

In Aberdeen, in 1506, the town's people were ordered to keep their back gates locked to restrict entry, the entrances to the town were to be guarded constantly and a licence was required for those who wished to provide lodgings. Aberdeen had fewer problems with many of the epidemics than did some of the other towns, and its regulations may have played a part in this.

Several towns, such as Edinburgh and Aberdeen, erected gibbets as a reminder that breaking the rules might have fatal consequences, but there were other penalties. In Edinburgh, on 25 June 1530, the Burgh records noted that 'George M'Turk and others [were] to be brynt on the cheik and bannist [burned on the cheek and banished]'. This was because they had failed to inform the authorities

of a child who had been ill in their house for three days and then died.

Apart from regulations restricting movement and encouraging the notification of disease, there were initiatives to improve hygiene and to isolate the infected from the healthy. Such measures made improvements by prevention rather than by specific treatment of established disease. Many of the burghs appointed cleansers, whose tasks included disinfecting houses and burying the dead. They were often well paid, as their duties were difficult and dangerous. Aberdeen was the first to appoint a burgh physician, James Cumming, in 1503. In 1570 Edinburgh appointed Robert Henrysoun, a surgeon, to advise the town on matters relating to the plague.

Areas outside towns were allocated for the care of those who were ill or who were thought to have been in contact with the disease. The Burgh Muir outside Edinburgh had two such areas, one at the clean or west end, for the isolation of those who had been in contact with those affected, and the other, at the foul or east end, where the sick were looked after. Clothes that were soiled were cleaned by boiling in a large cauldron on the Muir. In Aberdeen, during the 1514–16 epidemic, lodges were built on the Links area by the beach for the isolation and treatment of victims and contacts.

As outbreaks occurred, normal life in towns was often severely affected. Those not immediately afflicted usually tried to flee to a safer place. In 1545 the Court of Session was moved from Edinburgh to Linlithgow. Universities sometimes closed temporarily or moved to another site. In 1645, Glasgow University moved to Irvine, and King's College, Aberdeen, moved to Fraserburgh in 1647.

One of the best-known treatises in Europe on plague was that written by John of Burgundy, or John de Mandeville, at the end of the fourteenth century. Manuscript copies of this, translated from the Latin, are known to have existed in Scotland, one example being found in the fifteenth-century *Black Book of Paisley*. However, Scotland's first printed medical book in the vernacular was Gilbert Skeyne's *Ane Breve Descriptioun of the Pest* (1568).

Skeyne had been appointed mediciner to King's College, Aberdeen, in 1556 and his book described the signs that a victim of the plague might show.

Thair is mony notis quhilkis schausis ane mann infectit be pest. First gif the exterior partis of the bodie be caulde, and the interiour partis of the bodie vehement hait. As gif the hoill bodie be heauie with oft scharpe punctiounis, stinkand sueitting, tyritnes of bodie, ganting of mouthe, detestable brathe with greit difficultie, at sumtyme vehement feuer rather on nycht nor day.

[There are many signs which show a man infected by plague. First, the outside of the body is cold and the inside part very hot. The whole body is heavy with sharp pointing, stinking with sweat, weariness, gaping of the mouth, breathing with great difficulty and with detestable breath and high fever by night rather than day.]

The book also gave examples of ways in which infection might be avoided, such as:

Perfumand also al claithis in priuat lugeingis with the reik of sandal, rose vater or sic lyke materialis.

[Perfume all clothes in private lodgings with the smell of sandalwood, rose water and such like materials.]

There were directions on what to eat and drink and on medicines of various sorts to be taken or applied. (If the ingredients on the diverse list which follows were widely available, this confirms the existence of significant trading networks at this time.)

. . . fructis, feggis, bytter almondis, dry raisingis, sowr apill or peir, orange, citroun or limown, caperis, soure prunes, or cheryis, with daylie use of vinaigir or vergeus with all sortis of meittis.

[Fruits, figs, bitter almonds, dry raisins, sour apple or pear, orange, citron or lemon, capers, sour plums or cherries, with daily use of vinegar or verjuice, with all kinds of meats.]

Skeyne later moved from Aberdeen to Edinburgh, but his book was written in Aberdeen, bringing credit to the post that he held, that of mediciner to the University. The post of mediciner had been established at King's College, Aberdeen, for the teaching of medicine to students, but its purpose was to give some idea of medicine to those taking a general course at the University, rather than to provide teaching for those who would practice medicine as a career. In addition, it was not uncommon for mediciners, though doctors themselves, to take their academic responsibilities lightly, and Skeyne was one of the few to make a substantial contribution.

Leprosy

Returning crusaders probably brought leprosy to Britain from southern Europe and the East. The disease, caused by the bacillus *Mycobacterium leprae*, could produce marked facial and limb disfigurement in those affected, and this led to fear and exclusion from society of those with leprosy. Separate accommodation was provided for lepers and restrictive legislation was regularly enacted. In Scotland, there were, at various times, leper houses at Aldcambus (Coldingham), Aldnestun in Lauderdale, at Greenside in Edinburgh, Kingscase near Prestwick (thought to have been founded or endowed by Robert the Bruce), at the Gorbals in Glasgow, in Aberdeen and at Rothfan, near Elgin. There were also several small dwellings for lepers in Shetland.

A twelfth-century Act of the Scottish Parliament stated that those who had 'fallyn in lepyr that is callit mysal' should be put in the burgh's *spytaile* or hospital. If they had no means of paying, a collection from the burgh should be taken to the value of twenty shillings to allow them to be sustained and fed. Meat and fish that was old or otherwise unsaleable was given to those in leper houses, perhaps in the belief that those disfigured with *mysal* (measles) could eat measly food with impunity.

Although lepers had to live in specified places, their movement was not completely restricted. An Act of the Parliament of Scotland from 1428 allowed them to enter the town on Monday, Wednesday and Friday, between the hours of ten in the morning and two in the afternoon and, although they could not beg in kirk or kirkyard, they

The Bannatyne Manuscript

In 1568, while Edinburgh was affected by the plague, George Bannatyne escaped to the country and spent three months in Bannatyne House, Forfarshire, where he devoted his time to assembling and writing out by hand a collection of poetry. His manuscript, now in the National Library of Scotland, has bequeathed to us a treasury of medieval poems. It is the only source of some poems, which would, without his efforts, have been otherwise unknown. The pages above include part of Robert Henryson's *Ane Prayer for the Pest*. The first verse starts:

O Eteme God! of power infinyt!
To quhois hie knawlege na thing is obscure.
O Eternal God, of power infinite
To whose high knowledge nothing is obscure.

and ends

O Lord! that is to mankynd hail succure,
Preserve us fra this perrelus pestilens.
O Lord, who is mankind's whole and only help,
Preserve us from this perilous pestilence.

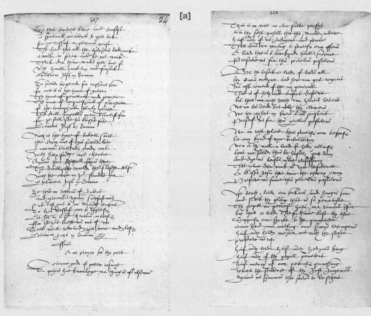

1.31a and b Pages 207 and 208 of the Bannatyne manuscript (*National Library of Scotland*).

could beg at the leper hospital at the town gate and at other places outside the town.

An extract from the *Records of the Burgh of Edinburgh* from 22 January 1527:

chairges all maner of lipper folkis that ar in lugeis and hospitals about this towne that thai convers nocht amang clene folks nother in kirk merkat or vther wayes bot hald thame be thame selffis in quyet vnder the payne of bannising the towne.

[charges all manner of leper folk that are in lodges (or shelters) and hospitals about this town that they converse not among clean folk, in kirk, market or in other ways, but hold themselves quietly to themselves, under pain of banishment from the town.]

Carole Rawcliffe's detailed and comprehensive 21st-century review of leprosy in medieval England suggests that attitudes to the disease varied considerably. Although

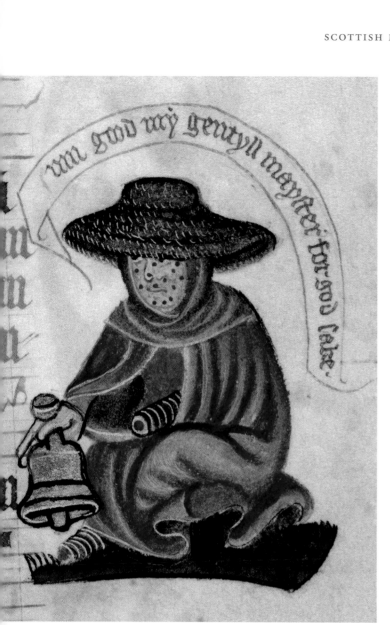

1.31 Early fifteenth-century music manuscript, with a marginal illustration of a leper. A hat partly covers the face and a robe covers up almost all of the body. A bell is used to warn passers-by of the disease (*British Library, Lansdown MS 541, f 127*).

The responsibility of deciding whether leprosy existed rested with the town's officers. On occasions someone designated as a leper might have had a different chronic skin condition altogether. In such cases, there might be improvement or recovery which could allow the sufferer to return to an unrestricted life.

As the centuries passed, the incidence of leprosy reduced in northern Europe. One factor may have been a greater awareness of other diseases, particularly affecting the skin, so that leprosy was less commonly diagnosed. Other significant factors were improvements in diet and general health and an increase in the numbers of those with natural immunity. Nutrition and genetics may be relevant in explaining why the disease persisted longest in Norway and Iceland and why the last indigenous case of leprosy recorded in Scotland was a man from Shetland, John Berns, who was a patient in the Royal Infirmary in Edinburgh in 1798.

Syphilis

Syphilis, a venereal disease caused by the spirochaetal bacterium, *Treponema pallidum*, spread rapidly through Europe after an outbreak related to the siege of Naples in 1494. It was known at first by names such as Grandgore or the sickness of Naples, before Fracastoro introduced the word syphilis as the title of his poem on the subject, published in 1530. The disease has been attributed to Columbus's sailors bringing the disease back from the New World, but there is increasing evidence that the causative organism, or one very like it, existed in the Old World long before Columbus's time.

The first major epidemic of syphilis in Scotland was in 1497, and was probably associated with the arrival, in 1495, of the pretender to the English throne, Perkin Warbeck, who brought with him a number of mercenaries from various countries. The rapid spread of the disease through all levels of society caused widespread alarm, and attempts were quickly made to stop its progress. A major feature of syphilis was the presence of genital ulcers. The disease was widely seen as a punishment for promiscuous behaviour and prostitutes were held responsible.

Aberdeen's Town Council Minutes of 21 April 1497 record:

restriction was one approach, the endowment of leper houses and financial and spiritual support for those who were designated lepers, were seen as worthy aims, or even obligations, for those who wished to demonstrate their charity. Matilda, who was the daughter of Queen Margaret of Scotland and King Malcolm Canmore, and married Henry I of England, provided a pious example of how to care for those afflicted with leprosy. Her biographer, Aelred of Rievaulx, described an occasion when, instead of avoiding contact with lepers, she washed and dried their feet and then kissed them.

Did Robert Bruce Have Leprosy?

Opinions have varied for many centuries as to whether Robert Bruce (1274–1329) had leprosy. The subject seems to have been raised firstly in the *Chronicon de Lanercost*, a history of England and Scotland from 1210–1346, which stated that Bruce was not able to take command of his army in 1327 because he had become leprous. However, it has also been suggested, and confirmed by documents of the time, that he deliberately left his army to go to Ireland, to create a diversion there. In addition, there is no evidence that his enemies, on either side of the Border, who regularly used terms of abuse when mentioning him, ever referred to him as a leper, although the word was often used, then, as an insult.

In 1818, during site clearance to build a new church at Dunfermline, on land that had belonged to the ancient cathedral, where it was believed that former kings and queens of Scotland had been buried, a structure, which appeared to be a Royal tomb, was found. Inside, encased in lead, was a skeleton.

The following year, in the presence of a number of witnesses, several of them eminent medical men, the remains were formally exhumed. The skeleton was thought to be that of Robert Bruce, as the breastbone had been sawn apart from top to bottom. (It was well known that his wish had been for his heart to be removed after death and taken to the Holy Land, though in its travels it had only reached as far as Spain, before a combination of events led to its eventual return to and burial in Scotland.)

The skeleton was examined and a plaster cast made of the skull, before the remains were re-interred. Numerous copies were made of the cast, four of which are still in the Anatomy Department of the University of Edinburgh. Comments from those who examined the cast subsequently have varied, from those who felt that it shows clear signs associated with leprosy, to those who remain unconvinced. In 2000 a comprehensive review, *Robert the Bruce and Leprosy*, by Kaufman and MacLennan, summarised available facts and concluded that there was no confirming evidence that he had had the disease.

Although this leaves the question unresolved, it is possible to detect

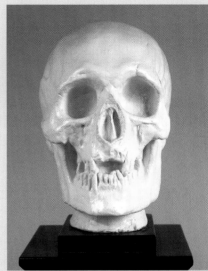

1.32 Model taken from a plaster cast of the skull of Robert Bruce. Examinations in the past suggested that the skull showed signs of leprosy, such as loss of the upper incisor teeth and of associated bone in the maxilla (upper jaw), but modern opinion is that these are not conclusive of the disease (© *Stirling Smith Art Gallery & Museum*).

leprosy in some archaeological specimens. In a study in 2000, unrelated to Robert Bruce, medieval skeletal remains from Orkney, which had shown bony evidence of leprosy, were found to contain DNA fragments of *Mycobacterium leprae*, the organism responsible for the disease.

The said day, it was statut ordainit be the aldermen and consale fro the eschevin of the infirmity cumm out of Franche and strang parties, that all licht weman be chargit and ordanit to decist fra thar vices and syne of venerie and all thair buthis and houssis skalit and thai to pass and wirk for their sustentacioun under the payne of ane key of het yrne one thar chekis, and banysene [banishing] of the toune.

[This day, a statute was ordained by the aldermen and council for the avoidance of the infirmity that has come from France and foreign parts, that all low women be charged and ordained to desist from their vices and sin of venery and all their booths and houses emptied and they work for their living, under pain of a key of hot iron on their cheeks and being banished from the town.]

In Edinburgh, six months later, in September 1497, attempts were made, under the heading of *Ane Grandgore Act*, to isolate those affected with the disease (and those who professed to be able to cure it), on the island of Inchkeith in the Forth. Any who did not go, but were subsequently found to have the disease, were to be branded on the cheek.

Robert Henryson: The Testament of Cresseid, *a Contemporary Description of Leprosy*

Among the poems of Robert Henryson, the Scottish poet writing in the second half of the fifteenth century, is the *Testament of Cresseid*, written as a sequel to Chaucer's Troilus and Cressida.

In the story of Troilus and Cressida, which was about the Trojan War, Cressida, who had been sent from her home in Troy to the Greeks besieging the city, forgot her promise of faithfulness to her lover Troilus and submitted to the Greek, Diomeid. She was subsequently discarded by him and became a prostitute in the Greek camp.

In Henryson's poem, Troilus survived, while Cresseid, blaming the gods rather than herself for her fall from grace, was cursed with the burden of disease associated with an immoral life. Henryson described her appearance as leprous and listed a number of the features associated at the time with leprosy, including facial disfigurement and voice changes.

Thy cristall ene minglit with blude I mak,
Thy voice sa cleir unpleasand hoir and hace,
Thy lustie lyre ourspred with spottis blak,
And lumpis haw appeirand in thy face;
Quhair thow cummis ilk man sall fle the place
This sall thow go begging fra hous to hous,
With cop and clapper lyka ane lazarous.

Thy crystal eyes I'll make bloodshot,
Thy voice so clear, unpleasant, old and hoarse,
Thy pretty cheeks o'erspread with blackened spots,
And livid lumps appearing on thy face;
Where thou walk, all shall flee the place,
Thus thou shall go a-begging from house to house,
With bowl and clapper like one who's leprous.

These attempts to limit the spread of the disease, by restriction of prostitution and by isolating those with the disease, had little effect, as did attempts to cure it. One of the substances used in the treatment of syphilis was mercury. For centuries this was the only treatment that was effective, but it had many side effects and could be dangerous, with its use sometimes ending in death. Mercury may have been implicated in Edinburgh in 1509, when Thomas Lyn was imprisoned for causing the 'slauchtir' of Sir Lancelot Paterson by negligent cure and medicine when treating him for the infirmity of Grantgor.

Medieval Hospitals

Many small hospitals were established in the centuries before the Reformation. MacLennan noted that 179 hospitals were founded between 1144 and the end of the sixteenth century in Scotland, and details of many of these can be found in Comrie's *History of Scottish Medicine*. Some were set up and maintained for their own use by various religious institutions, such as monasteries or abbeys. An example of this is the infirmary associated with the monastery of Inchcolm in the Firth of Forth. Some came into being to provide care for travellers or pilgrims in otherwise isolated places, for example in Stoneykirk, Wigtownshire, on the pilgrim route to Whithorn. Many,

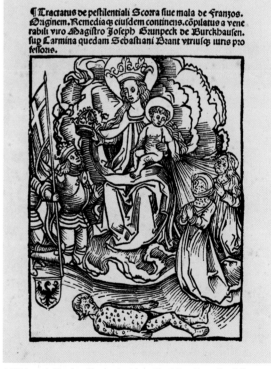

1.33 Joseph Grunbeck's woodcut from *Tractatus de pestilentiali Scorra sive mala de Franzos* (Augsburg 1496). This is one of the earliest illustrations relating to syphilis. Two women, covered with spots, are shown praying to the Virgin Mary. In the foreground lies a dead body also covered in spots (*Wellcome Library, London*).

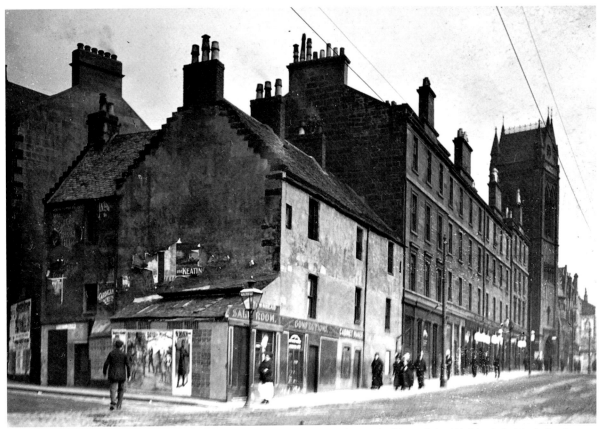

1.34 A photograph of Provand's Lordship taken in the late nineteenth century. The single-storey building on the end has since been demolished and the original three-storey building has been restored and is now a museum. All the other buildings have been demolished and the surrounding area landscaped (*University of Glasgow Library*).

such as the hospital of Maison Dieu at Brechin, were endowed by those with money, primarily for family or servants, and combined a desire to help those who were poor, chronically ill or elderly, with an act of generosity which reflected Christian ideals.

Although some hospitals existed for those with disease, for example for the isolation of those with leprosy, most medieval hospitals were not institutions dealing with the problems of ill health. They were usually small, but offered care, food and relative comfort when their funds permitted. Those cared for usually had to attend frequent religious services and pray regularly for the soul of the founder. Some hospitals owned property and land and were thus able to generate an income, which made their survival more likely. Many inevitably came to an end because they did not have continuing means of support. Others lost their originally charitable purposes and housed those who were not actually needy. Many others had their

funds misappropriated or otherwise taken over.

In 1424 and 1457, attempts were made by Act of Parliament to address the proper use of funds and to encourage the hospitals to return their founding aims. These met with little success, however, and, with the turbulence of the Reformation, most of these small hospitals came to an end, the buildings being demolished or put to other uses. Sciennes Hospital in Edinburgh was taken over by the town to isolate those suffering from plague, during an outbreak in 1575. One building that has survived in Glasgow on its original site, Glasgow's oldest house, is that which was founded as the Hospital of St Nicholas in 1471 by Bishop Andrew Muirhead. It had three storeys, with three rooms on each floor. After the Reformation it became the town house of William Baillie, laird of Provan, and was subsequently known as Provand's Lordship, the name it has today. By the nineteenth century it was surrounded by other buildings and increas-

Soutra Hospital

Sixteen miles south of Edinburgh, on the old road to and from England, (originally the Roman Dere Street), lay the Hospital of Soltray or Soutra, which was founded by Malcolm IV in 1164 for the relief of pilgrims, the poor, the old and the sick and infirm. Nearby was a well dedicated to the Holy Trinity. The hospital, perhaps initially because of its position on this much-travelled route, became important and the beneficiary of many grants, from the crown, the church and many individuals. In the 1460s, however, its funds were taken over to found Trinity Hospital in Edinburgh, and Soutra subsequently ceased to function as a hospital. All that can be seen above the ground now is Soutra Aisle, originally part of the church, but used after 1686 as a family burial place.

Archaeological work on the site, in the 1980s and early 1990s, identified the foundations of a number of buildings and found significant amounts of blood in the drainage systems, which would be consistent with bloodletting as a hospital activity. In addition, remains, either pollen or seeds or both, have been found of a number of plants of potential medical

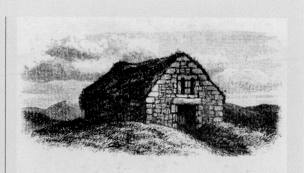

1.35 Soutra Aisle, on the site of Soutra Hospital. A stone above the entrance carries the date 1686, marking the date from which the small building was used as a burial place for the Pringles of Soutra (*Wellcome Library, London*).

significance, including flax, hemp, opium poppy, hemlock and henbane.

Soutra was run by Augustinian monks and, as at other religious establishments during the period, there would have been a good working knowledge of the use of herbals and plant-derived preparations, and it is likely that a number of the plants whose remains have been found were cultivated locally.

---

ingly threatened, but in the twentieth century steps were taken to preserve and then restore it.

The existence of such names as Spital, Spitalfield, Spitalhaugh, Spitalhill or Hospitalfield throughout Scotland shows how widespread medieval hospitals were. Though the names may indicate that an old hospital did exist nearby, they might also refer to land which provided revenue for a hospital situated elsewhere.

The Twelfth to Fourteenth centuries

With the coming of the Normans to Britain in the eleventh century, and the gradual spreading of their influence north, Scotland entered a period of growth and development, under Malcolm Canmore and Queen Margaret and their son David I and his heirs. The Abbeys of Dryburgh, Holyrood, Jedburgh, Kelso, Melrose and Newbattle were built. Small towns increased in number and in size. Lowland Scotland became a feudal society, based on the granting of land by the Crown and the assumption of the right to expect loyalty and homage in return. At times when the Crown was strong, this

produced a stability which allowed prosperity and relative peace, but if this central strength was absent, following the death of the king, for example, the resulting vacuum

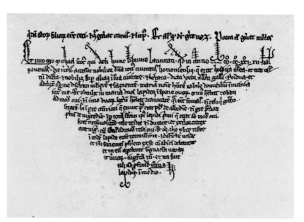

1.36 Original note of a consultation by Michael Scot in Bologna in 1221, from a thirteenth-century manuscript from Gonville and Caius College, Cambridge. One of his pills, known as 'Pilulae Magistri Michaelis Scoti', was noted to relieve headache, purge the humours wonderfully, produce joyfulness, brighten the intellect, improve the vision, sharpen hearing, preserve youth and retard baldness. The pills contained aloes, rhubarb and nine fruits and flowers (*Wellcome Library, London*).

Trinity Hospital, Edinburgh

Trinity Hospital in Edinburgh was
founded in 1462 by Queen Mary of
Gueldres in memory of her
husband James II, using funds
from several sources, including
Soutra Hospital. Records of the
Town Council in 1578 noted that it
was reorganised with twelve beds
for 'pepill seiklie and unabill to
labour for thair leiving'. The
hospital continued in its charitable
work until the 1840s, when, with
the coming of the railways, it was
demolished to make way for the
new Waverley Station.

Despite the disappearance of
the hospital, its funds continue
to be available in the twenty-first
century. The elderly of Edinburgh
who are on a low income may
apply for a grant of up to £240
a year.

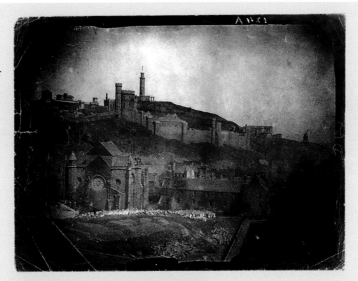

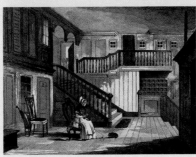

1.37 *Above*. Trinity Hospital (looking north-east towards Calton
Hill). This early photograph, taken in the 1840s before the
Hospital was demolished to make way for Waverley Station,
is one of a series of views of Edinburgh taken by the pioneer
photographers Hill and Adamson. The Hospital and Chapel
are in the foreground (*University of Glasgow Library*).

1.38 *Left*. Trinity Hospital, Edinburgh. This rather idealised
view of the Women's ward was produced in 1848, three years
after the building was demolished. It shows a quiet scene,
with an elderly woman knitting, in peaceful and spacious
accommodation (*Wellcome Library, London*).

might quickly lead to violence and the breakdown of law
and order.

The increasing communication with other countries
in Europe meant that Scots could travel to the continent
either for employment or, for those who could afford it,
education. Students and graduates who spoke Latin could
move readily from one centre to another.

One such traveller who made a name for himself in
the thirteenth century was known as Michael Scot. He is
known to have worked in Toledo in Spain and Salerno in
Italy and to have been tutor to the Emperor Frederick II.
He translated the works of various medical writers from
Latin and Arabic and wrote *Liber Physionomiae*, which
described how to recognise character and disease from a
person's appearance. The publication of his work in a
number of editions in later centuries, once the printing of
books had become established, meant that he had an
influence on generations of students.

How much his activities were concerned with medicine
is unclear, but the record of a consultation by him in 1221
in Bologna has been preserved in manuscript (Fig 1.29).

Gaelic Medicine

A distinctive feature of Scottish medicine existed for
centuries in Gaelic-speaking communities, sustained in
large part by the clan system. The leech (*ligiche* – Gaelic
for physician), had an important position, occupying one
of the senior roles in the community and in the retinue of
the clan chief, alongside those with skills in poetry and
music and those with knowledge of the ancient laws.
Certain families held hereditary appointments as physicians. These included the Beatons (or MacBeaths or
Macbeths), the McConachers (or O'Conachers) and the
McLeans.

Members of the wealthier families were sent abroad
for university education and, within the families, knowledge was passed on from one generation to the next, by
personal example, word of mouth and the use of written
text. Gaelic was the written and spoken language.

A number of Gaelic manuscripts still exist, mostly in
the National Library of Scotland. The majority date from
the sixteenth century, though some may be considerably
older. They show that translations of Greek, Roman or

Gaelic Medical Manuscripts

The National Library of Scotland has a comprehensive collection of Gaelic medical manuscripts, dating from the sixteenth to the eighteenth centuries. Most draw heavily on the works of earlier medical authors and usually contain Latin as well as Gaelic text.

In the mid-nineteenth century the Advocates' Library of Edinburgh made a special effort to bring together all Gaelic manuscripts that still existed in private collections, so that they could be preserved. Donald Mackinnon's 1912 catalogue of Gaelic manuscripts listed 21 of these as containing some medical material. They passed to the National Library of Scotland on its institution in 1925.

The shortest of the manuscripts, written on one sheet of paper, probably in the middle of the eighteenth century, contains a prescription for strangury, or difficulty and discomfort in passing urine. The longest has 476 pages and was written between 1611 and 1614, for the McConachers of Lorn. It must have functioned as a major source of reference, with summaries of medical texts, descriptions of disease and treatments for many conditions.

Figures 1.39 and 40 show the smallest item in the collection, a 6.5 by 4.5 cm vellum manuscript of 100 pages bound together. The front has a metal button for attachment to a leather thong to ensure closure. Other leather thongs hang down from the manuscript to allow it to be secured to the belt of the person using it. The

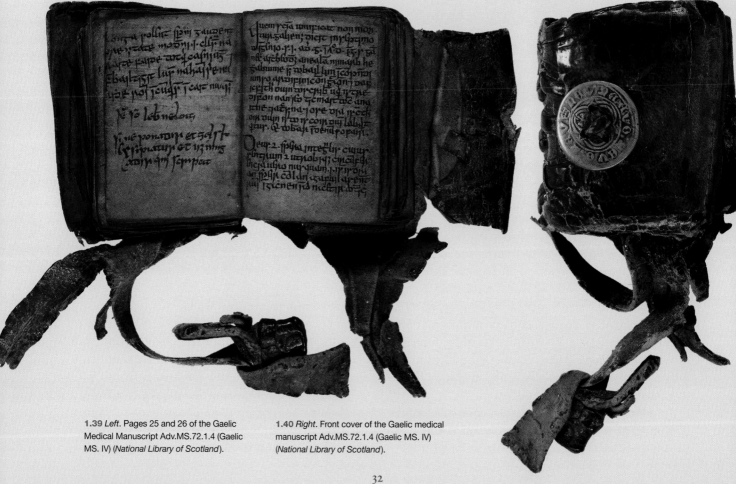

1.39 *Left*. Pages 25 and 26 of the Gaelic Medical Manuscript Adv.MS.72.1.4 (Gaelic MS. IV) (*National Library of Scotland*).

1.40 *Right*. Front cover of the Gaelic medical manuscript Adv.MS.72.1.4 (Gaelic MS. IV) (*National Library of Scotland*).

major part of the manuscript contains a collection of definitions of technical terms from medicine (and from philosophy and theology). Authors quoted include Hippocrates, Galen, Avicenna, Rhazes, John of Gaddesden and Bernard of Gordon, and definitions include the six non-naturals – entities not natural to the human body but necessary for life, which were noted as 'air, food, drink, movement, rest and depletion/repletion' and that of a contusion as 'a continuous bruise caused by a fall, or striking against something not sharp, like a blow from a stone or a stick, or striking against a wall, or a kick, or a blow from the foot, and the like.'

The manuscript belonged to the physicians of the MacBeath family, with the main medical part probably dating from about 1500–1550. It provided a repository of clerical and medical information for those whose profession ranged from looking after the ill to providing spiritual help for those in need.

Figure 1.40 shows the manuscript open at the beginning of the writings relevant to medicine. The right hand page is in Latin and Gaelic and the first two sentences are as below

Quem scientia vivificat non moritur, Galienus dicit in septimo de Ingenio Scientiae .i. adeir Galien in septimo de Ingenio Scientiae gach nech aithbeoduighes an ealadha ni marb he. Gurab uime sin dob áil lim in compendium so ar difinicion gach aon neith da ficfither dúin do scribadh, uair is tre difinicion na neithed ticmait dochum an aithne & a tuicaina; & ose Dia is cruthaighoir duin, is dó is coir duin labairt ar tús.

[Galen says in the seventh (book) of his (treatise) de ingenio Sanitatis that he whom science animates is not dead. Wherefore I desire to write this Compendium on the definition of everything we see, for it is by the definition of things that we come to know and understand them; and because God is our Creator it is of him we ought to speak first.]

Figure 1.41 shows one of the pages from a collection of manuscripts belonging originally to the Beatons of Mull. The collection is made up of thirteen different sections and includes descriptions of disease and of various treatments and prescriptions, as well as information on the planets and the signs of the zodiac. The text has been written by many different hands and charms and prayers have been frequently added to the margins of the pages.

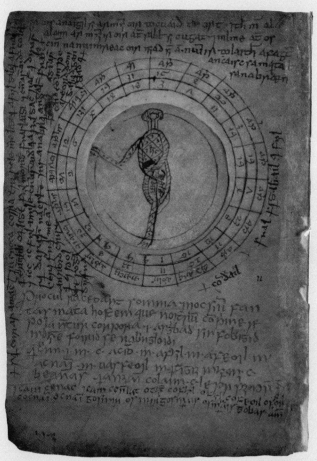

1.41 Page f 130v from the Gaelic medical manuscript Adv 72.1.2. Concentric circles show days and months and magic numbers and surround a roughly drawn human figure, attached by a leather thong to the page so that it can rotate. The device allows the calculation of the date of Easter. Around this are written a variety of medical charms, against urinary disease, against dreams and against worms. On the back of this page other charms are written, against menstruation, against fever, against violent death, poisons and demons of the air, and against bone failure (*National Library, Scotland*).

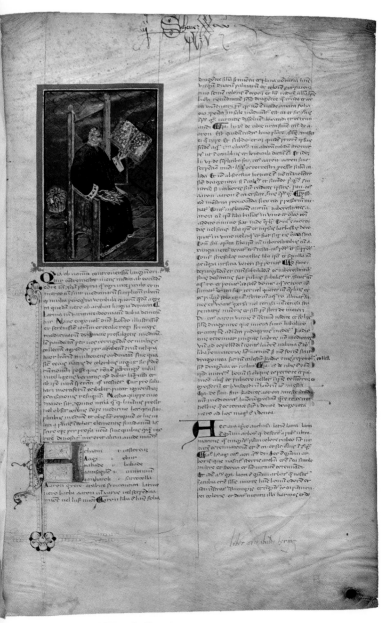

1.42 Part of a fifteenth-century manuscript, which has William Schevez's name inscribed at the top of the page. Schevez must have had a large income from his practice and his connections and he was able to spend much of it on his library. In 1493, for example, he paid 500 gold crowns for books to be sent from Flanders (*University of Glasgow Library*).

Arabic works, such as Hippocrates, Galen, Avicenna or Avenzoar, and work based on the writings of medieval authors, for example from Salerno or Montpellier, such as Bernard of Gordon, were available to Gaelic doctors. The manuscripts were produced in varying sizes, some of them small enough to be carried by the physician on his travels to see a patient. The nature of the country and the distribution of the population meant that travel to treat illness was regularly necessary and often took a considerable time. The manuscripts were valuable enough for special arrangements to be made, on occasions, for their transport. They might be sent by road, for example, rather than accompanying the physician on his quicker but riskier journey by boat.

Manuscripts such as these might have originally belonged to members of the family who had been to European universities in medieval Italy or France. As generation succeeded generation, many of the manuscripts acquired notes, written in the margins or at the end of the text, perhaps modifying certain treatments or adding new information.

While this family tradition of medicine meant that knowledge could be retained and formally taught, it might also inhibit progress and lead to physical and mental isolation from new ideas. However, the position is complex, as the practice of medicine often depended more on the practitioner and his experience than on the preservation of theories. Moreover, these healers were often known beyond their home communities, with many giving services to the Lords of the Isles and to the Scottish kings. When James VI of Scotland went to succeed Elizabeth in England, he took a Beaton with him to London as a court physician.

From the mid-sixteenth century onwards there were great developments in anatomy, physiology and scientific medicine. There was also an increase in the number of university centres at which to study medicine, particularly in Scotland. From the eighteenth century, as medical schools grew in size and importance, it became more likely that members of the medical families would study medicine formally. Those who remained within their communities still had considerable potential to contribute to local health.

In Gaelic-speaking, clan-based communities, as in other parts of Scotland, there also existed a strong culture of folk medicine. Alexander Carmichael's *Carmina Gadelica*, published at the end of the nineteenth century, records the existence of hundreds of traditional Gaelic charms, songs, hymns and incantations, dozens of which were specifically related to healing. Mary Beith's *Healing Threads,* published in 1995, lists more than a hundred plants which have been used in traditional medicine in the Highlands and islands. These include bog myrtle, meadowsweet, St John's wort, scurvy grass, sphagnum and various types of seaweed.

Medicine in the Fifteenth and Sixteenth Centuries
The continuing significance of the Church during this period and the importance of the relationship of Scotland with Europe can be seen by looking briefly at the careers of two Scots who studied medicine at university and at the illness and treatment of a Scottish archbishop.

At the beginning of the fifteenth century, Scots who wanted to study at university still had to go abroad. Of 230 Scottish graduates before 1410 whose European university has been identified, only five studied medicine. All five of these subsequently pursued a career in the Church, perceived, in those days, to be a more valued calling than medicine.

St Andrews University was established in 1413. William Schevez (*c*1428–1497) studied there and then went to the University of Louvain. Returning to Scotland he practised medicine, at one time as master of the hospital at Brechin, and subsequently as a physician at the court of James III. He combined his medical duties with those of a cleric, and in 1474 was appointed archdeacon of St Andrews, then archbishop in 1478 and, later, primate of Scotland. He had a great love of books, founding a library in the University of St Andrews and bringing to Scotland from Flanders a number of Latin medical manuscripts. Several of these still exist, and they give an idea of the treatments which might have been used by Schevez and his contemporaries in the fifteenth century. One of Schevez's books was Nicolaus's *Liber graduum*, which contained such information as:

Opium, cold in the fourth degree or in the second, when it is taken in the form of a chickpea,

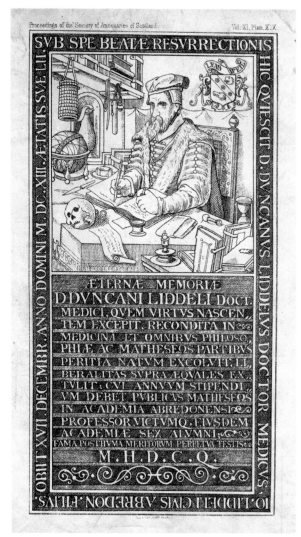

1.43 Memorial brass to the memory of Duncan Liddel, which is in the Kirk of St Nicholas, Aberdeen. In the portrait there are references to Liddel's varied career, including a skull, books, a pestle and mortar to represent medicine, a globe to represent his travels and other instruments to show his interests in science. The text notes his donation of funds to the University of Aberdeen for the salary of a professor of mathematics and for the support of six students (*Wellcome Library, London*).

it stupefies the sense of a man so that he cannot feel; it is useful for people with a cough, and it is given in modified doses for those showing added dissolution . . .

Sulphur . . . Aristotle said that sulphur water for washing the body was good against the pustules of scabies and impetigo.

Duncan Liddel (1561–1613) attended school and university in Aberdeen, but spent most of his professional life in

A Deathbed Scene from the Fifteenth Century

In 1859, during excavations in Mary King's Close, Edinburgh, associated with the construction of Cockburn Street, a sculptured stone was found face down in the foundations of a building. Since dated to the mid-fifteenth century, it appears to be a deathbed scene. On a couch, with hands in prayer, lies what seems to be a very ill person. Three figures in robes are at the bedside. One has a candle or a cross in one hand and a vessel which may have contained 'holy oil' in the other. A second has a candle in one hand and an open book in the other. Three smaller figures are kneeling, one at one side of the bed, one at the foot and another at a small cabinet nearby.

In addition, at what is probably

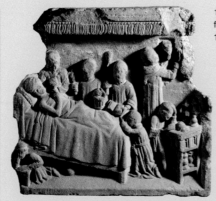

1.44 Fifteenth-century sculptured stone found in Mary King's Close, Edinburgh, in 1859 (*National Museums of Scotland*)

a window, there is a fourth standing figure. His position, arms raised, holding a vessel up to the light with head slightly tilted back, is one often seen in depictions of physicians of this period. Typical images show an ill patient in bed, with a physician holding up a flask of urine to the light to examine it. This procedure was known as

uroscopy, and from the appearance, colour, smell and sometimes taste of the urine, the physician gave his thoughts on the cause and expected progress of the disease.

Whether or not the stone shows uroscopy, it provides us with a striking and sombre image of life and death in the fifteenth century.

Europe. He studied at Frankfurt, Breslau, Rostock and Helmstadt, before being appointed a professor of medicine there from 1596 to 1607. He published a book on fevers and, after a successful career abroad, returned home to Aberdeen, leaving his books, instruments and a sum of money to Marischal College, on his death, for the support of students. His book on the conservation of health was published posthumously by Dr Patrick Dun in 1651.

In 1551, the archbishop of St Andrews, John Hamilton, who had succeeded Cardinal Beaton, had regular

episodes of severe difficulty with breathing. He had been working hard and had lost weight. His doctors wrote to Jerome Cardan, a celebrated physician from Milan, for help. The letter took two months to reach Cardan, and it was more than six months altogether before he was able to see the archbishop. They met in Edinburgh and, after examining Hamilton, Cardan was able to suggest treatment which brought about considerable improvement over the next six weeks or so. The archbishop was given a detailed explanation of what Cardan thought to be the cause of the illness. He was encouraged to rest and a sensible diet encouraged. His feather pillows were removed and he was encouraged to take regular shower baths.

Cardan was well rewarded for his success and during his stay saw many other patients. He returned to Milan, having asked to hear of the archbishop's progress over the following two years. After that interval, the archbishop wrote, saying:

I thank you for . . . my health, that is in great part restored, for the almost complete subjugation of my disease, for strength regained; in fine, I may say for life recovered. All those good

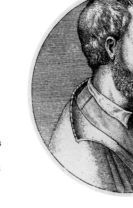

1.45 Jerome Cardan. From Joannes Sambucus's *Veterum aliquot ac recentium medicorum philosophorumque Icones* (Antwerp, 1574). That Cardan was one of the best known physicians in Europe is indicated by his appearance in Sambucus's collection of portraits of famous men from the Greek philosophers onwards (*Wellcome Library, London*).

things, and this body of mine itself, I hold as received from you . . . the accustomed attacks now scarcely occur once a month and sometimes once in two months; then too, they are not urgent and pressing, as they used to be, but are felt very slightly.

Cardan's involvement illustrates the renown that some practitioners of medicine enjoyed, the willingness to contact a doctor many hundreds of miles away, the length of time that travelling involved, the tact and common sense necessary to deal with a notable patient and the rewards that might follow success.

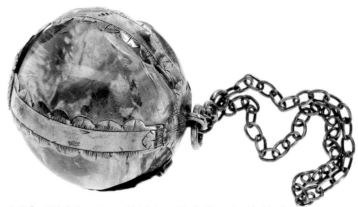

1.46 Crystal ball charmstone, which belonged to the Stewarts of Ardsheal in Argyllshire. The silver mounts enclosing it date from the sixteenth or seventeenth century. A chain is attached, which allowed the charm to be dipped into water, which would then be given to people or animals to cure disease or prevent illness (© *National Museums Scotland*).

Dealing with Problems of Ill Health –
Believing in Objects

Though Schevez and Liddel, Hamilton and Cardan illustrate some points of the practice of medicine during these years, they do not give us much insight into everyday life. There were so few practitioners of medicine that most people had no opportunity to be treated by them. Even if they were, they might very well use alternatives at the same time.

Attitudes to illness and disease meant that much ill health was accepted as an inevitable part of life. If recovery occurred, beliefs were reinforced in anything that had been used in treatment. In addition to food, drink and medicines, a variety of objects were associated with healing powers. One such was the Lee Penny, a stone brought to Scotland after the crusades in the fourteenth century, which had been mounted in a coin. There were also many charm stones, particularly in rural areas, which were usually in the possession of a family for generations. Anyone wanting to use them had to bring water specially for the purpose. The stone was dipped into the water, which then took on curative powers and could be used in the treatment of someone who was ill, or could be used for animals affected by disease.

While many of these charms may have had pagan origins, relics of the Christian saints were frequently venerated, inspiring pilgrimages and visits to shrines, wells, chapels and churches. Such relics commonly included bells and crosiers. Two relics associated with St Fillan are preserved in the National Museum of Scotland: a crosier, known as the Coigreach, and a bronze bell known as the Bernane, which was used to treat those who were believed to have problems in the head, such as disease of the mind or those with severe headache.

Conclusion

Throughout the medieval period there were major epidemics of disease. As time went on, those living in the towns showed an evolving ability to deal with the challenges which they faced. There was a difference between rural and urban life and between life on the mainland and life on the islands. Three universities were founded during this time in Scotland, but none of them was able to make a significant contribution, at this stage, to the teaching of medicine. The influence of the Church on medicine declined steadily, and its self interest caused wide disillusion. The Reformation brought hopes of equality and a new approach to education which proved difficult to deliver. The rise in the size of a few towns allowed the development of trade guilds and incorporations, and as professional groups began to exert their influence, the way was set for surgery and medicine to establish their separate identities. Notwithstanding these latter developments, there were so few practitioners with formal training that there was still a widespread dependence on traditional beliefs about the causes of disease, and most of the population depended on methods of treatment which changed little for many centuries.

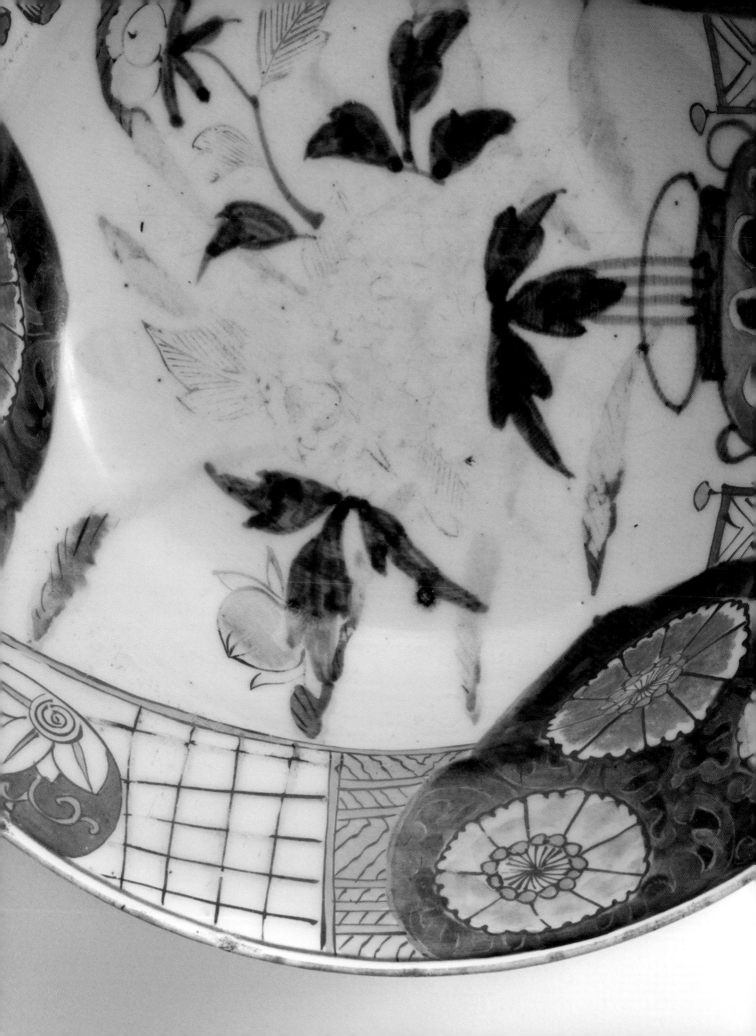

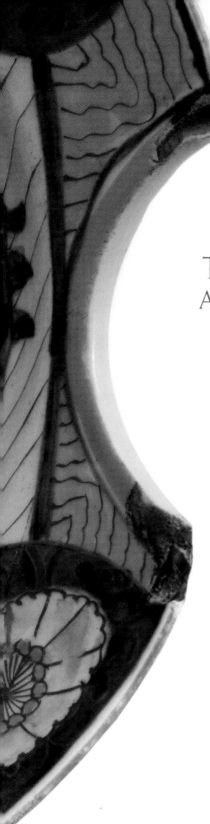

CHAPTER TWO

RENAISSANCE TO ENLIGHTENMENT: A PERIOD OF TRANSITION

Scottish Medicine *c*1600–*c*1750

Helen Dingwall

———

In the beginning of diseases, if there appears
cause for moving of any thing, move it.

HIPPOCRATES

39

INTRODUCTION AND HISTORICAL CONTEXT

By the early decades of the seventeenth century, both Scottish society and Scottish medicine were becoming more complex, though the patients' experience of consultation and treatment was relatively unchanged throughout the period covered by this chapter. By 1750 there was only one large hospital, in Edinburgh (Fig. 2.1, though there was an infirmary within the Town's Hospital in Glasgow). It would be well into the eighteenth century before medical hospitals became a significant feature of the medical sphere. The general social structure was changing, with growth of the urban network, but the majority of the population still lived in a rural or village setting. In the larger towns, merchants and craftsmen emerged as the dominant socio-economic groups, while more traditional social structures survived in the countryside, where livelihoods depended on the quality of the land and the actions of the landowners, rather than on trade or manufacture. By the end of the period Glasgow was growing rapidly in population, and in the importance of its trading routes with the Americas, the 'tobacco lords' emerging as a key influence on the economic prosperity of the town.

Politically, this whole period was one of considerable flux. The signing of the National Covenant in 1638 heralded the rise of the covenanting movement and a period of bitter civil war, followed by regicide, the Cromwellian occupation, the restoration of Charles II and the so-called Glorious Revolution of 1698-90. This latter event produced fresh conflicts in the form of the various Jacobite uprisings, culminating in the last major battle on British soil, which took place at Culloden in 1746. (Fig. 2.2). These turbulent times affected the lives of all, and provided much work for medical practitioners of all sorts, particularly those who served the army.

Relations between Scotland and England remained difficult throughout the rest of the period to 1750. The seventeenth century spanned the regal union, during which the two nations shared a monarch, but little else, and Scotland remained in some ways closer to Europe than to her southern neighbour, particularly in cultural terms, with consequent influences on the shaping of Scottish medicine. The parliamentary union of 1707 saw the establishment of rather closer links, but Scotland retained three of its most distinctive defining characteristics – and does so to the present day: law, education and the church, all of which had – and continue to have to some extent – effects on the shaping of Scottish medicine.

Once the Scottish parliament ceased to exist in 1707, what had been envisaged – by the Scots union negotiators

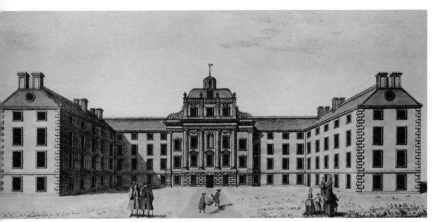

2.1 Royal Infirmary of Edinburgh. Engraving of the Royal Infirmary of Edinburgh, opened in 1741. The style is classical and ordered, very much in line with architectural tastes of the time, and given an imposing aspect (*LHSA*).

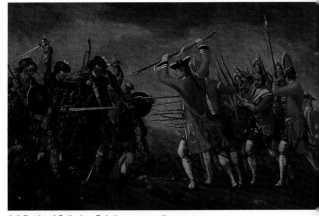

2.2 Battle of Culloden. Painting representing a scene from the Battle of Culloden. The Jacobite army faced bayonets for the first time – resulting in new types of injuries to be dealt with by the field surgeons (*The Royal Collection © 2011 Her Majesty Queen Elizabeth II*).

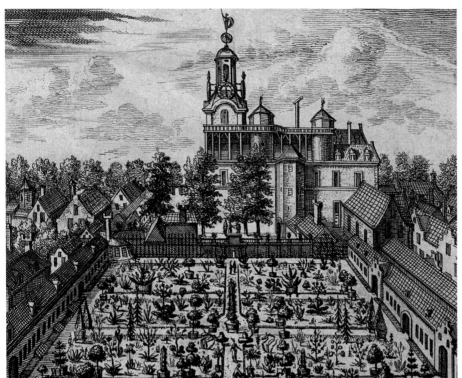

2.3 Leiden University. Line engraving of the old academy building at Leiden, also showing the medicinal botanical garden. One of the small canals at Leiden was named Schottendyke – the result of many Scottish students going there to study merchant trading and commerce as well as medicine (*Wellcome Library, London*).

at least – was that the Westminster parliament would be dissolved also, and the new parliament of Britain established *de novo*. The reality was very different, though, with 45 Scots MPs being 'grafted' on to the London parliament, together with 16 representative peers in the upper house. For most of the eighteenth century Scottish politics were managed on behalf of Westminster by a small number of powerful individuals, including the second and third dukes of Argyll.

It is difficult to assess the extent to which the new and different political background had an effect on the development of medicine in Scotland, but it is justifiable to claim that by the middle of the eighteenth century, the best medical education on offer was in Great Britain, and in Scotland in particular, following the foundation of the medical school in Edinburgh in 1726. The view has been put forward by some historians, particularly Emerson, that the foundation of the medical school owed as much to the influence of the Argylls as to John Monro or the long-serving Edinburgh political grandee, George Drummond.

This beginning of the period also saw the full flowering of the Renaissance, which had during the sixteenth century brought Scotland firmly into the mainstream of European culture, particularly in the arts and philosophy, and centred on the tenets of humanism. The period was subsequently one of transition, ending with the early years

of the Enlightenment. The historically strong contacts between Scotland and Europe had paved the way for this cultural transformation. European craftsmen had come to Scotland for generations in order to pass on their expertise (often because of religious persecution in their homelands), and the influence of humanist philosophy and the secularisation of learning meant that it was now possible to analyse man and the universe without the restraining and stifling hand of the Church of Rome. Scottish medical students continued to travel to Europe to study, and by the beginning of the eighteenth century Leiden had become the main centre of choice, though many students chose to take their final examinations at Reims, where the tests were reputedly easier. The choice of Leiden is not surprising, as there were already very strong merchant links with Scotland. Leiden university was a municipal institution like that of Edinburgh, and the medicine taught there reflected the aims of the Scottish students – to learn the 'best' medical philosophy and practice (Fig. 2.3).

The Christian faith remained a fundamental part of Scottish life – and indeed was the cause of much of the political and military turbulence of the period – but growing intellectual freedom enabled progress to be made in the acquisition of knowledge in general, and medicine in particular. The Reformation, which had begun in Scot-

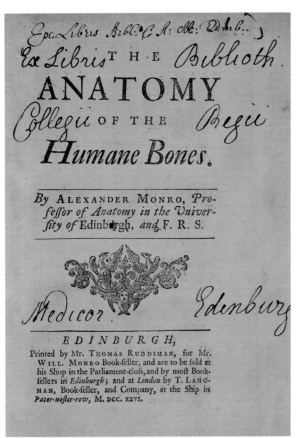

2.4 Publication by Alexander Monro *primus*. Title page of Alexander Monro *primus'* The Anatomy of the Humane Bones (Edinburgh, 1726). Monro was the first of a dynasty of Alexander Monros (though Alexander *primus'* father John Monro may be credited with its foundation), who dominated the teaching of anatomy in Edinburgh for most of the eighteenth century. The first and second of the dynasty, if not the third, made significant contributions to anatomical advances and the publication of their results. This was helped by the general push towards greater literacy levels and education for all (*RCPE*).

land in 1560, initiated fundamental changes in the Scottish church, though these took at least a generation to penetrate most parts of the country, and some remote areas, such as Barra and South Uist, remained largely unconverted. The *First and Second Books of Discipline*, issued by the new church, were essentially 'instruction manuals' for achieving a new, Godfearing and educated society. The *First Book* laid out requirements for church furnishings, including a bell, pulpit, baptismal basin and communion table. The second, published in 1578, set out the structure of the reformed church, including parity among the ministry. These things were difficult to achieve in all parts of the country, particularly in remote areas. The foundation of a school in every parish was encouraged, though again this took some time even to begin to be implemented, but would have clear effects on literacy levels

among the general population and potential medical practitioners in particular. There were certainly problems, such as the increasingly violent persecution of alleged witches, but the Reformation did have its benefits for medicine.

The increasing availability of printed books and gradual rise in general literacy levels allowed information and new knowledge to be spread more widely, and it was during this period that medical practitioners began to publish their own works as well as form corporations to protect their privileges (see Fig. 2.4 – an example from the works of Alexander Monro *primus*).

This chapter will look at a number of aspects of medicine in this period, including threats to health, general philosophical principles, the organisation of health care, the healers , the nature of health care, hospitals, medical and surgical practice, dentistry and mental illness.

Threats to Health

Agricultural techniques were improving by 1750, and the threat of famine receded, despite the population rising to over one million by the turn of the eighteenth century. Major famines in the 1620s and the so-called 'ill years' of the 1690s caused severe malnutrition, disease and loss of life, but apart from the effects of a particularly severe winter in 1739-40, there were no significant occurrences thereafter. Life expectancy was still low as compared to more recent times (in this period life expectancy was around 40 years, as compared with an average of 75 years for men and 80 years for women in 2010), and infant and child mortality was still a scourge, as were epidemic and endemic diseases similar to those suffered in prior centuries, such as plague, smallpox (Fig. 2.5), syphilis, leprosy and sibbens (Scottish yaws) – a bacterial affliction with similarities to syphilis, but probably non-venereal in origin.

Epidemics of plague continued to threaten Scotland during the first half of the seventeenth century, the last major attack coming in the 1640s. Outbreaks were dealt with by measures aimed at containment and isolation rather than treating or curing individual patients, though there was some awareness of the main proliferating factors. During the outbreak in Brechin in 1647, which claimed the lives of around one-third of the town's population, for

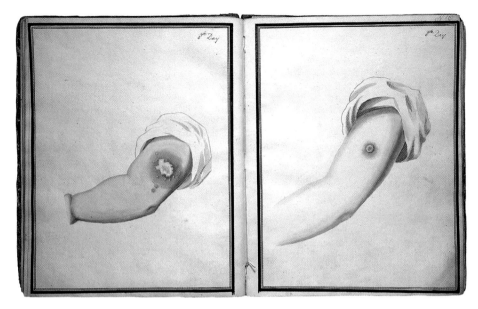

2.5 Smallpox/cowpox. Water-colour painting of eighth-day smallpox and cowpox by George Kirkland, demonstrating the lesions produced by these diseases (*Wellcome Library, London*).

example, the inhabitants were ordered to kill mice and rats. Scots were more likely to be attacked by the bubonic rather than the pneumonic form or variant of the disease, though both arose from the same pathogen *Pasteurella pestis* (now *Yersinia pestis*). This attacked the lymphatic system and produced painful swellings, or buboes, accompanied by purple spots. The outbreaks in the 1640s affected over 70 Scottish parishes, in all parts of the country, though concentrated rather more in the lowlands. As in earlier outbreaks, isolation was the principal measure taken to control the infection, and plague huts were built, such as those on Leith links in 1645, and at Kinnoul, in Perth. Smallpox was a consistent presence, not alleviated immediately by the innovations of inoculation from the early eighteenth century onwards, and vaccination from the 1790s. All of this provided much work for all sorts of medical practitioners.

Medical Philosophy

The philosophical basis of treatment for most conditions caused by these threats to health throughout much of the period was that of the revived tradition of classical, humoral medicine, based on the ancient teachings of Hippocrates (*c*460–377 BC) and Galen (*c*130–200 AD), added to by the Arabic physician Avicenna (*c*980–1037) and, later, Phillipus Aureolus Theophrastus Bombastus von Hohenheim (*c*1493–1541), who adopted the more easily-remembered name Paracelsus, and Jan Baptist Van Helmont (bap. 1579–1644). Over time a more monistic theory of humours was embraced, while iatro-mechanical and iatro-chemical explanations of the structure and func-

tion of the body were debated. Iatro-mechanists believed that the body functioned on a mechanical system, in accordance with the laws of physics, while those who favoured an iatro-chemical explanation considered that good health depended on correct chemical relations within body fluids, and that diseases could be explained in terms of chemical principles. These beliefs reflected the growing interest in, and knowledge of, science during this period. Despite the more 'scientific' inclinations of Paracelsus and Helmont, though, the people's experience of medical treatment would change very slowly.

According to humoral tradition, disease of any sort was thought to be the direct consequence of an imbalance in the four bodily humours – blood, phlegm, yellow bile and black bile (Fig. 2.6).

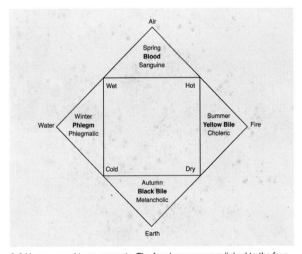

2.6 Humours and temperaments. The four humours were linked to the four seasons and the four temperaments (*Illustration by Susie Wright*).

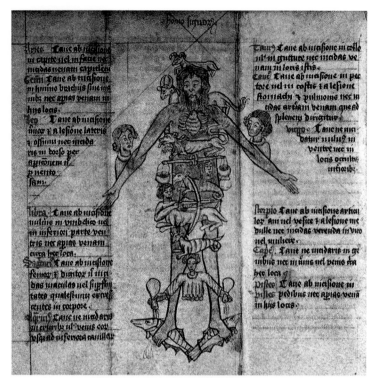

2.7 Zodiac Man. Fourteenth-century folding almanac showing Zodiac man with illustrations of astrological signs and their influence on the body. The zodiac images are related to the parts of the body thought to be affected during the astrological cycle. It has not been possible to find a Scottish image, but surgical apprentices were instructed to learn these signs and their significance, and would have used similar illustrations (*Wellcome Library, London*).

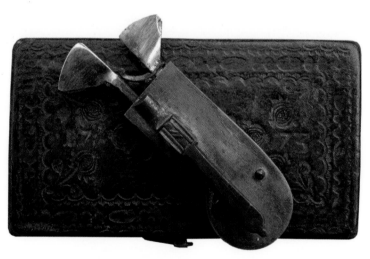

2.8 Bloodletting. Photograph of set of bloodletting implements used by Hugh McFarquhar, physician in the north of Scotland in the second half of the eighteenth century. The case is decorated by ornate tooling in the leather (*Courtesy of Tain Museum*).

Cure was in theory simple – eliminate the evil humours which caused the imbalance, and then restore the equilibrium of the body by herbal, or, later, chemical means. All of this was related to the time of year and the signs of the zodiac. So for any disease, be it smallpox or constipation, the basic regimen would be the same – first cleanse the body by means of emetics and/or purges, and then restore the correct balance of the body with tonics and medicines appropriate to the nature of the disease. Advice would also be offered about diet and general lifestyle. Galen followed Hippocrates in his holistic approach, but supplemented his advice with increasingly complex herbal preparations.

Paracelsus favoured the used of chemical preparations, including those derived from sulphur, iron, mercury, arsenic or antimony, and advocated individual remedies for specific diseases, though still owing something to the general principles of humoral medicine. The period was, therefore, one of philosophical transition as well as continuation of ancient beliefs.

For centuries physicians and healers of all sorts had consulted astrological charts, carefully observing the phases of the moon and the seasons of the year. There was a strongly-held belief that all aspects of life and death, illness and health were influenced by these cosmological factors just as much as by local causes. Localised medical conditions were connected to a systemic imbalance, particularly before advances in anatomy and physiology in the later-eighteenth and nineteenth centuries. Various versions of 'Zodiac man' were produced (see Fig. 2.7), with suitable illustrations demonstrating the parts of the body most likely to be affected during particular astrological and lunar phases. Wider issues were involved in the most apparently simple of medical complaints.

The types of cures and tonics offered to the sick were closely related to season and often region-specific. A commonly-used cure for jaundice involved an infusion of saffron (illustrating the relationship between colour of medicine and the yellow skin colour produced by jaundice), sheep's droppings and beer, drunk four times a day. It was believed that tying red silk round the waist would act as a prophylactic against rheumatism. The herbs and other substances used in the multifarious recipes in circulation depended on season and location. In coastal areas, for example, various types of seaweed featured prominently in cures, while this was much less likely in more inland areas.

Prophylactic bloodletting was usually carried out in the spring, to help rid the body of the malevolent effects of the long winter months and to restore the condition of the body for the period which required great physical activity for individuals working on the land, as most did at this time. Bloodletting was carried out by local healers as well as by qualified surgeons, and bloodletting tools (Fig. 2.8) were to be found in the equipment of most medical practitioners.

Other measures against the onset of disease included the taking of scurvy grass in springtime, together with seasonal bloodletting, the latter intended to keep the bodily fluids in balance and usually carried out in the spring also. Prophylaxis was a core feature of the holistic approach to health as well as to the treatment of ill-health. Preventative medicines were consumed in great quantities by a population which was greatly concerned with the state of its health. This is understandable, given the epidemic and endemic diseases which affected the population regularly, together with low life-expectancy and high rates of maternal, infant and child mortality. The first major step in the separation of authorised and lay medical practice came with the foundation of organisations of surgeons and physicians, though the philosophical basis of medical practice was similar across the whole spectrum of the medical marketplace.

Medical and Surgical Organisations

One of the major factors affecting both the provision and receipt of medical care in this period was the progress made in the organisation of medical and surgical training and supervision of practitioners, if not the treatment itself, and it is important to look at these before going on to assess the healers and how they healed their patients. The new institutions had considerable effects on how their members worked. Not surprisingly, lasting corporate institutions were founded in the largest towns of Edinburgh and Glasgow.

Scurvy Grass

Scurvy grass (*cochlearia*) comes from a genus of around thirty derivatives of the cabbage family. It was used as a prophylactic against scurvy – it has a high vitamin C content – and was consumed by sailors when they returned from often lengthy voyages, during which their diet was severely restricted and contained little or no fruit or vegetables. The plant has a peppery taste not unlike horseradish.

The unrelated species scurvy grass sorrel (*oxalis enneaphylla*), is a tuberous, perennial plant native to South America. It is also rich in vitamin C, and was eaten by the crews of ships rounding Cape Horn (there is evidence that sailors on Charles Darwin's ship consumed the plant).

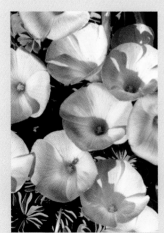

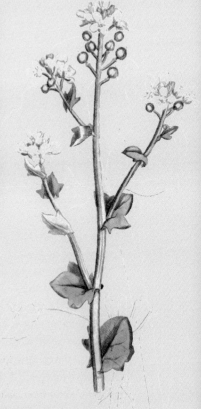

2.9 Right. Scurvy grass. Watercolour image of scurvy grass (© *Royal Botanic Garden, Edinburgh. Licensor www.scran.ac.uk*).

2.10 *Above*. Scurvy grass sorrel (*Royal Botanic Garden, Edinburgh*).

James IV

King James IV (1473–1513) was a Renaissance king. He was interested in all things cultural and artistic, and in science and medicine. It was said of him by a contemporary that he 'greedily imbibed an ancient custom of the nobility, for he was skilful in curing wounds'. The ethos of the Renaissance meant that it was now possible for a monarch to be 'cultured' as well as to show prowess as a military leader.

The royal household accounts contain a number of references to sums of money paid to individuals who allowed themselves to be treated by the monarch. These included: 2 shillings for the cost of dressings to 'John Balfour's sair leg quhilk [which] the king healit'; fourteen shillings given to the 'blind wif [wife] yat [that] had her eyne schorne' (probably means treatment of cataracts); or another payment made to an individual who had 'twa teeth drawen furth of his heid be [by] the king'.

James also participated in scientific experimentation. It is recorded by several commentators that conjoined twins 'with two bodies from the waist up' were brought up at the royal court and lived into their late twenties.

It is also alleged that James sent two infants to the island of Inchkeith, to be raised by a mute nurse, in order to determine what kind of language the children would speak. There is no record of the outcome.

In common with scientific thought at the time, James was also keenly interested in alchemy, setting up 'laboratories' at Stirling and Cambuskenneth, in order to pursue the search for a way of producing gold from base metals. He was encouraged in this by an Italian alchemist, John Damian de Falcius, known at the Scottish court as the 'French leech'. Damian also gained fame by attempting to fly from the walls of Stirling Castle.

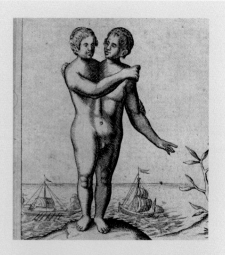

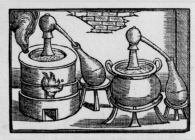

2.11 *Top.* Conjoined twins. (Engraving of 'two humans with abnormalities' from work published by Blasius and Liceti in 1665).

2.12 *Above.* Alchemy. Representation of alchemy equipment (*Wellcome Library, London*).

Edinburgh Surgeons

The Incorporation of Surgeons and Barbers of Edinburgh, which had been founded by a Town Council charter in 1505, and ratified by James IV (1473–1513) (Fig. 2.13) in 1506, was responsible for the training of surgical apprentices and overseeing surgical practice in the town. One difference between the Incorporation and the London barber-surgeons was that the latter were not required to be literate in Latin.

From the start, all Edinburgh surgical apprentices had to be literate in Latin and were required to study anatomy, with particular reference to the veins (for bloodletting) and also the astrological signs, this latter aspect being fully in tune with the prevailing philosophy. Apprentices were examined by the masters of the Incorporation at the end of their seven-year apprenticeship period, to confirm that they were fit to practise surgery. Advice was given to apprentices on the general condition and afflictions of the body, partly in the form of aphorisms, such as those of Hippocrates, one of which stated that 'those are to be let blood and purged in the Spring Time to whom the opening of a veine or purging may do good'. Initially the barbers were part of the Incorporation, but were considered much lesser beings by the surgeons, and by 1722 they had been detached from the Incorporation, forming their own society. It is more than likely, though, that some barbers continued to perform some surgical procedures such as bloodletting, despite the determined efforts of the Incorporation to prevent this.

The close study of anatomy was emphasised from the start. The Seal of Cause (charter of incorporation) was similar to those granted to other craft organisations, but also stipulated that apprentices must study anatomy and should have good knowledge of the veins, so that bloodletting could be carried out efficiently. The Incorporation was already almost half a century old when Andreas Vesalius' (1514–64) seminal work, *De Humani Corporis Fabrica*, which was published in 1543, promoted a revolution in

Hippocratic Aphorisms and Popular Axioms

Aphorisms – or short axiomatic statements on medical philosophy and practice – were at the core of medical philosophy and practice for many centuries, and this was no less the case throughout the early modern period. The Hippocratic aphorisms offered such gems of advice as:

It is better that a Feaver should succeed a Convulsion than a Convulsion a Feaver.

It is impossible to cure a vehement Apoplexie and very hard to cure a weak one – for all Apoplexies are caused by a stopping of the animal faculties from descending any lower into the body than the head.

Bodies extenuated and wasted with long sickness are to be restored and refreshed little by little, but those which have been brought low quickly and in short time are sooner to be restored.

Axiomatic advice appeared in commonplace books, in which the owners wrote down material of interest on all aspects of life and the world. These were based much more on superstition than medical philosophy and included the prescription and proscription of certain days in relation to bloodletting:

Thair be thrie days in ye yeir in ye quhilk no man sould latt him blude . . . these being the days following. The last day of Apryll, the first moneday of August and the last moneday of December.

This warning was accompanied by the dire prediction that 'if a women or man be latten blude on these dayis they sall dye within xv days'.

There were, however more auspicious days for prophylactic bloodletting, including 3 April, 18 April and 17 December.

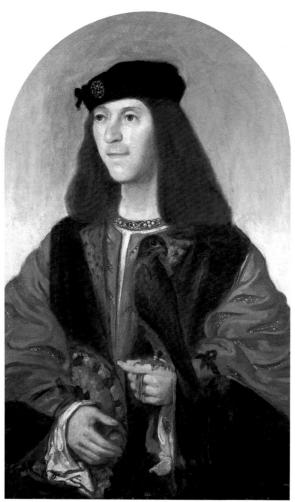

2.13 Portrait in oils of James IV. James was interested in all things scientific and medical, and was known to give money to individuals who had allowed him to let their blood or pull out teeth. He was also greatly interested in alchemy and spent much time and money on this and other scientific pursuits, though here the portrayal is of James' hunting interests (*RCSEd*).

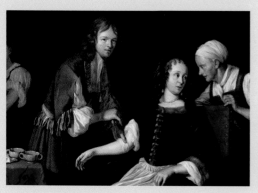

2.14 Bloodletting. Oil painting demonstrating bloodletting, seventeenth century (*Wellcome Library, London*).

anatomical study and knowledge (Fig. 2.15 and 2.16). With the Renaissance came the opportunity to dissect the human body rather than extrapolate from examination of animals, and although the practical effects on surgery and medical practice would not be widespread until the nineteenth century, the fact that the Edinburgh apprentices were able to read such works was at least a start in the long process of modernising human anatomy and, in turn, the medicine experienced by the patients.

One feature common to most developing institutions is the wish to offer an imposing visual impact, and most acquired a substantial meeting place as soon as they could. After a short period of residence in part of a tenement in Dickson's Close, the Edinburgh Incorporation bought

2.15 *Right*. Andreas Vesalius. Engraving of
Andreas Vesalius (1572) (*Wellcome Library,
London*).

2.16 *Far right*. Vesalius' *De Fabrica*. Image from
Vesalius' seminal work. The influence of classical
Renaissance art is seen clearly in the background against which the skeleton is depicted.
The illustration owes as much to images of
classical art in this period (including the typical,
imaginary idyllic background scene) as to correct
anatomy. The pose of the skeleton is perhaps
evocative of Atlas bearing the globe on his
shoulder – a sign of its great strength. Vesalius'
work was a significant step forward in the
elucidation of the structure and function of the
body, based on human dissection, which had
not been possible in the period when the Roman
Catholic religion dominated medicine as well
as general life and learning (*Wellcome Library,
London*).

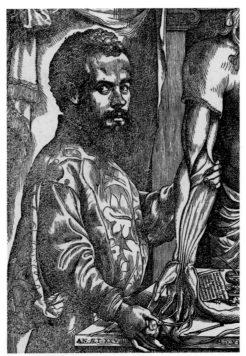

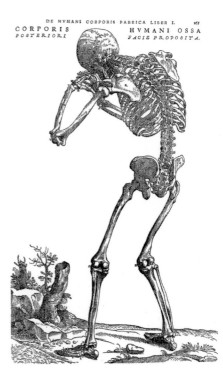

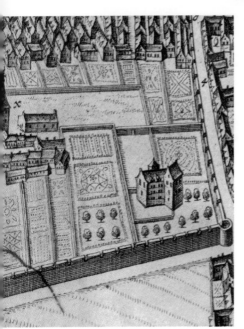

2.17 *Left*. Location of Curryhill
House. Section of Gordon of
Rothiemay's map (1647),
showing Curryhill House at
the south-east corner (*National
Library of Scotland*).

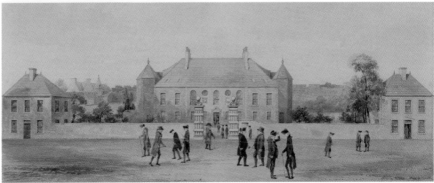

2.18 *Above*. Old Surgeons' Hall. Watercolour painting of Old Surgeons' Hall,
completed in 1697. The figures in the foreground are taken from Kay's
Portraits. The style of the building is very much in keeping with the view that
classical, orderly architecture would best portray the ideals of the Incorporation. Elements of a Scots identity are retained, though, with the towers at
either end of the main building reflecting the Scottish baronial style. There
are no female figures here, perhaps emphasising the 'male' nature of the
professions in this period (*RCSEd*).

Curryhill House in the south-west corner of Edinburgh,
in 1656 (shown in this section from Gordon of Rothiemay's map – bottom right, Fig. 2.17), and converted this
into a meeting house, which remained its home until the
construction of a new building on the same site. This was
completed in 1697 and contained an anatomical theatre,
as required by order of the Town Council (Fig. 2.18).

Following completion of the building, several annual
public dissections were carried out on the bodies of
executed criminals. The first recorded public dissection
took place in 1702 and involved examination of the body
of David Myles, who had been hanged for committing
incest with his sister – who also suffered the extreme
penalty as she had allegedly killed the baby produced as a
result of the relationship.

The building also contained a bagnio, or Turkish
bath, which was not intended to provide medical treatment. It was decorated with expensive Dutch tiles, and it

Dissection

During this period dissection became an increasingly important aspect of anatomical investigation. Dissections were carried out on the corpses of executed criminals, and following the construction of their new hall, the Edinburgh Incorporation of Surgeons performed annual public dissections. The intestines had to be buried within 48 hours of death, on Town Council instructions, so this influenced the order in which the various body parts were examined.

The event in 1702 was structured as follows, with a different surgeon demonstrating each day.

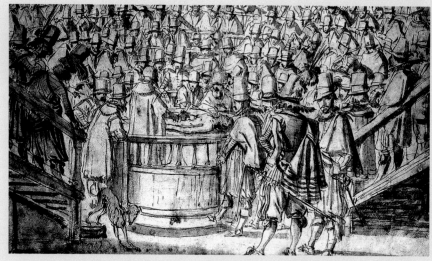

2.19 Dissection. Illustration of dissection taking place at the anatomy theatre in Leiden. Public dissections in Edinburgh would have been similar to this (*Welcome Library, London*).

DAY 1 – General account of body, muscles of the abdomen (James Hamilton)

DAY 2 – Peritoneum, stomach, intestines and pancreas (John Baillie)

DAY 3 – Liver, spleen, kidneys, ureters, bladder and reproductive organs (Alexander Monteith)

DAY 4 – Brain and its nerves, with an account of the 'animal spirits' (David Fyfe)

DAY 5 – Muscles of the extremities (Hugh Paterson)

DAY 6 – Skeleton and head (Robert Clerk)

DAY 7 – Joints and remainder of skeleton (James Auchinleck)

DAY 8 – Epilogue (Archibald Pitcairne)

The discussion of the animal spirits on day 4 reflects the transitional nature of the period, with close examination of the body coupled with discussion of long-held beliefs about the nature of the body and the senses.

was hoped that this would provide the Incorporation with much-needed income from its customers. There were many problems, including difficulties with the individuals appointed to attend the bathers and dubious activities in the upstairs bedrooms, and the bagnio eventually fell into disuse.

In due course the Incorporation established a library and a collection of curiosities, which would eventually form the basis of an important museum collection. This contained a set of cock's spurs 'prodigiously long', a box containing 'six German lancets' and, most curious of all, 'an Italian padlock for women' – presumably some sort of chastity belt. None of these has survived, but this collection was the start of what would become a very significant museum collection. The core library collection was transferred to Edinburgh University in 1763, during one of the Incorporation's recurrent financial crises.

It was thought vital to the image of the learned society

for the Incorporation to have a library and museum, and strict rules were set out regarding consultation and borrowing books, including a ban on smoking, which seems very much ahead of its time. The surgeons and their apprentices thus had access to most of the important medical and surgical treatises of the time, including the crucial work of William Harvey (1578–1657) on the circulation of blood (see Fig. 2.20).

The list of books donated to the Incorporation's library when it was established in 1699 confirms that Vesalius' work was in the collection as well as that of Harvey. Another equally important book in terms of improving the surgeons' work was Peter Lowe's *The Whole Art of Chirurgerie*, first published in 1597. This offered detailed guidelines on performing the surgical operations that were possible in theory at least (see fuller discussion of Lowe below).

The Incorporation enjoyed royal patronage through-

2.20 Plate from Harvey's *Exercitatio Anatomica De Motu Cordis*, first published in 1628. Harvey's claims were not unopposed, but in the long term his discoveries were crucial to medicine. (*RCPE*).

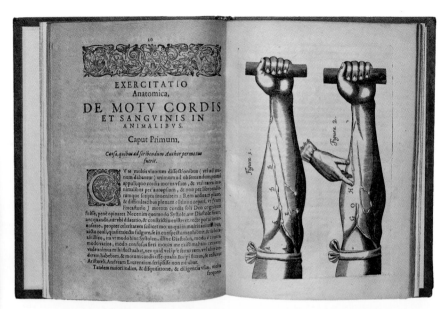

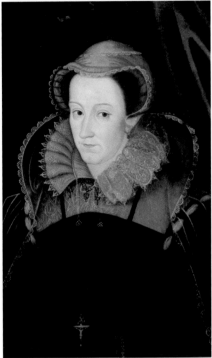

2.21 *Above*. Mary, Queen of Scots. Oil painting of Mary, Queen of Scots (*National Galleries of Scotland*).

2.22 *Right*. Letter of exemption to the Incorporation of Surgeons of Edinburgh. This was granted by Mary, Queen of Scots, in 1567, only a few months before she was forced to demit the throne. This document is important not only for its physical attractiveness in terms of early-modern manuscripts, but also for its significance in emphasising the importance of royal patronage for the progress of the Incorporation (*RCSEd, GB799RCSEd7/1567*).

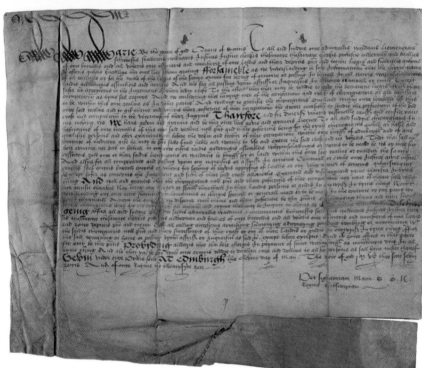

out its long history, and in 1567 Mary, Queen of Scots (Fig. 2.21) granted the surgeons exemption from bearing arms in battle, provided that they agreed to treat the wounded of both sides in any conflict (Fig. 2.22).

This was a key concession which allowed the surgeons to treat the wounded rather than risk their own death – and consequent decline in their numbers – on the field of battle. In the 1690s, after a protracted battle with the physicians concerning rights of supervision over Edin-

burgh apothecaries, the Incorporation's privileges were confirmed by means of a royal patent from William and Mary. This reliance on royal and gentry patronage was a key factor in the survival of many institutions at this time. The Royal College of Physicians (RCPE) (see below) and the Advocates' Library were established as a consequence of royal patronage, and institutions and individuals would continue to rely on this kind of help for a considerable time to come. Scottish surgeons acted as royal surgeons

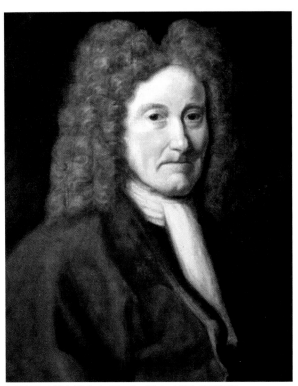

2.23 Robert Sibbald. Portrait in oils of Robert Sibbald (*RCPE*).

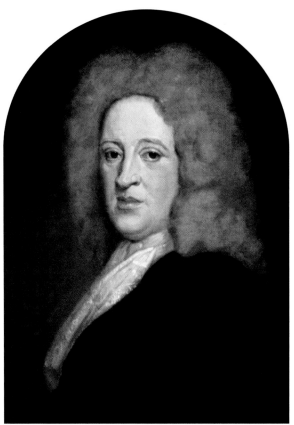

2.24 Archibald Pitcairne. Portrait in oils of Archibald Pitcairne (*RCSEd*).

and served royal and noble houses at home and abroad for generations. It has been claimed that Scottish surgeons were on the whole more highly regarded than their English counterparts, and the available evidence would seem to confirm that this was indeed the case.

By 1750 and the dawn of the Enlightenment, the Incorporation was well-established. The range of surgical procedures the members could perform was very limited, partly because of the lack of anaesthetics, but also because of the problems caused by significant blood loss and infection. Surgeons were mainly concerned with the treatment of injuries caused by violence or accident, together with attempts to cure cataracts or treat infections and administer therapeutic enemas and draw blood. The following century would see significant changes in the status and operation of the Incorporation, but for the moment it was firmly rooted in the tradition of the urban craft. One difference between the Incorporation and the other crafts, though, was that, while the Town Council could interfere

and dictate standards, such as the weight of a loaf of bread or the quality of a candle, it could not have the same influence in the day-to-day work of the surgeons. This was one aspect which helped to raise it above the status of the 'standard' craft guild.

Edinburgh Physicians

In 1681 the Edinburgh physicians finally achieved their long-held aim of establishing a college. Their attempts had been thwarted by the surgeons on several occasions, but with the backing of prominent physicians such as Robert Sibbald (1641–1722) (Fig. 2.23) and Archibald Pitcairne (1652–1713) (Fig. 2.24), and the patronage of the Duke of York, the future James VII and II, success was achieved eventually.

The final push to success has been attributed to Robert Sibbald in particular, but the background circumstances also played a part, with the presence in Scotland

Robert Sibbald (1641–1722)

Sir Robert Sibbald was one of the most notable physicians in early modern Scotland. After study at Edinburgh University, he travelled to Leiden, which was to become one of the key centres of medical education in Europe. Further study in Paris followed, and Sibbald gained his MD degree in Angers in 1662. He returned to Scotland in 1662, and helped to set up a botanical garden in Edinburgh. Sibbald was also a key figure in the foundation of the RCPE in 1681, being elected president in 1684. Besides medicine, Sibbald pursued interests in geography and natural science, being appointed Geographer Royal with a remit to produce a natural history of Scotland. He did publish widely, including his *Scotia Illustrata* of 1684, but was never able to complete his proposed Scottish Atlas.

Sibbald's medical practice was very much in the old humoral tradition, but he did favour more modern approaches to observation also, studying Scottish plants and herbs in order to improve treatments. His pamphlet entitled *Provision for the Poor in Time of Dearth and Scarcity*, published in 1699, offered potential solutions for the severe famines occurring at the time, using available natural resources more efficiently.

Sibbald was a typical polymath of his time, interested in many subjects in addition to the philosophy and practice of medicine and the foundation of a physicians' college.

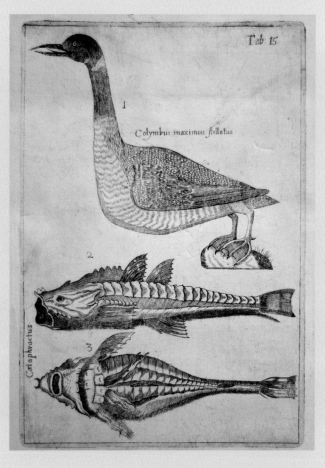

2.25 *Scotia Illustrata.* Image from Sibbald's *Scotia Illustrata*, published in 1684 (*RCPE*).

of the Duke of York, whose patronage of arts and sciences was not wholly – or possibly even partly – altruistic. It was characteristic of the Scots that they were extremely reluctant to depose the legitimate monarch, despite major shortcomings, and James was well aware of this. Patronage was important to the progress of medical institutions, and the Edinburgh physicians owed a great deal to the support of the Duke of York, future James VII. James' driving purpose was to gain political support in the wake of the exclusion crisis in England, which threatened to deprive him of the succession.

The efforts of Sibbald and his predecessors eventually bore fruit when the College charter was signed on St Andrew's day, 1681 – this date probably offering yet another coincidence (1681 may be seen as a 'golden year' in cultural terms, as the Advocates' Library was founded that year, and Stair's *Institutes of the Laws of Scotland* provided the first comprehensive account of Scots Law).

One clause in the charter would prove somewhat problematic, though – the physicians agreed that they would not undertake any teaching, which rather limited its activities and also caused tensions between the College and the University. In the tentative early years the College also experienced problems in dealing with the prevailing religious controversies, particularly following the accession of James VII and II to the throne in 1685. Sibbald was apparently persuaded to become a Roman Catholic, though he had previously signed the Test Act, which prevented Roman Catholics from holding any public office. The inevitable consequence of this was his resignation as President of the College, having been elected to this office only the previous year. Despite his eminence in the College, Archibald Pitcairne defected to the Incorporation of Surgeons, probably partly for political reasons and partly because of disagreements over his views on such matters as the arguments over chemical or mechanical explana-

Archibald Pitcairne

Archibald Pitcairne (1652–1713) was a significant figure in medicine, both in Edinburgh and abroad. He graduated MA from Edinburgh University in 1668 and then undertook medical studies in Paris, obtaining his MD from the University of Reims in 1671.

Pitcairne was one of the best-known medical men of his generation. He was instrumental in the foundation and early years of the RCPE, but defected to the Incorporation of Surgeons, possibly for political reasons, because of his alleged Jacobite sympathies.

He was appointed professor of medicine at Leiden in 1692, but returned to Scotland to marry in 1693. He did not return to Leiden, perhaps, it is suggested, because his wife (the daughter of another eminent Edinburgh physician, Sir Archibald Stevenson) did not care to live abroad.

Pitcairne can in some ways be seen as a proto-Enlightenment man and proto-scientist (in the modern usage of the term), as he was engaged in the debate over new mechanical or chemical theories of how the human body was structured and functioned. He also met, corresponded with, and debated scientific matters with Isaac Newton, his letters covering many topics such as weighing a corpse or the appropriate surgical procedure for emphysema, as well as discussing his problems with other members of the medical fraternity in Edinburgh. He published many of his thoughts and theories in his *Dissertationes Medicae* (1701).

Pitcairne had a lucrative medical practice in and around Edinburgh, and surviving records give an insight into his medical philosophy and approach to individual patients.

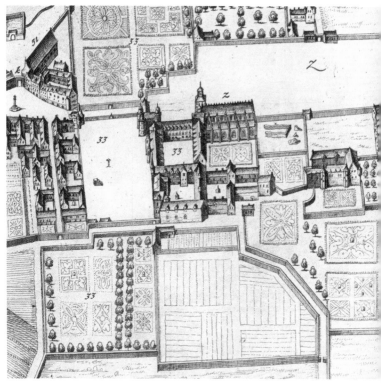

2.26 Physic Garden. Location of the physic garden at Holyrood in Gordon of Rothiemay's map of 1647 (*National Library of Scotland*).

tions for the structure and function of the body, or the treatment of fevers.

The organisation developed in some ways along the lines of the crafts, with aims to protect the interests and privileges of the members, though the Fellows would not have wished such a comparison to be made. The initial membership comprised some 20 physicians, all of whom had gained their medical qualifications outwith Scotland. A six-man council was elected, and two censors charged with the oversight of practice within the city and suburbs. Royal approval was confirmed by the fact that knight-hoods were conferred on Sibbald, Archibald Stevenson (1629–1722) and Andrew Balfour (1630–1694). The usual offices, such as treasurer and secretary, were filled, and entrants were obliged to possess an MD degree, mostly gained at European universities. From 1705 the College was involved in the examining of candidates for the MD degree at Edinburgh University before the Medical School was established in 1726. A physic garden was also established near Holyrood to produce medicinal plants (Fig. 2.26)

Taking its responsibilities seriously, the new college undertook from the start to offer free medical care to the poor – this task being undertaken by two physicians,

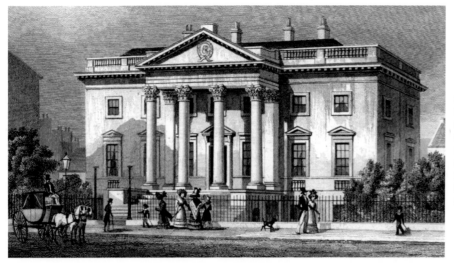

2.27 Physicians' Hall, Edinburgh. Engraving of Physicians' Hall, George Street, Edinburgh. The classical architectural style was in keeping with the New Town, and reflected the ambitions of the College to be seen as an important and influential body in the medical sphere and in the town in general (*RCPE*).

appointed yearly. Recompense would be claimed from the Town Council (there is direct evidence that the Town Council did fund treatment for the poor), so it is probable that at least some compensation for expenses was received by the 'rota' physicians for their efforts. In line with the trappings of the intellectual society a library was begun in a 'presse [cupboard] with three shelves of books' which had been donated by Sibbald himself. It was also decided that a Fellow should make a presentation monthly, either an exposition of one of the Hippocratic aphorisms (which were still a core element in medical philosophy at the time) or a topic of the speaker's choice.

The early years of the College's life were characterised by bitter and protracted triangular disputes among physicians, surgeons and apothecaries. These centred on rights of supervision over the apothecaries, who for most of the period had no discrete organisation. In general, the Incorporation of Surgeons could rely on the support of the Town Council, whereas the Physicians were more likely to gain political support from the Privy Council. In essence the arguments were about supervisory rights over the apothecaries. These had been held by the Incorporation of Surgeons, but were transferred briefly to the College of Physicians in the 1680s. Matters were settled finally with the award of a Patent to the Incorporation of Surgeons by William and Mary in 1695, which upheld its previous rights and privileges and returned responsibility for pharmacy and the apothecaries to the Incorporation. There was ongoing tension between the physicians and surgeons, partly as the physicians considered themselves to be superior intellectually, given their abstract, philosophical training, their 'hands-off' approach to the patients, and their possession of university degrees, in

contrast to the more practical apprenticeships undertaken by surgical trainees.

In keeping with the desire of emerging institutions to portray an impressive visual aspect, the College sought to acquire suitably impressive premises, and following a period of residence in Fountain Close, and a fifteen-year period in 'temporary' accommodation provided by the Royal Infirmary, the Fellows moved into their imposing new hall in George Street in 1781 (Fig. 2.27), by which time the College was well established as a key player in the politics and practice of Edinburgh medicine.

Glasgow Physicians and Surgeons

Things developed rather differently in Glasgow where, in 1599, a joint Faculty of Physicians and Surgeons (FPSG) was chartered by the town as a result of a petition submitted by Peter Lowe (*c*1550–1610) and Robert Hamilton (dates uncertain, may have graduated MA at Glasgow University in 1584 (see Fig. 2.30a and b)), complaining that poor supervision of medical practitioners was having a detrimental effect on the reputation of doctors and surgeons, and claiming that such an institution could rectify this and ensure standards and proper practice in future. Apothecary William Spang was at the same time appointed to inspect the drugs being sold in the town. The return of Peter Lowe from his long stay in France (many Scottish physicians and surgeons served long periods abroad in royal houses and armies) provided the main stimulus, against a backcloth of increasing concern on the part of the city fathers about the lack of reliable medical care. A petition was submitted subsequently to James VI, and Lowe and Hamilton were granted supervisory rights over medical and surgical practitioners in

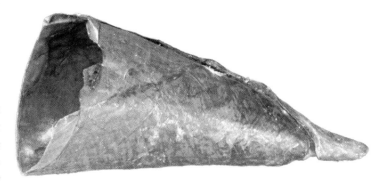

Glasgow and large areas of south-west Scotland. Although Lowe did not act alone, is it probably correct to claim that his was the dominant influence, bringing as he did the combined advantages of strong European contacts, experience of surgery in France and his contribution to surgery in his published works.

From the start, the Faculty (subsequently Royal College) was unique in Britain, as physicians and surgeons formed and still share a combined institution. This did not necessarily mean that relations between the two groups of members were harmonious. Physicians were few in number and, though growing rapidly, Glasgow was much smaller than Edinburgh, and therefore housed fewer practitioners. The initial membership of the Faculty comprised two physicians and six surgeons, so it was perhaps sensible to have this joint body in order to maintain the strength of the organisation, which did not enjoy the kind of support from the Town Council that was the case in Edinburgh. Later, in 1656, the Glasgow Town Council issued a charter founding an Incorporation of Surgeons, which was both separate from, and part of, the Faculty, referred to as a 'pendicle' of the Faculty. In the case of all three Scottish medical corporations, it is clear that their foundations owed as much to patronage and high-level social contacts as they did to the wishes of practitioners to organise themselves.

In most ways the Glasgow Faculty operated on very similar lines to the Edinburgh Incorporation in terms of the surgeons at least, though one interesting difference is that for a time in Glasgow partial licences were awarded to surgeons who were not considered good enough to undertake the whole range of surgical procedures. The licence often allowed the holder to perform barber duties and a limited range of surgery. The minutes of the Faculty show, for example, that in 1628 Alexander Lyes was declared able 'only to draw blood with a horn and such things as pertain thereto alone' (See example of such a horn in Fig. 2.28). It was possible to upgrade licences, and in November 1672 Gilbert Wilson of Strathaven was deemed competent to let blood and perform cautery 'beyond what he is formerly admitted to', while in July 1673 Allan Kirkwood from Darnley was permitted to undertake the cure of fractures in addition to the terms of

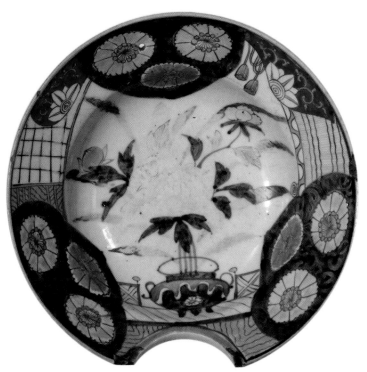

2.28 *Top.* Cupping horn. Horn for cupping or drawing blood, made of parchment or skin. The horn demonstrates the continued use of natural materials in medicine (*National Museums Scotland*).

2.29 *Above.* Bleeding dish. Painted bleeding dish with notch cut out in order for the dish to be positioned close to the veins (*RCSEd*).

his original licence allowing him to cure simple wounds. In this way it was hoped that standards could be maintained and individuals deemed incompetent prevented from practising within the jurisdiction of the Faculty.

The more famous of the two main founding fathers of the Glasgow Faculty was Peter Lowe. Details of his early life are scarce, but it is known that he left Scotland for France in the mid-1560s, and remained there for over 30 years, serving the French armies and royal houses as surgeon before returning to Scotland and taking up resi-

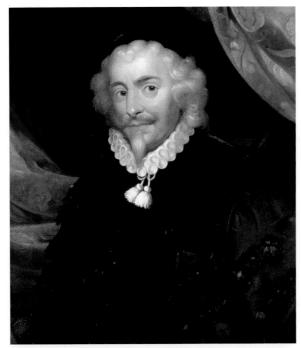

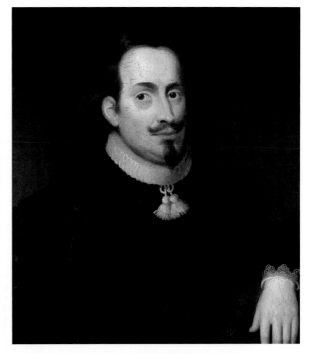

2.30a *Left*. Peter Lowe. Portrait in oils of Peter Lowe (nineteenth-century copy of original) (*RCPSG*) and 2.30b *Right*. Robert Hamilton. Portrait in oils of Robert Hamilton (nineteenth-century copy of original). Lowe and Hamilton were joint founders of the FPSG. The images suggest that Lowe may be seen as the 'senior partner', given the much more sumptuous background to his portrait. The similarities in dress suggest that this was typical formal attire for practitioners at the time. (*RCPSG*).

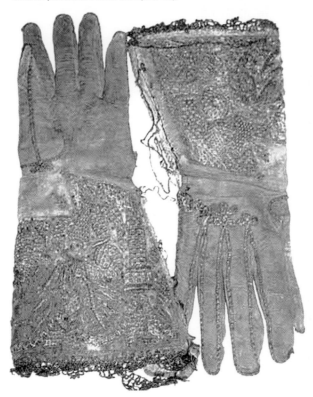

2.31 Lowe's gloves. Pair of leather gloves owned by Lowe. Their apparent high quality and ornate decoration confirm his high status (*RCPSG*).

dence in Glasgow around 1598. This contact with royal establishments would serve Lowe well, as it did most other medical practitioners who became sufficiently well known to be remembered down the centuries.

As well as being instrumental in establishing the Glasgow Faculty, Lowe is remembered for the publication of an important surgical textbook, *The Whole Course of Chirurgerie,* written in the vernacular rather than Latin, and aimed specifically at apprentices and young surgeons (see Fig. 2.32). It contained detailed instructions on surgical procedures, and also on the holistic care of patients, which was a key facet of medical practice and philosophy at the time. The book was published initially in London in 1597, and reprinted several times during the following century.

The first edition was not illustrated, but all subsequent issues were. The operations covered included amputation, cutting for the stone, trepanning, repair of hare lip and the treatment of cataracts. It is clear that many of the illustrations in the book were copied from the works of the eminent French surgeon Ambroise Paré (Fig. 2.33a and 2.33b).

Copying images from other publications was common practice at the time, and seen as a compliment to the author, rather than bad academic practice. Although Lowe's work was written in the vernacular, he did not trouble to alter some of the French annotations to some of the illustrations (Fig. 2.34).

The overall structure of each edition is similar, the

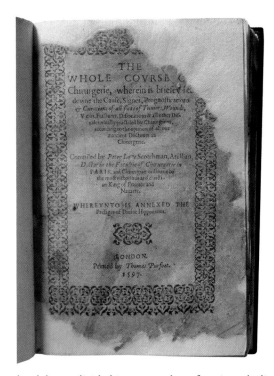

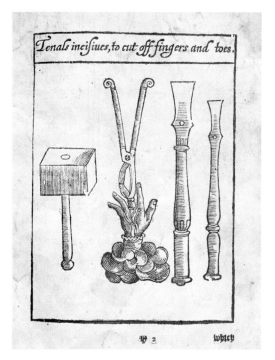

book being divided into a number of sections dealing with various aspects of surgery, general health and medication. Interestingly, many of the early chapters take the form of catechisms (a list of questions and answers). In the first edition the questions are asked by Lowe himself, and the answers attributed to Jean Cointret, Dean of the Faculty of Medicine in Paris, possibly as a tribute by Lowe to his French teachers. In subsequent editions Lowe is the questioner and his son John the respondent. In response to a question about the purpose of surgical procedures, the following responses are given:

> 'to take away that which is hurtfull and
>   superfluous' such as 'tumours against nature'
> to 'bring forth a child being dead out of the
>   mother's wombe'
> 'to help and add to nature that which it
>   wanteth' [prosthetic eye or limb]
> 'to put in the naturall place that which is out of
>   his place' [reducing dislocations] or means
>   to 'putt in guttes' [reducing hernia]
> 'to separate that which is contained' (as in
>   tongue-tie); 'to join that which is separated'
>   [fractures]. [Lowe 1634, 6-7].

Lowe died in 1610, but his surgical legacy lasted for many generations. The inscription on his gravestone is appealing:

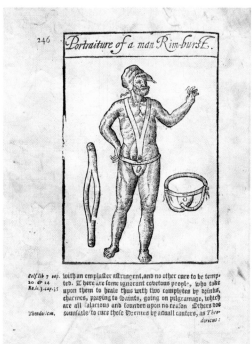

2.32 *Top left*. Lowe's *'Discourse'*. Title page of the first edition of Lowe's work, published in 1597 (*RCPSG*).

2.33a *Top* and **2.33b** *above*. Illustrations from Lowe's *Discourse*. Plates from Lowe's work, illustrating instruments for amputation of digits, and supports used for the treatment of rymburst [hernia]. Again the decoration and style reflect Renaissance classicism. It was not enough just to illustrate the basic implement; embellishment was expected (*RCSEd*).

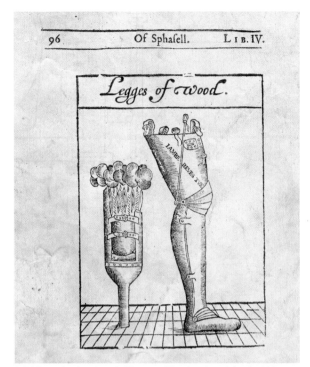

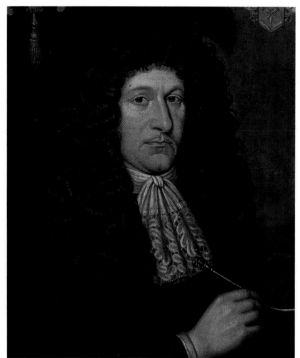

2.34 Illustration from Lowe's *Discourse*. Plate from Lowe's book with image taken from the works of Paré, with the annotation on the leg in French. The leg is styled to look like armour, possibly reflecting the significance of warfare as well as producing a sturdy limb. The simpler version may have been intended either as a temporary measure before the final limb was prepared, or the type of limb provided for the poor (*RCSEd*).

2.35 Matthew Mackail. Portrait in oils of Matthew Mackail (1678). He is holding a surgical instrument to demonstrate his profession (*University of Aberdeen*).

Stay, passenger and view this stone,
For under it lyis such a one who cuired many
    whill he lieved,
So gracious he noe man grieved,
Yea when his phisicks force oft failed, his
    pleasant purpose then prevailed,
For of his God he got the grace to live in mirth
    and die in peace,
Heavin hes his soul, his corps this stone,
Sigh passenger, and soe be gone.

Lowe was careful to emphasise the holistic aspects of his philosophy, and his explanations of the various types of 'qualities' of medicine and the types of treatments which should be employed, confirms him to be firmly in the humoral mould. It is clear that most of the substances he mentions would be readily available to the amateur as well as the trained practitioner, and that of necessity cures would depend to a certain extent on the seasons of the year and also on geographical location. Lowe can be said, therefore to be both a man of his time and a man ahead of his time.

As in Edinburgh, the Glasgow Faculty did not have a permanent home from the start, and it was not until 1708 that the first building was completed. Eventually, in 1781, the Faculty moved into a new hall in St Enoch Square, which was, in common with the aspirations of these institutions, an impressive building.

Aberdeen Medical Practitioners

In Aberdeen there was a loose organisation of surgeons, though not a formal incorporation, from at least 1494, when the 'barbouris' are noted in Town Council documents, and a Seal of Cause appears to have been granted in mid-sixteenth century. Further confirmation of privileges came in 1647, but this was apparently related to barbers and wigmakers only, and thereafter there seems to have been no discrete surgeons' organisation. The first medical practitioner to appear on the Aberdeen Burgess Roll was one Mr Walter Prendergast, admitted in 1444, while later additions to the roll included Mathew MacKail [1691/2–1733] (Fig. 2.35), appointed Professor of Medicine, in 1717. Between 1604 and 1760 only 25 physicians can be found on the burgh taxation rolls, while in the same

Qualities of Medicine as described by Peter Lowe

Lowe's descriptions of the qualities of medicine are interesting and entirely in line with the dominant medical philosophy of the time. He describes four degrees – hot, cold, dry and humid. Cures for each of the four types are described here, with one example for each category. Some items appeared in more than one group.

FOUR DEGREES OF MEDICINE

The first degree medicines *produce scarcely any alteration in the senses*

Second degree medicines *produce somewhat more noticeable effects*

Third degree medicines *offend the senses but not extreamly*

The fourth degree medicines *maketh a scar and corrupteth the senses*

HOT

1st degree – mercurialis

2nd degree – cardamom

3rd degree – iris

4th degree – anacardus

COLD

1st degree – hepatica (herbaceous plant from buttercup family)

2nd degree – pulmonaria (lungwort),

3rd degree – tormentil (rich in tannins, used to stem blood)

4th degree – papaver (opium)

HUMID

1st degree – viola (vitamin A and C, antioxidant)

2nd degree – ammoniacum

3rd degree – fragaria (woodland strawberry)

4th degree – argentum vivum (mercury)

DRY

1st degree – castanea (chestnut)

2nd degree – aristolochia

3rd degree – hellebore

4th degree – anacardus

period some 48 surgeons are noted. These numbers were not enough to sustain a corporate organisation. Similarly, no other Scottish town was large enough to have sufficient numbers of physicians or surgeons to warrant a corporate organisation, so in terms of developing medical institutions over the period, this was clearly a process confined to the largest towns. Most of the physicians to be found in the institutions had trained in Europe, and the next step was to make it possible for medical students to acquire their education in Scotland.

The Logical Next Step –
The Establishment of Medical Schools in Scotland

Once the institutions were established it was perhaps logical that the next step should be to provide the means whereby physicians could study and qualify in Scotland in order to become members of these institutions, rather than having to travel to European medical schools, which were not inexpensive. It was also logical that the lead was taken by Edinburgh, given its size, political importance and the number of resident practitioners.

Edinburgh Medical School

The opportunities for would-be physicians to train in Scotland were very limited before the foundation of the Edinburgh Medical School in 1726. In Aberdeen a mediciner had been appointed since the foundation of the university in 1495, but this post was often treated as a sinecure by the incumbent, rather than a serious appointment, though a few individuals such as Gilbert Skene (?1522–99), did make a significant contribution (discussed in Chapter 1).

The Edinburgh Town Council had made some attempts to boost the teaching of medicine and anatomy with the appointment of Robert Sibbald, James Halket (1655–*c*1710) and Archibald Pitcairne as professors of physic in 1685, though there is no evidence that they offered any formal teaching. Robert Eliot (n.d.) was appointed Professor of Anatomy in 1705, but without university accommodation, and again it is not clear if he provided any teaching. A number of MD degrees were conferred by Edinburgh University from 1705, the examinations of the candidates being conducted by Fellows of the College of Physicians, but there were only around 20 in total.

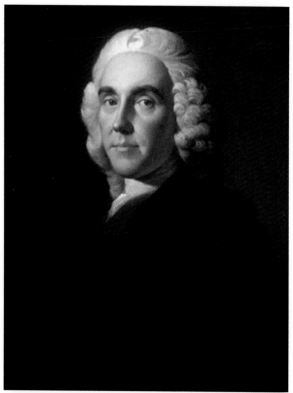

2.36 Alexander Monro *primus*. Portrait in oils of Alexander Monro *primus* (*RCSEd*).

by historians, who variously cite factors such as the need for a new cultural focus following the union of 1707, or the individual efforts of John Monro, George Drummond and Archibald Campbell (1682–1761), Earl of Islay (later third Duke of Argyll), who had studied chemistry in Leiden with Boerhaave and who largely managed Scottish politics on behalf of the Westminster government. All of the four initial medical professors – Andrew Plummer (1697–1756), John Rutherford (1695–1779) (maternal grandfather of Sir Walter Scott), Andrew Sinclair (d. 1760) and John Innes (d. 1733) had studied at Leiden and experienced the growing emphasis on clinical teaching at the bedside, which was an important new direction in medical practice and training. The noted Dutch physician Herman Boerhaave (1668–1738) advocated more direct contact with the patients, including some limited physical examination (Fig. 2.37).

It was a start. The physic gardens provided further opportunities to study the plants from which most treatments were still derived, and from that point Edinburgh began to attract large numbers of students from all parts of the globe. It has been claimed, though, that in the later years of the eighteenth century there was a certain stagnation in the Medical School, which caused some of the students to complain that their teachers merely regurgitated what they had learnt at Leiden, rather than being innovative or embracing new science and mathematics. This was perhaps to be expected, given that most of the early professors were grounded in that system, and unlikely to bring in radical change. That would have to await the next generation, but there is no doubting the importance of the events of 1726.

A further development in Edinburgh was the Royal Medical Society, founded in 1737. This was the earliest medical students' society in Britain – and the only student society to hold a royal charter. It provided a forum for debate and discussion among medical students, and continues to this day. Many eminent medical men – and women – have served as its president, and much research has been produced and debated by its members, who included Sir Stuart Threipland (Fig. 2.38), physician to Charles Edward Stuart during the 1745 Jacobite uprising, Benjamin Franklin and Joseph Lister.

Alexander Monro *primus* (1698–1767) (Fig. 2.36) acquired the chair of anatomy in 1722, primarily as a result of political manoeuvring by his ambitious father John Monro (1670–1740), who had himself studied at Leiden, and the wily and experienced *doyen* of Edinburgh politics, George Drummond (1688–1766). In 1725 Monro moved his teaching to within the walls of the University, possibly following a grave-robbing scandal in the town. Once there, he enlisted the help of royal botanist Charles Alston (1683–1760), who had gained his royal appointment with support from the Duchess of Hamilton, and James Crawford (1682–1731), professor of chemistry (who was also a qualified physician) in providing a *de facto* prototype medical curriculum, though this may not have been their primary intention.

The culmination of these developments was the foundation of the Medical School in 1726. The complex combination of circumstances and causes is still debated

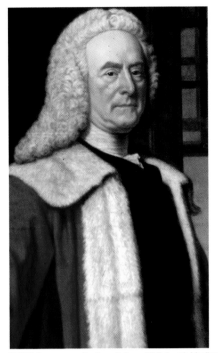
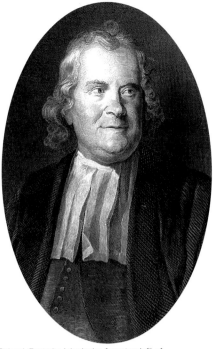
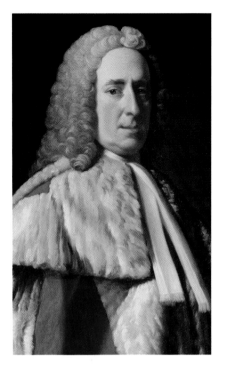

2.37 Influences on the foundation of Edinburgh Medical School. Portraits (*clockwise from top left*) of George Drummond (*LHSA*), Herman Boerhaave (*Wellcome Library, London*), Archibald Campbell, third Duke of Argyll (*National Galleries of Scotland*) and John Monro (*RCSEd*), all of whom had some influence on the foundation and operation of the Edinburgh Medical School.

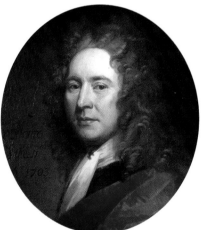

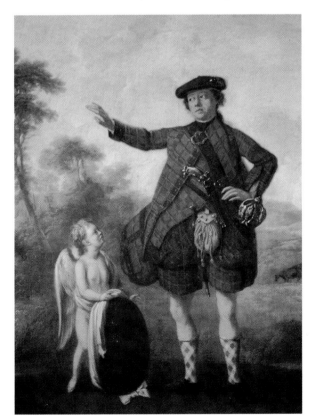

2.38 Sir Stuart Threipland. Portrait of Sir Stuart Threipland, physician to the Young Pretender and member of the Royal Medical Society (*in a private collection*).

Glasgow Medical School

In Glasgow the prospects for a medical school were hampered by ongoing friction between the University and the FPSG. In 1637 the University had appointed Mr Robert Mayne to act as professor of medicine, at an annual stipend of 400 merks (£266 13s 4d Scots), but the appointment lapsed only a few years later. Around 1704 a further tentative step was taken when a piece of University ground was given over to be used as a physic garden, and a Glasgow surgeon, John Marshall, was appointed as supervisor. By 1713 a chair of medicine was re-established, and one of anatomy set up in 1720. Teaching, though, depended on at least five students requesting classes, and it was not really until the 1740s that there was an effective medical faculty. One of the most notable teachers was William Cullen (1710–90) (discussed fully in Chapter 3), who made significant contributions to chemistry as well as medicine in general. Cullen, and his equally important colleague, Joseph Black (1728–99) would eventually be head-hunted eastwards, but their early medical work was centred in Glasgow.

Aberdeen Medical School

There were also problems in Aberdeen, the conflict here being between the two colleges, King's and Marischal, with the result that formal, corporate medical training was delayed until the nineteenth century. Some of the mediciners did make significant contributions, though, and dynastic factors were important, including James Gregory (elder and younger) and John Gregory. James Gregory the younger (1753–1821) was also a practising physician, and was effectively the elder statesman of the physicians in Aberdeen, while his brother John (1724–1773) was one of the first surgeons to operate in the Aberdeen Infirmary. He subsequently sojourned briefly to London and was then appointed to the Chair of Medicine in Edinburgh in 1766. He is also remembered for his publication in 1722 of *Lectures on the Duties and Qualifications of a Physician.*

The medical schools in the major Scottish towns originated at different times, and were shaped by different factors, but there is no doubt that these institutions formed a key part in the development of Scottish medicine, though not of the experience of the patients at that time. What they aimed to produce was physicians who could be set apart from the complexity of the medical marketplace and recognised as the main authority, in the mould of what is seen in modern times as professional.

Professions

Historians are divided on the issue of when it can be claimed that the medical profession existed, but it would seem that in this period at least the foundations were laid. All of the medical and surgical institutions claimed to be acting for the good of medicine and the well-being of the patients, and the advent of clinical medicine would be complemented by much greater understanding of the structure and function of the body and its various systems,

especially from the second half of the eighteenth century. Even though qualified practitioners prescribed very similar cures to those offered by amateur healers of all sorts, this does not detract from their efforts to act professionally as individuals and as groups. By the second half of the eighteenth century many medical practitioners were publishing their own works, thus adding directly to the growing pool of opinion on the nature of diseases and the methods of their treatment.

Some historians take the view that professions could not exist until the industrial revolution had helped to free individuals from the bonds of patronage, in other words when professionals could act independently of any obligation to a benefactor. In earlier times members of the legal profession, perhaps more than physicians, had relied heavily on the influence of wealthy patrons in order to achieve their positions. Similarly, university chairs had been – and continued to be – political appointments, and this would be the case well into the nineteenth century. It may also be claimed that a profession could not exist until it was regarded by society as a whole in that light, or until it was able to apply exclusive knowledge and maintain possession of that exclusive knowledge. The medical marketplace was still very broad, and individuals from all walks of life offered medical treatments of various sorts. This perhaps separated the medical profession from the other learned groups. It was rather more difficult for lay individuals to offer legal or religious services, but very easy in terms of health care. The fact that the available knowledge was shared or possessed by qualified and unqualified practitioners perhaps delayed full recognition of medicine as a profession, but it does seem fairly clear that the foundations were being laid, in terms of self-policing bodies, acquisition of knowledge, imposition of qualifications by examination, and the more difficult to assess facet of altruistic intent, together with powers of expulsion and control of fees, however imperfect some of these were. The application of this proto-professional model was of more importance to the patients, perhaps, than internal rules and regulations. Members of the institutions aimed to heal, and did this in a variety of ways and against a backcloth of a complicated, broad, and open medical marketplace.

HEALERS AND HEALING

Although medical professionals were beginning to separate themselves from the rest of the healing sphere, in a sense the whole adult population in this period could be seen as deliverers of health care. Self-treatment was often the only option, and long traditions of local and regional healing had evolved over the centuries. Large tracts of the country had no qualified medical practitioner – one observer noted that there was only one 'medical man' for 50 miles north of Aberdeen at the start of the eighteenth century. This was Dr Beattie of Garioch, who did his rounds 'on a shaggy pony'. By 1750 there were certainly many more qualified physicians in Scotland, some of whom were famous both in their own day and since, and time-served master surgeons in the lowland, urban areas, but this kind of service was only available in remoter areas to gentry households who could afford to give hospitality to a physician and stable his horses for the duration of the consultation and treatment. There were no nurses in the modern sense of the word, and most women designated as nurse in written records were in fact wet-nurses at this time.

'Official' Healers and Healing

Professional medicine developed in an urban setting, practised by physicians, surgeons and apothecaries, but there was no clear barrier between folk medicine and 'legitimate' medical practice, and many of the plants and remedies advised by lay healers were used by official practitioners. The particular substances used to treat any condition were related partly to location and season, and there were few items in the qualified physician's medicine chest that could not be acquired by the lay public except, perhaps, non-plant-based substances such as mercury. By the middle of the eighteenth century chemical medicines were more readily available, and required more than the domestic setting for their production. Scotland was rather slower than England to embrace medicines produced by formal chemical processes. The designation of categories of healers was vague in the minds of most individuals, but attempts were made by the institutions to enforce demarcation. This section will consider the three main groups

of official practitioner – physicians, surgeons and apothecaries, and also the establishment of hospitals as a further key aspect of the medical sphere.

Physicians

The consultation was at the heart of medical practice at whatever level of society, and although its nature changed with the advent of clinical examination and the availability of stethoscopes and other instruments, the exchange of information and ideas between doctor and patient did not. In this period, though, it was perhaps the case that, at least at high social levels, the views of the patient carried more weight than they did in subsequent periods. The patients were entirely free to consult as many practitioners

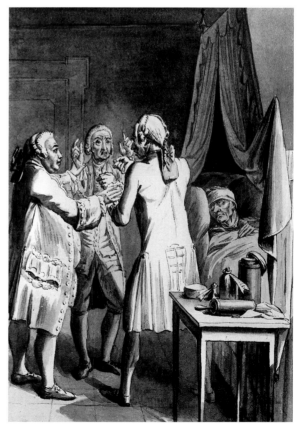

2.39 Eighteenth-century medical consultation. The patient is somewhat peripheral to the proceedings, while the assembled physicians indulge in an animated exchange of views (*Wellcome Library, London*).

as they pleased, and in high status cases the physicians themselves would call in their colleagues to opine on the symptoms. High-status patients residing at their country estates often consulted their medical attendants by letter. Fig. 2.39, though not a Scottish work, does illustrate what might be a typical consultation in this period.

During the consultation the physician took a careful history of symptoms, but also, importantly, of general lifestyle, as a holistic approach was necessary. He observed the mood and condition of the patient, and perhaps examined a specimen of urine, but in the main relied on his interpretation of the patient's description of his or her symptoms, relating these to general disease templates. By 1750 more attention was paid to the specific, local symptoms described by individual patients, but in general similar symptoms were thought to relate to similar causes. Watches with second hands were available by 1707, pioneered by Sir John Floyer (1649–1734), author of *The Physician's Pulse Watch*, published that year. Before that it was difficult to count the pulse accurately, though its quality could be assessed, and it was likely that quality was deemed more important than frequency at this time.

Once the history had been taken, standard forms of treatment were advised. In the vast majority of instances this involved purges, emetics or enemas in the first instance, in order to clear the body of evil matter so that it could then be restored by means of medicines and possibly changes to lifestyle. Many prescriptions for the first phase of treatment involved senna or antimony, which was

used in various forms as both purgative and emetic, as were rhubarb and turpentine and blackthorn flowers. Purging was frequently administered in the form of an enema (clyster). Hellebore was used as a powerful emetic, and bloodletting also featured in this 'clearance' package (Fig. 2.40). The commonplace book of Sir John Wedderburn, an early-eighteenth-century physician, includes advice given to one of his patients that 'bloodletting [would have] been more beneficial at the beginning of your first course [episode of illness] than now, yet in the spring it may be done to great advantage if no crosse emergent symptome do forbid, especially for the itch it may be used' [National Library of Scotland, MS 6504, f. 74]. There were many similar instances of venesection being used routinely as well as seasonally or prophylactically.

The next step in treatment was the prescription of restorative agents for whichever body system was deemed to be the cause of the patient's symptoms. Scurvy, for example, was treated with substances thought to counteract the disease, including fumitory (herb used to rid body of impurities), mountain sage, juniper berries and rosemary. Dietary advice was to avoid beef, pork and fowl, also cheese and fish roasted in salt. Archibald Pitcairne gave detailed advice to a woman apparently suffering from rheumatism. After the expected clearance regimen came concoctions involving millipedes (crushed) – which may in fact have been wood lice – and the patient was advised to travel to Bath to take the waters – an option open only to those enjoying high social status. Clearly the Bath

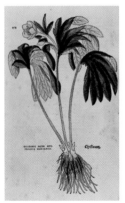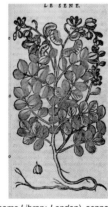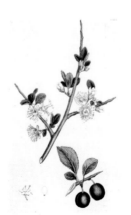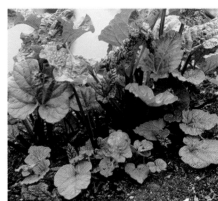

2.40 Purgatives. Hellebore (*Wellcome Library, London*), senna (*RCPE*), blackthorn (*Wellcome Library, London*) and rhubarb (*Wellcome Library, London*), used as purgatives throughout the period.

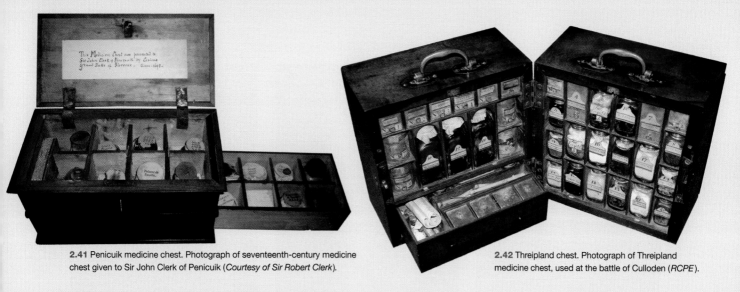

2.41 Penicuik medicine chest. Photograph of seventeenth-century medicine chest given to Sir John Clerk of Penicuik (*Courtesy of Sir Robert Clerk*).

2.42 Threipland chest. Photograph of Threipland medicine chest, used at the battle of Culloden (*RCPE*).

Penicuik and Threipland Medicine Chests

Sir John Clerk of Penicuik's Medicine Chest

Sir John Clerk (1676–1755), second baronet of Penicuik, was given the medicine chest by Cosimo, Grand Duke of Florence, in 1698. Clerk may well have met the duke on his European grand tour, a traditional part of the education of a gentleman in the period. Following his return from Europe, Clerk would make his name in politics and cultural affairs, being a prolific author and composer as well as one of the most prominent politicians of his day. He was one of the commissioners who negotiated the Act of Union in late 1706 and early 1707.

The medicine chest, though Italian in origin, is typical of its period, and the bottles, which appear to contain many of the original contents, are labelled in a mixture of Italian and Latin. Among the labels which can be deciphered with confidence are:

> *Elixir proprietatis.* A widely-used substance containing aloes, saffron and tincture of myrrh.
> *Ess. Di Contraeirua* (Essence of Contayerva), derived from a plant found in Mexico and the West Indies. It was used as a stimulant and mild tonic, and for treatment of fevers.
> *Olio da Stomaco.* An oil for the stomach.
> *Poluer da Renella.* A powder used for treating kidney disorders. 'Renella' denotes a deposit in the kidneys or bladder, so this was most probably used to treat kidney stones.
> *Giulebbo Gemmato.* A syrup or sugar solution of precious stones. Inclusion of precious stones in powder form was not uncommon at this time, but was confined to the more wealthy patients, given the cost. (*Information on these substances from Peter Worling.*)

The Threipland Medicine Chest

Sir Stuart Threipland (1716–1805) undertook his medical studies in Edinburgh and was a founder-member of the Royal Medical Society. He volunteered for the Jacobite army during the uprising of 1745 and acted as physician to Charles Edward Stuart, the Young Pretender, both during the conflict and after Charles had deserted the battlefield at Culloden.

This medicine chest is said to have been used by Threipland. There are over 150 medicinal items, together with a number of miniature instruments, including scales for measuring out the ingredients for medical recipes. The items include balsams, elixirs, powders, tinctures and ointments. Whereas the much smaller Penicuik chest comprised prepared substances, there were only three prepared mixtures in the Threipland chest, which were used as treatments for fever, toothache and scurvy, all of which could affect the fighting abilities of soldiers to a considerable degree. Among the substances which had been in use for many years prior to this time were Peruvian bark (cinchona), opium, ipecacuanha and myrrh.

The contents of the Threipland chest were very much in line with the contents of the *Edinburgh Pharmacopoeia*, the first four editions of which had listed many outlandish items such as dog's gall, goat's blood, warts from a horse, or the urine of a pre-pubescent boy. Folk remedies often included crushed snails, earthworms or sheep's droppings, and in some ways the inclusion of such ingredients in the physicians' official *Pharmacopoeia* is not surprising, but by 1745 it does seem a little outdated, and indeed the 1745 edition was stripped of many such substances.

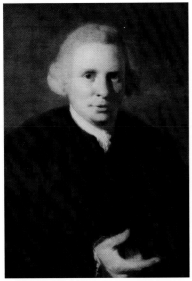
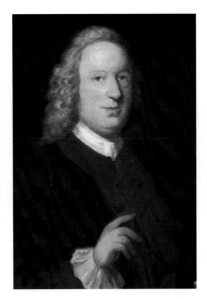
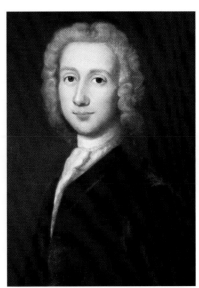
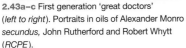

2.43a–c First generation 'great doctors'
(*left to right*). Portraits in oils of Alexander Monro
secundus, John Rutherford and Robert Whytt
(*RCPE*).

waters were regarded as superior to any healing waters in
Scotland. Millipedes were also prescribed to a young girl
with menstrual difficulties, together with asses' milk and
mercury, while the views of the patient held some sway in
the case of another patient who was advised to take
laudanum and sarsaparilla (a perennial plant imported
from South America and used to treat a variety of conditions, including syphilis) as she did not like mercury. The
particularly unpleasant side-effects of mercury, including
excessive salivation and mouth ulceration were well
known, though it continued to be prescribed in various
forms until well into the nineteenth century.

The 'Great Doctors' – the First Generation
Though most physicians treated their patients in a similar
fashion, towards the end of the period covered here, a
group of physicians who have become known as the 'great
doctors' emerged. These men would make significant
contributions to the science of medicine, far beyond what
might be expected from a small nation. The efforts of this
elite group must be given due prominence in any historical analysis, but care must be taken not to take too much
of a Whiggish, 'grand sweep of progress' view. These men
were of course important, but the consumers of medical
treatment noticed little change, and would not do so until
well into the nineteenth century. Among the key individuals in this period were Alexander Monro *primus*, his son

Alexander Monro *secundus* (1733–1817), John Rutherford
and Robert Whytt (Fig. 2.43a–c). The 'great doctors' of
the eighteenth century may perhaps be divided into two
groups – those who developed the medical school and
began clinical teaching, and the second group, whose
members built on these organisational foundations and
began to find out much more about the structure and
function of the human body.

The first-generation 'great doctors', many of whom
had been bred on the 'Dutch model', provided the teaching in the early years of the medical school – though as
time passed they began to be criticised for not embracing
the new philosophical perspectives of men of reason such
as Francis Hutcheson (the father of moral philosophy) –
in other words, for not moving with the times. The
Monro family dominated academic anatomy and surgery
for the best part of a century (see Chapter 3), while the
Hamiltons turned their attentions to midwifery – early
indications of future specialisations. Father and son
Alexander (bap. 1739–1802) and James (1767–1839) Hamilton may be credited with the establishment of academic
midwifery, the precursor of the specialty of obstetrics.
Alexander Hamilton was one of the rare individuals to
have qualified as both surgeon and physician (serving as
Deacon of the Incorporation of Surgeons) and to be
appointed subsequently to a university chair – that of
midwifery – jointly with Thomas Young in 1780. Hamil-

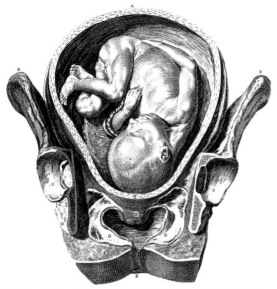

2.44 Alexander Hamilton. Plate from Alexander Hamilton's *Anatomical Tables with Illustrations* (Edinburgh, 1787) showing the uterus with a fully-developed foetus. The clarity of the image is impressive. Illustrations were produced by Charles Grignion (*c*1721–1810), an English engraver (*Wellcome Library, London*).

2.45 Notebook. Notes on bones from a notebook on surgery and anatomy compiled by Robert Whytt (*Wellcome Library, London*).

ton was succeeded by his son James in 1800. Though it would take until the 1830s for midwifery to be confirmed as a core subject in the medical curriculum, the early efforts of the Hamiltons and Thomas Young helped to further the cause considerably.

Robert Whytt (1714–66) was perhaps the first of the new wave of scientific physicians to be associated with eighteenth-century Edinburgh medicine. He followed the 'old' route of peripatetic training, culminating in the award of an MD from Reims in 1736. He became a fellow of the RCPE in 1738.

Whytt's initial interest lay in the treatment of the endemic problem of bladder stones (Fig. 2.46), and he advocated the use of lime water and soap, given by catheter. This treatment continued to be given well into the nineteenth century, but eventually was shown to be ineffective. Interestingly, he had derived this treatment in part from his analysis of a secret cure by one Joanna Stephens, which had aroused national interest and had even been mentioned in parliament. This juxtaposition of amateur and professional medicine was rooted in the past, but at the same time looked to a more scientific future.

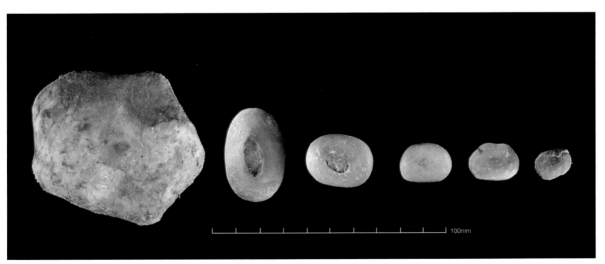

2.46 Bladder stones. Showing the variety of size and shape (*Wellcome Library, London*).

Whytt eventually turned his thoughts to the structure of the body and the nature and function of the soul – which again demonstrates elements of old beliefs and attempts to produce new scientific explanations. Whytt believed, *inter alia*, that the body could not function – particularly the heart – without the direct influence of the soul in every particle. By the time his *Essay on the Vital and other Involuntary Motions of Animals* was published in 1751, Whytt was Professor of the Practice of Medicine at Edinburgh University. His ideas were derived from a complex combination of factors, including past tradition, new science and contacts with European thinkers and physicians. He can in many ways be seen as a typical transitional figure, bridging the gap between old and new science and medicine.

Perhaps an essential precursor to the practical application of the efforts of the great doctors was the introduction of bedside teaching for students, and John Rutherford is generally credited as being the pioneer in this field. It has been claimed, though, that in fact a considerable amount of teaching was carried out in the Infirmary attached to the Glasgow Town's hospital by a succession of physicians, including William Cullen. Rutherford started out as a surgical apprentice before moving to London, then Leiden. Following graduation with his MD from Reims in 1719, he came back to Scotland and, as mentioned, was one of the founding professors of the medical school. Following the opening of the second Infirmary, Rutherford was allowed to give a course of clinical lectures, and also discussed and examined patients brought by his students in order to emphasise that the particular set of symptoms displayed by the individual patient were just as important as broad axiomatic statements on the nature of illnesses in general. The popularity of this kind of teaching was such that in due course a ward was set aside for Rutherford's use. Thus began a key feature of medicine in Britain, and one which marked the start of a sea-change in medical philosophy – the importance of the individual, rather than relating symptoms to 'standard' explanations.

The heyday of the 'second generation great doctors' came in the latter part of the eighteenth century and early-nineteenth century, and is dealt with in detail in the following chapter. There is no doubt, though, that these earlier doctors made significant individual contributions to the development of new medical theories, but their achievements must be viewed in the context of a number of other factors, including the availability of medical hospitals and the changing social, political and economic background.

Many of the physicians who made up the membership of the RCPE or FPSG had lucrative medical practices in the towns. They were consulted by the highest in the land and offered medical advice which was a heady mix of new science and old-fashioned superstition. Some of Archibald Pitcairne's case books survive, for example, and they contain some interesting advice and prescriptions. Despite being one of the foremost physicians in Scotland (though he would defect to the Incorporation of Surgeons), he was not above prescribing such things as the fastening of live doves to the soles of the feet as a last resort for a patient *in extremis*.

Surgeons

For all of the period under review here, the opportunities for performing complex surgical procedures successfully were few, given that speed was of the essence in the absence of anaesthetics apart from alcohol or strong herbal potions. The surgeons of Edinburgh and Glasgow made strenuous efforts to prevent unqualified individuals from performing anything other than the most basic treatments and dressings, but in the rural areas this was not possible. Surgery was performed in the main to try and save life, not to improve deformity, or for reasons other than necessity. Apprentices learned human anatomy in as much detail as was known at the time – for example, one Edinburgh apprentice was asked in his examination to describe the brain and its eleven pairs of nerves, whereas there are in fact twelve pairs.

It was also becoming more common – though not routine – for post mortem examinations to be carried out occasionally to try to establish the cause of death. These examinations were carried out mostly on the bodies of the gentry, but the whole body was not necessarily examined. In this example from 1702, the head was not opened as the medical attendants (Fig. 2.47) were confident of

Post Mortem Examination of Lady Polwarth (1702)

My Lady having dyed on the 11th of December her breast and the upper pairt of her belly were opened the next day by Patrick Telfer chirurgeon in presence of Sir Archibald Stevenson and Doctor Archibald Pitcairn doctors of medicine. So much opening being thought sufficient for discovering the cause of her ladyships lingering and tedious disease to inform her relations. Her body was found to be emaciate to the utmost degree. The chist of her breast was the narrowest and of the smallest capacitie that could be expected to be seen in one of her build and talness and was full of extravasat purulent mater. The right lobe of the lungs was wholely exulcereit and soe attach'd to the pleura with a great inflammation that it could not be separat without lacerating the whole membrane. The substance of the lungs in both right and left side was wholelie stuff'd with evident purulent mater in all the little cavities and cells thereof. The heart was firm and in a good condition. The liver being in several parts cut was not found to any degree ill affected. The stomach was not opened nor the intestines but lookes very well. No other part was inspected.

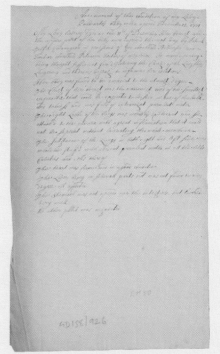

2.47 Post mortems. Report of post-mortem examination carried out on the body of Lady Polwarth in 1702 (*National Archives of Scotland, GD158/296*).

finding the cause of death without the necessity to invade the body more than necessary, and permission had not been given to carry out a more extensive examination.

Some evidence as to what surgical procedures were more likely to be carried out comes from the topics allocated to surgical apprentices in Edinburgh for their final examinations to become masters of the Incorporation (they were also required to become burgesses of the town before they could practise in their own right. This could be achieved *gratis* by the sons or sons-in-law of burgesses). These included amputation of the leg and arm, removal of cataract, repair of hare lip and trepanning of the skull. Most procedures were necessitated by violence, war or accident. As mentioned, cutting for the stone was normally avoided by surgeons, though this was a common problem in the general population. The *Caledonian Mercury* reported on 27 February 1725 that a post-mortem on the late Lord Chief Justice had revealed four bladder stones, the largest of which weighed 'seven ounces and a half', though there is no indication of whether he had been operated on, or by whom. The prevalence of this

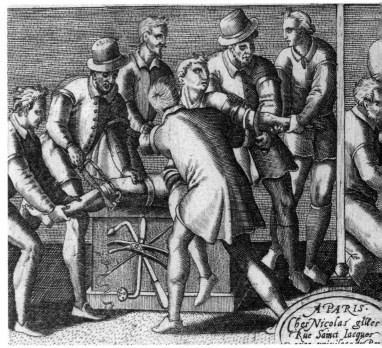

2.48 Amputation. Engraving of amputation – not a Scottish image, but typical of the period (*Wellcome Library, London*).

2.49 Archibald Pitcairn's medical practice. Letter to Archibald Pitcairne on the right-hand page, with his reply on the left-hand page (*University of Edinburgh, Special Collections Department, Dc.1.62, Praxeos Pitcarnianae*).

Archibald Pitcairne's Medical Practice in Edinburgh

The evidence from surviving case records suggests that Pitcairne was consulted both by patients directly and by other physicians seeking a second opinion. Pitcairne appended his advice to these letters, as the following example illustrates. This advised some treatments which may not have been available to the population at large.

The letter on the right hand page is from John Hay of Haystoun, written in 1703, twenty days after his wife had given birth to a son. She is complaining of a return of symptoms which she had suffered previously:

> . . . vomiting and looseness as formerlie was her custome. And now she spits blood thir thrie or four dayes bygane. And no great pain but comes up with couching [coughing] and when she couchs it comes up clear.

A postscript notes that

> she has no stich in her stomach but the blood comes easillie away. She bloods now at the nose as formerllie was her custome.

Pitcairne's advice, written on the facing page, comprised prescriptions for the following:

Aluminis liquor (alum, used to treat vomiting and diarrhoea)
Sang. drac. (dragon's blood – used as a colouring)
Aqua cinnamoni (cinnamon water, used as a mild astringent)
Laud. Liq. (Laudanum liquid – often associated with Tincture of Opium, but also could be made with opium, saffron, cinnamon and cloves)
Tinct. Antiphthisica (tincture for phthisis or consumption)
Syr. Coral (syrup of coral, known to have been used in early modern medicines and believed to have an antibiotic effect)
Aq. Calc. (Lime water – used very commonly in all sorts of conditions).

Interestingly, there is evidence that in the nineteenth century such post-partum symptoms were treated with almost exactly the same types of medicines.

(Edinburgh University Library, Dc.1.62, Praxeos Pitcarnianae) (*Interpretation of the prescribed items provided by Peter Worling*)

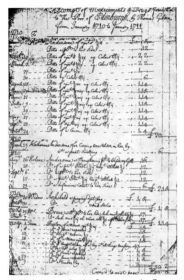

2.50 Accounts for the Surgeon to the Poor of Edinburgh, 1710, showing amputation and subsequent provision of 'timber leg' (*Edinburgh City Archives, Moses Bundle 136/5321*).

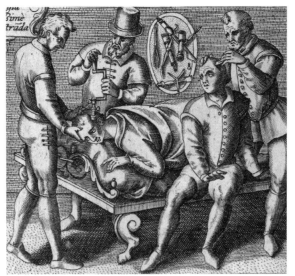

2.51 Trepanning. Image of trepanning operation (the image is French but the experience of Scottish patients would have been very similar) (*Wellcome Library, London*).

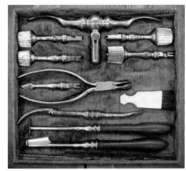

2.52 Trepanning. Set of eighteenth-century trepanning instruments (produced by Stanton of London) (*RCPSG*).

problem resulted in the advertisement of many alleged cures, including one which appeared in the *Edinburgh Evening Courant* on 7 August 1732, and comprised an infusion of marshmallow leaves, mercury (the herb) and saxifrage, to be drunk twice a day.

Amputation was often performed because the surgeons could not undertake procedures aimed at salvaging a limb. Surgeons prided themselves on performing the operation at great speed, to try to ensure that the patient did not die of blood loss or shock (Fig 2.48). The fact that illustrations of prosthetic limbs featured in contemporary surgical treatises confirms that at least some of the patients did survive long enough to require to be fitted with an artificial limb. One such was a woman in receipt of poor relief in Edinburgh in 1710. The accounts for the surgeon appointed by the Town Council to provide free treatment for the poor include the case of Jean Beaton, who had a leg amputated at a cost of £40 Scots in April (at this time £1 sterling was equivalent to £12 Scots). In October of the same year the town also paid out £3 for 'a timber leg', confirming that it was possible to survive this heroic procedure despite living in poverty and probably squalid conditions (Fig. 2.50). Many amputations were performed on battlefields as a result of combat and individuals did survive, despite the conditions.

Trepanning was one of the earliest surgical procedures to be performed (see Chapter 1) (Fig. 2.51 and 2.52), and indeed the Edinburgh surgical apprentices were asked questions on the subject in their examinations. There are, though, few references to trepanning in the surviving records, and Peter Lowe advised a cautious approach, being of the opinion that 'it is not meet to trepan in all fractures as ye have heard, or to discover the brains without necessitous and good judgement, so that the young Chyrurgion may not so hastily, as in time past, trepan for every simple fracture'. This is only one opinion, however, and there is no doubt that the operation was carried out, but perhaps by this time not quite on the same scale as in very early times, despite the prevailing importance of 'spirits' to the holistic view of the body and its relationship with the universe. In 1792 the Royal College of Surgeons of Edinburgh received the gift of a set of trepanning instruments for use in battlefield surgery – they had been specially prepared so as to be 'secure against injury from motion or the weather' and 'may even be carried in the pocket'.

The work of military surgeons had been changed greatly by the need to learn how to deal with the effects of gunshot wounds, which were very different from the injuries inflicted by other sorts of weapons. Fig. 2.53

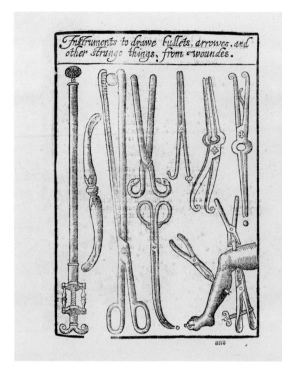

2.53 Bullet removal. Plate from Lowe, *Discourse*, illustrating instruments to be used for removing bullets from various parts of the body. As with most surgical instruments of the time, they were works of art as well as practical implements (*RCSEd*).

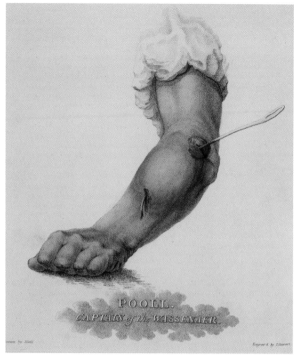

2.54 Coloured engraving showing treatment of gunshot wound, from John Bell's *Principles of Surgery* (Edinburgh, 1801–8), showing the bullet track being kept open for drainage (*Wellcome Library, London*).

shows the kind of instruments in use in the late sixteenth century.

Gunshot injuries produced severe tissue damage, and contained fragments of clothing as well as the bullets or shot, and presented different kinds of surgical problems to those produced by the effects of human power, such as lances, pikes or swords (Fig. 2.54). Battlefield surgeons thus had to rethink their treatment methods and try to deal with the increased risk of infection caused by foreign materials within the wounds. Bones shattered by gunshot were much more difficult to deal with than the flesh wounds or fractures caused by falling from horses and the like. War surgery is certainly one area where technological advances enforced change in medical and surgical treatment.

It is clear that many Scottish surgeons owned the works of Ambroise Paré (1510–90). Paré was concerned to alleviate the suffering of gunshot victims, especially given the practice of applying boiling oil or tar to treat the wounds. He had found himself without any oil on one occasion and had instead used a 'digestive made of egg yolk, rose oil and turpentine'. On examination the following day he found that patients who had been treated with oil were 'feverish, with great swelling and inflammation', while those who had received the much gentler prepara-

tion had 'little pain in their wounds, without inflammation and swelling, having rested well through the night'. Lowe had served as a military surgeon in France, and gave very detailed instructions on the correct technique for treating gunshot wounds; so it is likely that at least some Scottish gunshot victims would avoid the torture of boiling oil. Military surgery is a case in which the background context was crucial to both doctor and patient, and where political disputes and technological advances could stimulate developments in medical and surgical practice.

More complex surgery would be possible with the advent of anaesthesia, but some attempts were being made to push the boundaries a little, in an attempt to reduce the appallingly high levels of maternal and child mortality. By the second half of the eighteenth century Caesarean sections on live mothers were being attempted. Eight documented cases from Edinburgh have been described by Kaufman, the first procedure being carried out by Robert Smith in 1737, and the others at intervals till 1800, the surgeons involved including Alexander Wood, William Chalmer, Thomas Young, and the more famous John and Charles Bell. Of the eight patients, all of the mothers perished, but three of the infants survived.

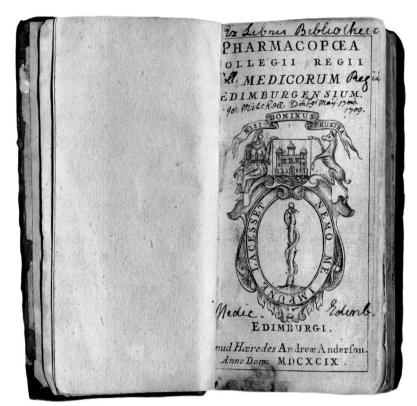

2.55 Title page of first edition of *Edinburgh Pharmacopoeia* (1699) (*RCPEd*).

Apothecaries

Often rather neglected in the great scheme of medical history, but just as important in many ways as the physicians or surgeons were the apothecaries, who played a key role in the delivery of medical care in most Scottish towns. Precise designation is difficult, as at this time it was common to refer to any medical practitioner as 'the apothecary'. The poet William Dunbar (1460–1520) was apparently able to make the distinction clearly in his eulogy of the glittering court of James IV (*c*1505):

> Kirkmen, courtears and craftisman fine
> Doctouris in jure and medicine
> Divinouris, rethoris and philosophours,
> Astrologists, artistis and oratouris . . .
> Musicians, menstralis and mirrie singeris . . .
> Prytouris, payntouris and potingaris [apothecaries].

As there were no longstanding, discrete groupings of urban apothecaries in Scotland, information about their apprenticeship training is very sparse. In Edinburgh a Fraternity of Apothecaries and Surgeon-Apothecaries was in existence for two decades in the second half of the seventeenth century. Its origins and demise are obscure, but the few surviving, fragmentary pages of minutes give some flavour of its activities. It was linked to the Incor-

poration of Surgeons, but the precise nature of the link is unclear and it was apparently the case that members had to choose which body to ally themselves with. Some evidence of their end-of-apprenticeship tests comes from a single example in 1685.

Hugh Paterson was examined by the Fraternity and by some physicians (who held supervision rights for a short period). He was ordered to 'read several receipts', and was asked to make up items which appeared frequently in prescriptions – *unguentum apostolorum* (used to treat sores and comprising twelve ingredients, hence the reference to the apostles) and *emplastrum diachylon* (a poultice, originally plant-based but later made of lead oxide and oil – it is not clear which version is referred to here). Paterson was able to satisfy his examiners, as the minutes note that he was found *sufficientlie qualifiet*. He took an oath to the effect that he would be 'faithfull in his dispensing, compounding and administrating of medicaments of all printed and written receipts.'

Once approved, the apothecaries provided services on a number of levels. They sold individual substances, made up recipes as required, and also provided many of the complicated prescriptions requested by medical practitioners. Some of the latter contained many substances – the more complex the prescription the more significant it would seem to the receiver, and it would also impress upon the patient the superiority of the qualified physician over the lay healer, who would often advise much simpler concoctions, with only one or two main ingredients. The first edition of the *Edinburgh Pharmacopoeia* (Fig. 2.55), published after much consultation in 1699, contained many of the seemingly outlandish items stocked by the apothecaries, such as cantharides (beetles). There would be several subsequent editions of the work before the most unlikely items were removed from its contents.

By the seventeenth century, though, apothecaries were, especially in the towns, becoming more distinctive practitioners in the medical sphere. They prepared and dispensed the often extremely complicated cures prescribed by physicians, or requested by the patients themselves. There was a strong network for circulating popular recipes, both for illness and for prevention. In the larger coastal towns in particular, some apothecaries were also functioning as merchants, importing goods in their own names rather than trading through a merchant, so they were of considerable economic as well as medical importance. Their shops were stocked with multifarious substances, including some fairly exotic items brought in from all corners of the globe. There are a few surviving inventories of Edinburgh apothecaries' shops from the earlier part of the period, mostly found in testaments, and these give vivid illustration of the stock held by these establishments.

Thomas Davidson (d. 1575) ran what seems to have been a successful business until his death. His testament contains a detailed inventory of the contents of his shop, and lists a great variety of ingredients, including tamarind, cardamom, lupin seeds, opium, almonds, roses, cloves, mint, frankincense, myrrh, capers, beetles, millipedes, arsenic, antimony, borax and mercury, in readiness for making up receipts provided by physicians or requested by the patients themselves (Fig. 2.56).

It appears that Davidson also had a thriving business in supplying ready-made items, as his shelves contained supplies of a number of popular medicaments, including *unguentum apostolorum*, *pilulae aromaticae* (aromatic pills), *unguentum althea* (ointment made from marshmallow plant) and *emplastrum melilot* (plaster or poultice containing honey).

Unfortunately no indigenous Scottish images of apothecaries' shops exist, but given the very close links and similarities between Scotland and Europe at this time, it is fair to claim that a reconstruction based on European illustrations will give a fairly good impression of what was occurring in Scotland (Fig. 2.57).

Port records from the period also indicate that large quantities of medical glassware and other necessities were coming into Leith. A few examples will illustrate the variety of goods involved in the work of the urban apothecary. In September 1690 John King signed for a mixed consignment of medicinal goods, including senna, cumin, dragon's blood (resinous juice of the calamus tree, originating in the East Indies), cantharides (beetles used as a vesicator or blistering agent), and mastic. Not unsurprisingly, perhaps, the largest component was the senna. Most of the apothecaries' requirements came in to Scotland by

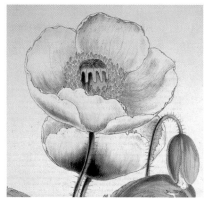 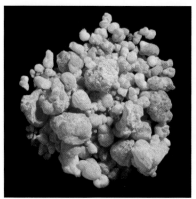 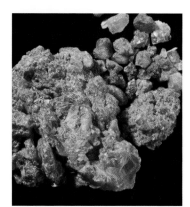

2.56 Opium, frankincense and myrrh, which formed part of the stock of Thomas Davidson's shop (*Wellcome Library, London*).

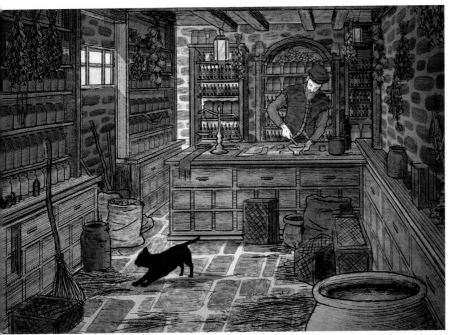

2.57 Reconstruction of early-modern apothecary's shop. The image is slightly stylised but gives a fair impression of what such a shop would have contained (*Illustration by David Morrow*).

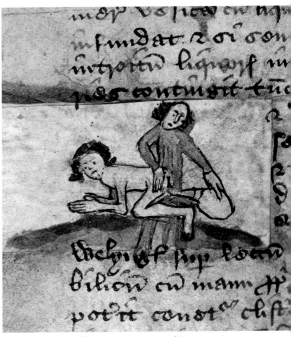

2.58 Enemas. Early fifteenth-century manuscript image of administration of an enema using a pig's bladder. The proportions of the image, particularly the size and position of the hands, suggest that the power of prayer was just as important as the treatment itself (*Wellcome Library, London*).

sea, but one large consignment recorded in the overland customs books in 1691 included *aristolochia longa* (often used after childbirth), *terra sigillata* (a mineral used as toothpaste), rue, Chinese cinnamon, hellebore (a strong emetic), verdigris (copper oxide, used to cleanse wounds), Peruvian bark and prunes. Cargoes also included vessels, pots and other containers, often referred to as 'pigs'.

Since most people were deeply concerned about matters of health, those who could afford it spent large sums of money on apothecaries' accounts and it is clear that at least some urban apothecaries could run extremely lucrative enterprises. One account submitted to the Earl of Tweedale by Patrick Hepburne, a well-known Edinburgh apothecary, amounted to some £377 Scots, covering the period 1665–70. It contained many items, some of which appeared frequently on the list, such as rose water, oil of almonds, pectoral ointments and various purging concoctions. Enemas were often given using a pig's bladder with a pipe attached, and one of the first items on

the list is 'ane glass wt a purgative and cooling Glister [enema]' and 'ane mounted blather [bladder] and canone to give it with'. It was not only family members who endured frequent purges – similar equipment was issued 'to the footeman' (Fig. 2.58).

These accounts confirm that in large houses the servants were provided with medical care at the expense of the householder. Among the more unusual items were 'a pott with orange flower butter' and scorzonera root (used as a diuretic). Interestingly, there were very few non-plant-based substances, apart from 'ane glass with spirite of sulphure'.

The above account is of 'general practice' in the early modern period. Towards the end of this period a new dimension began to affect the dynamics of the medical marketplace – this was the advent of new, and increasingly large, hospitals meant primarily for medical treatment rather than hospitality in the broader sense.

HOSPITALS

Till the early decades of the eighteenth century most people were still treated by the various practitioners at home, but this period saw the start of a significant process in official medical practice – the establishment of medical hospitals in which patients could be treated and observed. Though the proliferation of large voluntary hospitals would be mainly a product of the nineteenth century, one major medical hospital did come into being in this period. Hospitals had existed for several centuries, but, as discussed in the previous chapter, these offered general refuge and hospitality as well as some medical care. Others, mainly in the towns, provided shelter for indigent burgesses and respectable poor, and the Infirmary of the Glasgow Town's Hospital (Fig. 2.59), founded in 1733 and mainly providing a workhouse, was probably the first to offer medical treatment as well as accommodation or work. Indeed, it has been claimed that clinical teaching was first offered at the Town's Hospital, and not in Edinburgh.

Edinburgh had a number of institutions, including Trinity Hospital and the Merchants' and Trades' Maiden Hospitals, while Aberdeen had St Thomas' Hospital, the Guild Brethren Hospital and the Poor's Hospital, which was opened in 1741. Bishop Dunbar's Hospital, demolished in the late eighteenth century, was used to house plague victims (Fig. 2.60).

Given the very close connection between the early voluntary hospitals, which were financed by public contributions and sponsorship, and the perceived problems with destitute and itinerant poor, it is not surprising that the first hospitals with a medical as well as containment focus came into being in the larger towns, which had to cope, particularly in times of dearth, with the influx of large numbers of rural poor. The philanthropy of the early hospital patrons was tinged with a clear desire to maintain order in society, and it was assumed that any disorder or social upheaval would stem from the lowest levels. Admission to the voluntary hospitals depended on recommendation from a subscriber or sponsor.

Medical hospitals began on a very small scale, and, following Glasgow's Town's Hospital, the first Edinburgh Infirmary was established in 1729 in the wake of the opening of the Medical School (Fig. 2.61). There were only six beds, so there were severe limits to what could be done. By 1736 the surgeons were becoming frustrated with the lack of facilities available to them, and when negotiation with the Infirmary managers failed, a separate surgical hospital was set up in College Wynd, to the west of

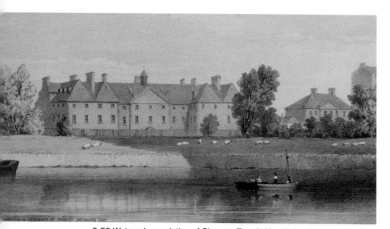

2.59 Watercolour painting of Glasgow Town's Hospital, which gives a rather romantic impression, though the reality may have been very different in terms of the experiences of the inmates. The softness of the colours and the quiet, almost rural scene belies the reality of life in a rapidly-growing town (*By courtesy of the Mitchell Library, Glasgow City Council*).

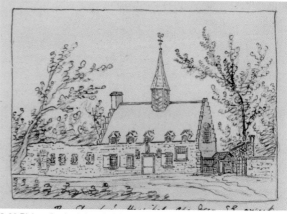

2.60 Bishop Dunbar's hospital. Line drawing of Bishop Dunbar's hospital in Aberdeen before its demolition in the early nineteenth century. The image is clearly that of a church, with the implication that religion and healing were closely linked (© *National Library of Scotland. Licensor www.scran.ac.uk*).

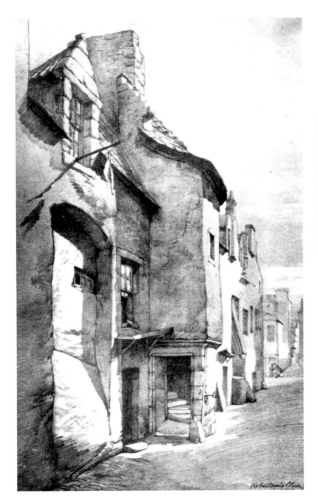

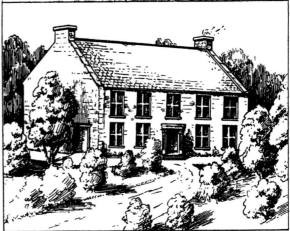

2.61 *Left.* Robertson's Close, Edinburgh. This was the site of the first infirmary, opened in 1729. It was not purpose-built, and the six patients it could care for were housed in cramped accommodation. There is no classical architecture here (*RCSEd*).

2.62 *Above.* Line drawing of Aberdeen Infirmary *c*1749. From D. Rorie, *Book of Aberdeen* (1939). This gives an impression of the relatively small size of the building, as was the case with most of the early medical hospitals. The architecture of the early hospitals suggests something rather different from the much larger voluntary hospitals which appeared later in the period (*courtesy of British Medical Association*).

Robertson's Close. However, by 1738, agreement had been reached with the managers, and the surgeons' hospital became part of the new Royal Infirmary, its beds continuing to be occupied till around 1743.

It soon became apparent that the town and its medical community needed a much bigger establishment. A royal charter was granted by George II and a subscription list opened, with contributions coming in from all over Scotland. The second infirmary opened its much more opulent doors in 1741 (see Fig. 2.1 above), and this was the true foundation of a large-scale hospital with the capacity for clinical teaching. The first listed patient came from Caithness, so the benefits of the infirmary were not restricted to locals – the subscriptions came from all over the country. The first group of patients suffered from such diverse – and vaguely-described – conditions as thigh pain, cancer in the face (which did not necessarily mean a malignancy at that time), hysteric disorders, bloody flux, tertian ague, consumption, dropsy and leg ulcers caused by scurvy.

Aberdeen Infirmary – A Case Study

Much has been written about the Edinburgh and Glasgow hospitals, but perhaps less has been said about Aberdeen. The first medical infirmary in Aberdeen was opened in 1742 (Fig. 2.62). It was built in what was then a green area 'on account of the goodness of the air', and was designed to function 'for the benefit of the diseased poor in all the northern parts of the Kingdom'. The hospitals may have been changing their focus slowly, but the patients still came almost universally from the lower social levels. Higher-status patients would not deign to go into a hospital – medical practitioners attended and treated them at home. There was also a considerable element of social control in the minds of those who founded such establishments.

As with most such projects, control of the Aberdeen Infirmary lay in the hands of managers drawn from the great and good of the town. Dr James Gordon of Pitlurg and Straloch, who was Professor of Medicine at Marischal College, agreed to act as both physician and surgeon, at a

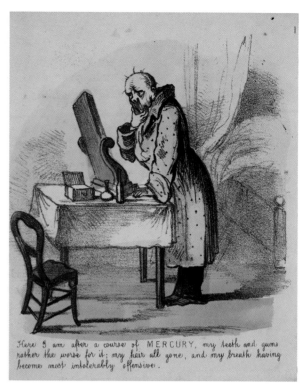

Here I am after a course of MERCURY, my teeth and gums rather the worse for it; my hair all gone, and my breath having become most intolerably offensive.

2.63 Case note. Part of case note of patient 89 from Aberdeen Infirmary in the 1750s. It is likely that the hospital treated many seafarers. The note also confirms the use of mercury and the need for separate rooms for patients undergoing this treatment (*Northern Health Services Archives*).

2.64 Effects of mercury treatment. Colour lithograph illustrating the effects of mercury treatment by James Morison, *c*1850. The portrayal is satirical, but the reality may have been little different (*Wellcome Library, London*).

fee of ten guineas. Drugs were to be purchased as cheaply as possible – at the 'lowest price at sight of the physicians in the town'. Dr Gordon started out by keeping detailed records of the patients admitted, though these became rather more sketchy with time. One of the first patients was William Davidson, from the workhouse, suffering from a fractured arm. Another patient, Alexander Davidson, illustrates very well the core attitudes and philosophies of these early medical hospitals, where concern for good statistics was just as important as in later times. This patient, who suffered from 'universal rheumatic pains and palsie of one of his limbs', was deemed unsuitable because he was incurable, and therefore 'not a proper object for the infirmary'. It needs to be remembered that patients not likely to recover were not normally admitted to the infirmaries, whose priority seems to have been to deal only with patients likely to recover, however long that took. The hospitals were also slow to admit accident cases for the same reasons. This may be due in part to the fact that these institutions depended on the contributions of subscribers, who were more willing to support individuals likely to recover sufficiently to make an economic contri-

bution in the future, as a return for the support given by the hospital benefactors.

As with the Edinburgh Infirmary, the Aberdeen hospital was pressed into service as a military hospital during the Jacobite conflicts of 1745–6, particularly for the treatment of casualties from the battle of Inverurie in December 1745. It was then commandeered by the Duke of Cumberland's forces. Following this the infirmary grew steadily, and one indication of the widespread use of mercury in treatment is that in 1744 two rooms were set aside for 'patients under salivations'. The extreme side-effects of mercury were well known, but it continued to be used until well into the nineteenth century (Fig. 2.64). It was used to treat a multiplicity of conditions, including those of three Aberdeen patients, who suffered variously from sore throat, warts and scrofula (tuberculous glands, usually in the neck). One interesting patient was admitted in the 1750s with joint pains following a voyage to Virginia. He was treated with 'mercurial medicines' (Fig. 2.63).

Also in common with the other hospitals of the day, the patients were admitted from all parts of the north-east, not just from the town itself, and often after other treatments had proved unsuccessful. If a patient could secure the support of a subscriber and could make the journey, there were no geographical barriers to admission and no designated catchment areas.

Perhaps surprisingly, the majority of patients admitted to the Aberdeen hospital were surgical rather than medical, despite the general reluctance to admit serious accident cases. Records show that the surgical procedures carried out included amputations and cataract operations, the claim being made that of 20 leg amputations 'not one died of the operation'. Despite this success, though, the Aberdeen surgeons, in common with their colleagues elsewhere, avoided operating for the stone – a very common and painful affliction, which affected adults and children alike. Dr Thomas Livingston, appointed in 1752, was said to be the first surgeon to attempt the procedure in Aberdeen. The exact reasons for the frequent occurrence of stone at this time are unclear, but are thought to be related to diet and environment. The incidence in developed countries nowadays is much less, but the problem is still fairly severe.

In all cases, hospital patients were removed from their homes and from the direct influence of relatives, but the treatments they received differed little from those which they might have received before the hospital was established. What was new, though, and what would be of great importance for the future of medicine was observation. Patients were often confined for lengthy periods, and meticulous notes were taken of their general condition, symptoms and response to medication or other treatments. In many cases, though, it is more than likely that any improvement owed as much to better nutrition as to any prescription, however complicated. The hospitals may have had few beds and treated a narrow range of conditions, but the importance of the systematic observation and recording of patients' histories which was carried out cannot be overestimated. It was perhaps fortunate for the patients that the most eminent physicians and surgeons of their day were eager to offer their services to these establishments. The next development in the evolution of medicine was the very early beginnings of specialties and special interests.

THE BEGINNING OF SPECIALTIES

For most of the period covered here, practitioners and healers were 'general' in the broadest sense of the term. They offered treatments and cures for all sorts of diseases and conditions. By the middle of the eighteenth century, though, the beginnings of what would become specialties were beginning to appear. Two of these 'proto-specialties' were in the areas of mental illness and dentistry.

Mental Illness

For much of the period under consideration here, disorders of the mind were not considered to be set apart from afflictions of the body. This is understandable, given the prevalent views on the holistic nature of man and his relationship with the universe. Mental illnesses were treated with many of the same measures as organic disease, including mercury. Individuals with what are nowadays termed learning difficulties were accepted as an integral part of their local communities.

By the mid-eighteenth century, some physicians believed that the origins of mental illness were very different from those of 'ordinary' diseases. This may have coincided with changes in social attitudes, so that the 'village idiot' now became something of an embarrassment rather than a fully-accepted member of the community. In rural areas the situation was naturally much slower to change, but in the more rapidly-developing and increasingly sophisticated large urban centres, attitudes began to harden somewhat. In addition, the progress which was being made in the description of bodily structures and functions was beginning to convince some physicians that perhaps mental illness was derived from different causes, and, in consequence, might require different kinds of treatment. In addition, no real distinction was made at that time between mental illness and congenital mental deficiency. (Fig. 2.65)

In earlier times most conditions of madness were described variously as 'melancholia', 'furiosity' or 'possession'. Some rather violent cures for these afflictions had been tried, including immersing, binding up and leaving the afflicted individual overnight in a religious location.

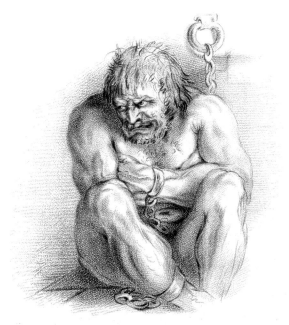

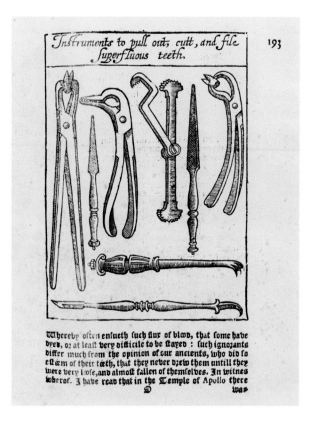

2.65 *Above.* Madness. Image from Sir Charles Bell's *The Anatomy and Physiology of Expression*, published in 1844. This demonstrates both the perception of the insane and the restraint used to deal with such individuals. It suggests that the public viewed sufferers as dangerous rather than ill (*Wellcome Library, London*).

2.66 *Right.* Plate from Lowe's textbook showing instruments to 'pull out, cutt and file superfluous teeth' (*RCSEd*).

If the victim had freed him or herself by the next day, a cure was deemed to have been achieved. This is somewhat redolent of 'tests' to confirm witchcraft. (Unexpected immersion was also tried in cases of tetanus, or lockjaw, despite the hydrophobia produced by these conditions. The aim was clearly to shock the senses into correcting themselves).

Towards the end of this period ideas began to change slowly, and the question of offering different treatments for mental disorders was mooted, in particular the separation of those with mental illness from their communities (see discussion of Andrew Duncan in Chapter 3). There is also some correlation here with the emergence of medical hospitals. More people – at least from lower levels of society – were admitted to hospitals, so the fact of physical separation from relatives was now accepted as part of the medical sphere. This separation reduced influence wielded by family members, and also to some extent that of the patient, who had hitherto had a more direct role as agent as well as patient. The plans for the second Edinburgh Infirmary included restraining cells for the insane, and this was the first part of the building to be completed (the Town's Hospital in Glasgow also incorporated padded cells). By the mid-eighteenth century, increasing numbers of physicians were showing an interest in the consideration

of mental illness as a series of conditions which did not necessarily fit into the old holistic-humoral philosophy. Eventually, as will be discussed in subsequent chapters, the trend towards isolating the insane or temporarily mentally-compromised in large asylums gathered pace. One of the main initiatives came from Andrew Duncan, whose proposal for a public lunatic asylum in Edinburgh came to fruition eventually in 1807. These institutions would indulge in new treatments with electrical and other equipment – at this period the treatment of mental illness and deficiency was at something of a crossroads.

Dentistry

Dentistry as a profession separate from medicine is a comparatively recent development. Medicine and surgery were developing rapidly in terms of organisation and teaching, but dental problems were not deemed to merit fully separate treatment. Dealing with painful teeth had long been part of the sphere of the local, amateur healer, rather than the trained practitioner. Remedies to deal with toothache and other oral problems were circulated widely, and various ingenious methods used to pull out rotten teeth. Cavities were filled with mastic (a resinous paste) and often alcohol was suggested to deaden the pain. Even the highest in the land took an interest – perhaps from

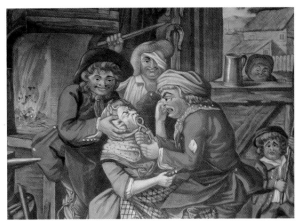

2.67 *Above*. Eighteenth-century satirical image of amateur tooth-pulling, which may not be far from a true representation of what did happen in real life. This is very much in the satirical genre, but does portray the physical force needed. The eighteenth century was the heyday of the satirical portrayal, and this image is in the style of 'Tim Bobbin' (John Collier [1708-86]), who styled himself as the Lancashire Hogarth, and whose satirical poetry and images were well known.

2.68 *Right*. Cures for toothache from sixteenth-century commonplace book. The recipe on the bottom half of the pages is as follows: 'For ye toothache or wormes in ye teith. Take peper and stampe it and temper it w' gude wyne and supe th'of warme and hauld it in thy mowth till it be cauld and than spit it out, and do this oft and thow salbe delyverit of angwysh and greif.'

personal agonies – as evidenced in the household accounts of James IV, which, in 1503, included the cost of an 'irn to byrn sair teeth'. Replacement teeth of various sorts had long been produced, including the use of transplanted teeth which had been retrieved from casualties of battle.

Peter Lowe covered dental problems in his surgical textbook, but as part of the treatment of the body as a whole, and not as something that would require specialisation. His recommendations for dealing with tooth cavities included dietary advice, including avoidance of milk, green fruit, and 'hard things'. The next stage was to rinse the mouth with claret boiled with tormentil and marrubium (horehound, a herbaceous perennial plant which was used to treat a variety of illnesses). Following that, the affected part should be treated with a mixture of oil of vitriol, sage and cloves, taking care that the caustic oil should not touch any other part. A cauter of hot iron was the next step, though 'for great personages' the cauters should be made of gold or silver (Fig. 2.66).

Though this advice was available to any practitioner who had access to a copy of Lowe, pulling teeth remained very much within the ambit of the local blacksmith, or other tradesman or itinerant practitioners, with muscular strength and experience being the main qualifications (Fig. 2.67). Because of the excruciating nature of toothache,

many folk remedies were circulated, often involving alcohol. A commonplace book dating from the late sixteenth century contained several pages of advice, including the use of a concoction of vinegar, mustard powder and pepper applied to the tooth cavities. Another recipe involved holding a mixture of hot vinegar and wine in the mouth till it cooled, repeat several times and 'thow salbe delyv^{rt} of all angwysch and griefe' (Fig. 2.68).

The individual most often cited as being the first real dental professional was James Rae (1716–91), a Fellow of the Royal College of Surgeons of Edinburgh, who began in the early 1780s to publicise a course of lectures which included 'diseases of the teeth'. He also offered a dental service to patients, claiming to be expert in all dental problems and to supply high-quality false teeth, as well as performing transplantation of teeth. Rae was, technically, the first Fellow of the College, it having achieved a royal charter in 1778. His brother William also pursued an interest in dentistry, though he relocated to London. The emergence of dentistry as a discrete sector of the medical profession would come in the nineteenth century, but the start made by the Rae family and others was nonetheless important.

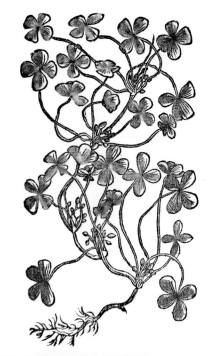

OUTSIDE THE INNER CIRCLE

In addition to the efforts of the various groups of licensed practitioners discussed above, many other groups and individuals offered treatments which were consumed by people at all levels of society. These included itinerant practitioners, witches, charmers and folk healers, all of whom worked within the broad medical marketplace, where demarcations between qualified and unqualified individuals could not be enforced. Many people continued to visit healing wells. All of these groups must be given due consideration in the broad analysis. In addition to all of this, in many homes the lady of the house kept a commonplace book, containing items of general and domestic interest, including recipes for medical cures as well as for cooking. Some of these recipes may have been provided originally by a physician or other medical practitioner, and if they were found to be efficacious, were circulated round family and friends. Veronica, Countess of Kincardine, for example, wrote to the Earl of Tweeddale in 1686, requesting information on the 'dyet of steel', as some of her household were 'much affected w^t the scurvie' – this condition did not spare the elite. One rather unpalatable concoction doing the rounds of the gentry in the same period comprised multifarious ingredients, including garden snails, sorrel, rue, rosemary and 'two quarts of great earth worms'. The remainder of this chapter will consider these areas, including Highland medicine, itinerant practitioners, witchcraft and other types of lay healing.

Highlands

Despite the lowland focus of licensed medicine and surgery, there was a 'professional', but very different, tradition in the Highlands. Medicine in the north-western areas of the country, roughly equivalent to the Gaelic-speaking parts of the country at the time, was dynastic, passed down from father to son within a few key families, particularly the Beatons. Successive generations were sent to study abroad, many at Montpellier, so that Highland 'official' medicine shared a common philosophical core with lowland medicine, and Highland physicians cannot be designated as lay practitioners. The surviving manu-

2.69a *Right*. Lentille d'Eau (Duckweed). Sea plants used to combat colds, measles and urinary problems.

2.69b *Below*. Kelp, North Uist. This was used frequently in Highland cures. Kelp was used in the manufacturing of alkalis, but was also considered to be of great medical value, in particular in nourishing the nervous system (© *Colin McPherson. Licensor www.scran.ac.uk*).

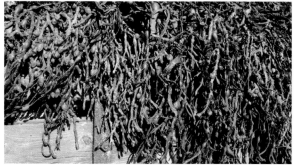

scripts used by these physicians consist mainly of Gaelic translations of Hippocrates, Galen and Avicenna. A key work of the Beatons was based on the *Regimen Sanitatis* of Salerno, which has been discussed in Chapter 1.

Gaelic medicine in this period was entirely conventional in many ways, as it was rooted firmly in the tradition of Western humoral medicine. In line with this, the advice given was holistic, with strong exhortations to follow a healthy lifestyle and good diet as a means of maintaining health and preventing the onset of illness. Detailed advice was offered in the *Regimen* on daily routines, though the recommendation that teeth should be cleaned with a melon leaf betrayed its origins in warmer climates. This advice may have been rather difficult to follow in the remotest corners of the Highlands or western isles. Religion remained at the heart of the matter also, as it was deemed important to say a Hail Mary daily as part of the holistic health package. Remedies were prescribed according to what was available in these areas, and thus seaweed

Remedy for Colic from a Commonplace Book

An excellent Receipt for the Gout in the stomach or Cholic by Doctor Ratcliffe

Raisins – two and a half pounds
Rhubarb – half a pound
Snake root – one ounce
Senna – two ounces
Coriander seed – half an ounce
Cochineal - one ounce
Saffron – half an ounce
Seville orange – yellow rind

Ingredients to be infused in two gallons of best French brandy in a chimney corner in a large stone jug, then left for ten days, stirring each day, then strained and a further five quarts of brandy added and left for six weeks. (18th century)

Many such recipes were based on considerable quantities of alcohol, from brandy to ale and wine.

2.70 Commonplace book. Eighteenth-century recipe for colic, taken from a commonplace book (Ms. 10282, p.35) (*By kind permission of the Trustees of the National Library of Scotland*).

was a common ingredient in many cures (Fig. 2.69).

Further evidence about the nature of Highland lifestyles, medical conditions and superstitions in this period comes from the writings of Martin Martin (d.1718), who travelled extensively in the north of Scotland at the end of the seventeenth century, and published a number of works detailing his observations. He visited Skye in the 1690s, met several members of the Beaton family and commented on one of these, Neil Beaton, with a combination of admiration and some disdain:

[T]he illiterate empiric Neil Beaton in Skye, who of late is so well known in the isles and continent, for his great success in curing several dangerous distempers, though he never appeared in the quality of a physician until he arrived at the age of forty years, and then also without the advantage of education. He pretends to judge of the various qualities of plants and roots by their various tastes . . . he extracts the juice of plants and roots after a chemical way, peculiar to himself, and with little or no charge. He considers his patient's constitution before any medicine is

administered to them . . . He treats Riverius's Lilium Medicinae, and some other practical pieces he has heard of, with contempt; since in several instances it appears that their method of curing has failed, where his has had good success.

Some of the diseases cured by him are as follows; running sores in legs and arms, grievous headaches; he had the boldness to cut a piece out of a woman's skull broader than a half-a-crown, and by this restored her to perfect health . . . The success attending this man's cures was so extraordinary that several people thought his performances to have proceeded rather from a compact with the devil, than from the virtue of simples. To obviate this, Mr Beaton pretends to have had some education from his father, though he died when he himself was a boy. I have discoursed him seriously at different times and am fully satisfied that he uses no unlawful means for obtaining his end.

It is clear from Martin Martin's work that, as in lowland areas, medicines and treatments were integral parts of life and health, not just in temporary periods of disease. His

Highland Incantations

Alexander Carmichael's collection of Highland incantations in *Carmina Gadelica* contains a number of interesting medical prescriptions and rituals, including the following:

The 'Gravel Charm' for curing bladder stones

I have a charm for the gravel disease,
For the disease that is perverse;
I have a charm for the red disease,
For the disease that is irritating.
As runs a river cold, as grinds a rapid mill,
Thou who didst ordain land and sea,
Cease the blood and let flow the urine.
In name of Father, and of Son,
In name of Holy Spirit.

(Red disease probably refers to blood in the urine.)

A cure for seizures comprised several similar stanzas:

I trample on thee, thou seizure
As tramples whale on brine,
Thou seizure of back, thou seizure of body
Thou foul wasting of chest.
May the strong Lord of life
Destroy thy disease of body
From the crown of thine head
To the base of thy heel.

2.71 Charm stone. The hole indicates that it may have been suspended in water using a rope (© *National Museums Scotland*).

accounts of cures and illnesses form part of the general description of the particular location in which they were found, and not as something separate. Martin's account of the Isle of Jura, for example, notes that it was the 'wholesomest plot of ground either in the isles or continent of Scotland', and, consequently, the people were much healthier than those in neighbouring islands. Inhabitants did not suffer from 'convulsion, vapours, palsies, surfeits, lethargies, migrains, consumption, rickets, pains of the stomach or coughs', and bloodletting and purging were not used regularly – very much in contrast with most other areas of the country. Colds were treated by nothing more exotic than 'brochan' (a thin mixture of oatmeal and water). On the Isle of Skye, a cure for 'twisting of the guts' was to give the patient cold water and oatmeal and then hang him or her upside down. Application of sea dulse to the abdomen was said to 'take away the afterbirth with great ease and safety'. Many of the substances used seemed to have a place in cures for a variety of illnesses and afflictions, and animals were often treated with similar substances. The situation in the Highlands was different, but similar to that in the lowlands. Indeed, Highland culture in general was in some ways more sophisticated than elsewhere in the country.

The effects of the Reformation took several generations to reach the furthest corners of the country, and there remained a significant Roman Catholic minority in Scotland in general, and in the Highlands in particular, throughout the period. Medical practitioners were advised not to resort to bloodletting too frequently, and particularly in individuals over the age of 40, as to do so might cause blindness or loss of memory. There were close similarities between the *Regimen* and William Buchan's *Domestic Medicine*, published initially in 1769, and discussed in Chapter 3, despite the 150-year span between their publications. Buchan's work in turn would see multiple editions produced until well into the twentieth century, a good example of the genre of 'home doctor' books being written by qualified medical practitioners.

Itinerant Practitioners

Itinerant practitioners, sometimes referred to as quacks or mountebanks, travelled round the more accessible parts of the country, offering entertainments and lectures as well as allegedly infallible cures for all sorts of ailments. One of the most infamous of these was James Graham (1745–94), who visited Edinburgh in 1780s, proclaiming magic powers for his 'celestial bed' and advocating electric therapy. Itinerant stonecutters, who claimed perfect success rates in dealing with bladder stones were another part of this extremely complex medical marketplace. In earlier times the itinerant practitioners were frequently accompanied by circus acts such as tightrope walkers, and medical advertising was part of an entertainment package.

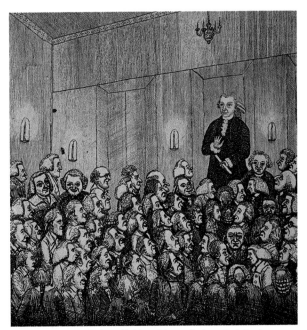

2.72 *Above.* James Graham. Etching of James Graham, lecturing in Edinburgh – his presence caused controversy in the town and led to protests from the Royal College of Surgeons and attempts to drive him out of the town. Graham was one of the 'new breed' of itinerant practitioners – he had undergone some medical training and used this as justification for his activities and claims. He made good use of the rapidly-developing newspaper press to advertise his claims and activities. The image here suggests that his lectures and demonstrations were popular with the general public, if not with medical practitioners (*Wellcome Library, London*).

2.73 *Right.* Work by James Graham. Title page of one of Graham's publications, indicating the sweeping nature of his claims to knowledge. The format is similar to the title pages of many 'legitimate' medical publications at this time, and the intention was clearly to show that Graham's claims should be taken seriously (*Wellcome Library, London*).

A

DISCOURSE,

DELIVERED ON SUNDAY, AUGUST 17. 1783,

AT

EDINBURGH,

WHEREIN

The nature, and manner of the Resurrection of the human Body, and the immortality, or future modes of existence, and progress of the Soul! are Philosophically, Medically, and Religiously explained,

BY

Doctor JAMES GRAHAM,

OF THE

Temple of Health,

In *Pall-Mall*, near the KING's Palace, London.

THE FIFTH EDITION, Corrected.

HULL:

PRINTED BY T. BRIGGS, IN CHURCH-LANE.

MDCCLXXXVII

Buffoon-like characters, known as Merry Andrews, acted as the practitioners' assistants, helping to entertain the crowds. Later, though, these itinerant practitioners adopted a much more serious image in order to gain credibility. (Fig. 2.72 and 2.73)

Claims about cures were often advertised in the local press, and a number of the individuals involved had undergone some formal medical training. Francis Clerk, 'oculist', came to Edinburgh in 1710 and advertised his visit in the *Caledonian Mercury*, while in 1726 James Black claimed in the same publication that he had power to cure people of 'flying pains', stating that he did not use vomits, purges or 'common dyet', unlike the methods used by the qualified practitioners (Fig. 2.74).

Some itinerant practitioners concentrated on a single procedure, particularly in areas such as lithotomy (cutting for bladder stones), a procedure generally avoided by qualified surgeons, or the treatment of cataracts, which was attempted more frequently by the official surgeons. The importance of eyes to life and the economy is confirmed by the close attention paid to eye diseases and injuries from earliest times.

Witchcraft, Charming and Folk Healing

In all areas of Scotland, urban as well as rural, certain beliefs and superstitions were shared, and many ailments and conditions related to binary opposites – well and ill, light and dark, winter and summer, hot and cold, good and evil. This meant that explanations for many conditions were complex. This connection between illness or accident and these binary forces was not just a Scottish phenomenon, and the close links between illness and superstition, and the fact that much of the local healing work was in the hands of women, meant that accusations of witchcraft were very easy to make, particularly in the most concentrated phases of the witch-hunt in the first from Stirling, that a Woman of the Name of Monteith was lately hang'd there for the same unnatural Crime.

Yesterday died in the Tolbooth William Arthur, said to have been concerned in the late Riot at Glasgow, where he has continued ever since.

ADVERTISEMENTS.

¶*¶ That I JAMES BLACK, Professor of Pyrotechny, for present at Glasgow, have found out Medicines of singular Vertue, (studiously concealed by all Artists hitherto) by which Medicines, I profess, (Deo juvante) to Cure, in general all Fevers : Now, under Fevers I comprehend Calentures, Small Pox, Measles &c. and likewise all Fluxes, &c. and the King's Evil, which so bafles Physicians, that it seems to deride their Medicines, and all Rheumatisms, altho of a long standing, and mostly all other flying Pains thro' the Body; and the Lues Venerea, tho' never so gone, &c. All Coughs and Pains of the Stomach, and all without torturing the Body with noxious Poysons, such as Vomits, &c. I practice all my Cures without hindering the Patient from common Diet, a Cruelty used in common Prescriptions. This I do in no long Time, N. B. I sell no Medicines, but to those who inform me personally of their Case, or who gives me a full Account by Writ ; and am to be found at the Coffeehouse at Glasgow, or Daniel Montgomery's Postmaster there, &c.

¶*¶ There is to be exposed to Sale, by Way of Publick Roup, at Robert Colquhoun's at the Milburn of Touch, within two Miles of Stirling, upon Tuesday the second Day of August next, betwixt the Hours of ten and twelve Forenoon, Two black Horses, and a black Mare of the Coach Kind, two Horses for a Sadle, a Mare at the Foaling for a Sadle, and a two year-old Fillie, which belonged to the deceast Laird of Touch.

[¶] That there is a convenient Dwelling House, consisting of four large Fire Rooms, with Garrets and Pantries, a Malt Barn, Kill and Coble, with a Corn-Barn, Stables, Cellars, Lofts, a Dovecoat and large Garden, all newly built, called SUNNYBRAES, lying within a Short Ridgelength of Dumfermling, upon the King's High Way, and upon the Post Road from the Queensferry to the Highlands ; to be feued or set in Tack, for long or short Space. The En-

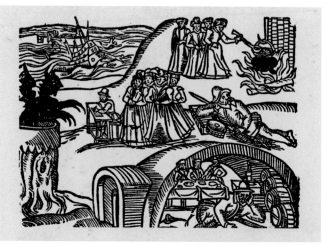

2.74 *Left.* Newspaper advertisement from *Caledonian Mercury*, 21 July 1726. This proclaimed the powers of James Black, 'Professor of Pyrotechny,' claiming the ability to cure all sorts of conditions, including smallpox, measles and the King's Evil (*By kind permission of the Trustees of the National Library of Scotland*).

2.75 *Above.* Witchcraft. Plate from *Newes from Scotland*, a pamphlet published in London in 1591. Illustration of the North Berwick witches, who were accused of causing a great storm when James VI and his bride were sailing to Scotland, forcing them to seek shelter in Norway for several weeks. The devil is shown in deep black, as is the witches' cauldron, emphasising the diabolic pact associated with black witchcraft (© *University of Glasgow. Newes from Scotland 1597 (London, Bodley Head, 1924). Licensor www.scran.ac.uk*).

half of the seventeenth century, sparked by the close interest shown by James VI (Fig. 2.75).

White witches – as opposed to black witches who were accused of a diabolic pact – and charmers were consulted in cases of illness to humans or animals, and in many cases provided innocuous cures. Many of their potions, though, were linked to the performance of a ritual, or specific action such as walking backwards round a well or other place of significance. Physical charming objects, such as stones, were also incorporated into the 'treatment package' (Figs. 2.76 and 2.77).

As most healers, charmers and white witches were female, it is not surprising that all but ten percent of those accused of witchcraft were female. Though incantations were to be found in all areas performed either by the sufferer or the healer, they were potentially more dangerous to the utterers in lowland parts, as it was easier for rumour to spread in these parts and to turn into accusations of witchcraft. In her book *Healing Threads,* Mary Beith notes one case in Edinburgh in 1643, when Marion

Fisher was called before the Kirk Session of St Cuthbert's, accused of charming and using spells, and advising the use of an incantation:

Our Lord to hunting red,
His sooll soot sled;
Doun he lighted,
his sool sot righted
Blod to blod
Shenew to shenew
To the other sent in God's name.
In the name of the Father, Son, and Holy Ghost.

The inference here is of an injury or fracture. The first line may refer to riding (i.e. the 'red' may mean 'rode' rather than red), the horse subsequently slipping or becoming unshod (sled) and then 'righted'. The 'sool sot' may be a misrepresentation of 'foal foot', which was again common to this type of verse, which was probably based on a charm which mentions St Peter – the 'other sent in God's name'.

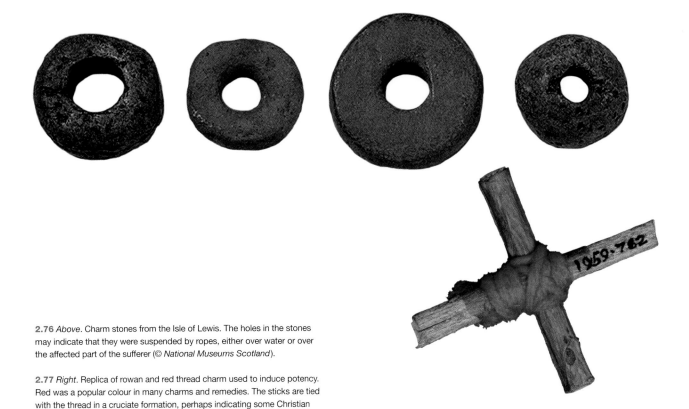

2.76 *Above*. Charm stones from the Isle of Lewis. The holes in the stones may indicate that they were suspended by ropes, either over water or over the affected part of the sufferer (© *National Museums Scotland*).

2.77 *Right*. Replica of rowan and red thread charm used to induce potency. Red was a popular colour in many charms and remedies. The sticks are tied with the thread in a cruciate formation, perhaps indicating some Christian influences (© *National Museums Scotland*).

(Information on interpretation given by Joyce Miller.)

Of the 3398 individuals involved in witchcraft cases in Scotland between 1500 and 1740 (and documented in the Scottish Witchcraft Project (2000–2003)), some 140 involved folk healing. This is a very small number in comparison to accusations of black witchcraft, but it shows that the barrier separating witchcraft and healing was very thin indeed. In 1612 Elspit Scott was accused of using rituals such as collecting south-running water in silence, which seems a fairly innocuous action and undeserving of witchcraft accusation, while in 1659 Issobell Bennet was accused of using a horseshoe, a hook and a piece of raw meat in one of her cures. Bessie Aiken, tried in 1597, was said to use red nettles, fresh butter and salt water to cure pains in the loins. These seem quite unremarkable remedies, but she was also accused of roasting kittens and using the drippings to rub on a sick person.

The interface between witchcraft and folk healing was just as permeable as that between witchcraft and charming. In Morayshire in the 1770s, for example, wreaths of woodbine were used as a cure for certain fevers, it being stipulated that the afflicted person should walk under the wreath during the full moon in March.

Healing Wells

People still regarded themselves as being integrated fully with the seasons, agricultural cycles and the weather, as well as holding a complex mixture of beliefs in Christianity, witchcraft and other superstitions, and demonstrated a degree of what might be termed sophistication in this ability to embrace multiple belief systems. There was no perceived conflict between worshipping in a Christian church every Sunday and travelling to a healing well or other shrine which was alleged to offer cures or disease prevention on another day of the week. As discussed in the previous chapter, some wells were significant for their association with the legendary exploits of early Christians, some of whom were canonised subsequently, but the reputation of others came from more pagan origins.

Among these places were the Culloden Wishing Well,

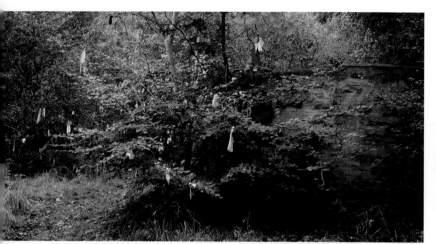

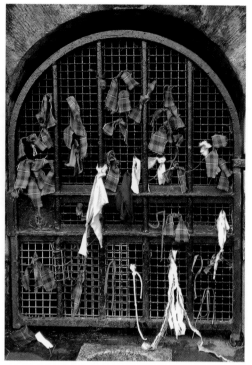

2.78 *Above*. Photograph of Culloden wishing well. Like the Munlochy well near Inverness, a feature is the hanging of cloths and other objects around it in the belief that, as they decayed, the disease or other problem would disappear (© *Jim Thomson, Culloden*).

2.79 *Right*. Recent photograph of St Margaret's Well, Holyrood, Edinburgh. The tradition continues (*I. Macintyre*).

2.80 *Opposite*. Brow on the Solway. Chalybeate spring visited by people from the Dumfries area to drink the water and also to bathe in the Solway (© *Dumfries and Galloway Museum Service. Licensor www.scran.ac.uk*).

and St Margaret's Well, Holyrood (Fig. 2.78 and 2.79). As these pictures show the practice of hanging objects near these wells continues to the present day. A description of events in 1890 by David Rorie gives a vivid impression of visits to the Culloden well:

> Despite the protests made by prominent figures in the Free and Free Presbyterian Churches against the annual pilgrimage to the Wishing Well at Culloden Moor, the numbers taking part in yesterday's trek were greater than ever. The brilliant weather was no doubt largely responsible for the record crowd which took part in the centuries-old custom of dropping coins in the well, drinking the water, wishing a wish, and tying a rag to one of the nearby trees. The pilgrimage started at an early hour . . . As midday approached the numbers grew, and by early afternoon the crowd reached unprecedented proportions. The trek continued until sunset, when the trees round the well hung heavy with 'clouties', and a big heap of silver and copper coins lay at the bottom of the well, to be collected later and handed over to local charities . . . Hundreds came by car, motor cycle, push bicycles, and even on foot, and bus companies which provided special services from Inverness and Nairn reported that they never had a bigger demand for transport to the well. A conservative estimate is that 12,000 people took part in the pilgrimage. The money found at the bottom of the well amounted in value to £27 7/-.
>
> (D. Rorie, *Aberdeen Press and Journal*, 3 May 1937)

Later on, the use of chemical wells increased, and these tended not to have the exotic or ritualistic overtones which had characterised the earlier 'legendary' wells. The particular chemicals related to individual wells could be smelt, and the water might be coloured by these chemicals, so there was no need to dress up the cure in tradition or ritual. The chalybeate (iron) well at Whitehills in Aberdeenshire is known as the Red Well, presumably because of the chemical composition of the water. Similar chalybeate wells are to be found at Peterhead, Fraserburgh and Moffat (see Fig. 2.80). Whatever the characteristics of any particular well, the benefits hoped for by pilgrims in this period were similar to those in earlier times. Some beliefs were, naturally, region or location-specific, but were all related to good or bad outcomes – this was a central aspect of medicine, particularly in rural or isolated areas.

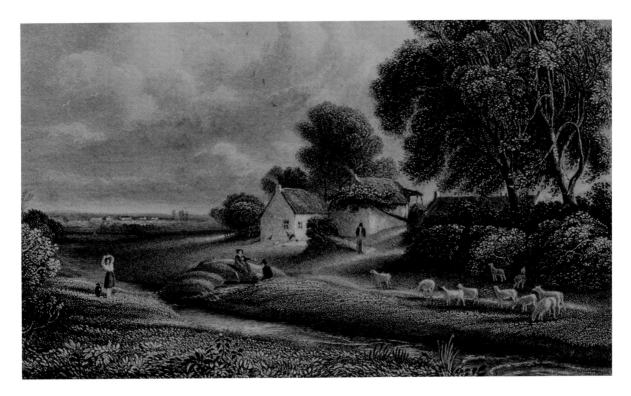

CONCLUSION

The period encompassing the whole of the seventeenth century and the first half of the eighteenth can be seen as one of consolidation and transition in terms of Scottish medicine and the experiences of the patients. In some ways the period was a bridge between the medieval period, with the all-pervading influence of the Roman Catholic church, and the start of the Enlightenment period, which would see a great release in terms of intellectual freedom, attitudes to the human race and the universe, and a growing focus on experiment and reason. The latter part of the eighteenth century would see the start of a new phase in medical knowledge – though not necessarily in medical practice. The early modern period showed much continuity as well as considerable change. The growth of the urban network allowed medical and surgical organisations to be established and consolidated, and the gradual rise in literacy levels and growing culture of print allowed information to be circulated more widely. In terms of the patients' experiences, though, little changed. The medical marketplace continued to offer all sorts of medicines and treatments, and in the more rural areas folk medicine and superstition still played a major part in the medical sphere.

It is also possible to consider the period in terms of concentric circles. Within the central core, in the lowland large towns, predominantly Edinburgh and Glasgow, the medical sphere was perhaps at its most complex. A wide variety of possibilities existed, including the qualified physicians, time-served surgeons and apothecaries, medical schools and the first medical hospitals. In terms of an identity, that of early-modern Scottish medicine was very much a conglomeration of circumstances and opportunities, but still with the Hippocratic, Galenic and Paracelsian traditions at its core, modified by regional and seasonal variations.

The further away a patient was from the more advanced urban centres, the less likely he or she was to be able to consult a qualified practitioner, and the more likely that an amateur healer would be the main port of call (though of course amateur healers were very much to the fore in the towns also – it was the element of choice that was different). Despite the emergence of qualified physicians and surgeons, though, the reality of medical practice was slow to change. The next chapter deals with the explosion of knowledge, experiment and reason, which were major characteristics of Enlightenment philosophy, though the day-to-day experiences of the patients were slow to change. The early modern period was clearly one of transition in the organisation and training of medical practitioners, but more static in terms of the day-to-day experience of patients.

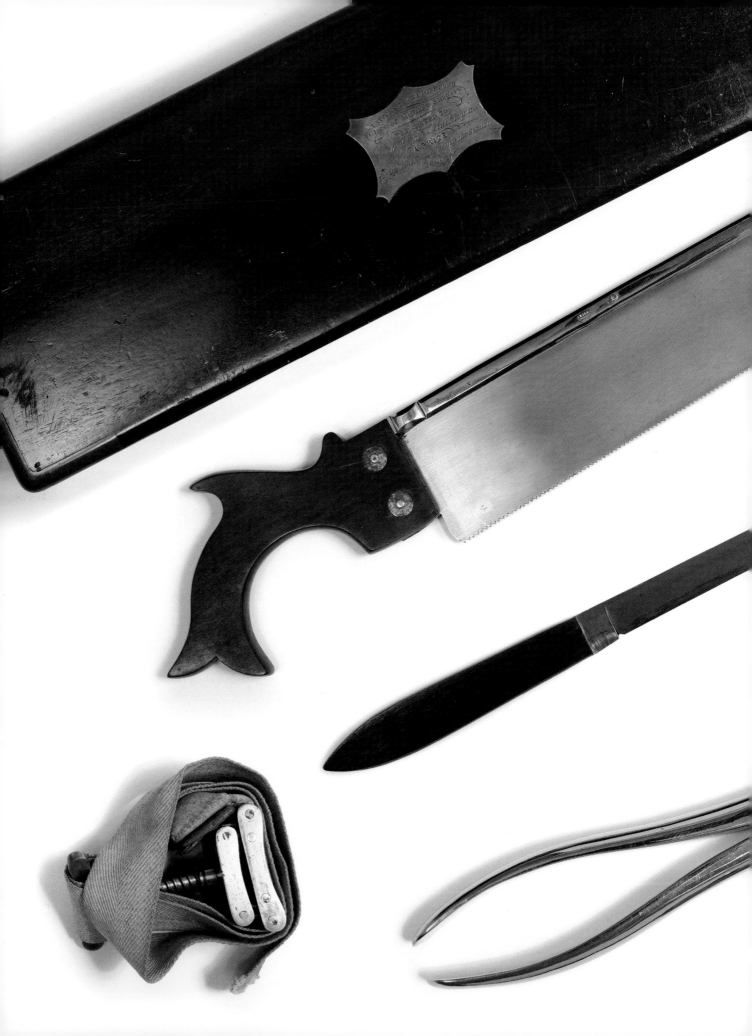

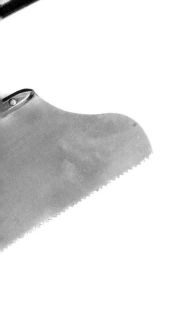

CHAPTER THREE

ENLIGHTENMENT
AND SCIENCE
Scottish Medicine *c*1750–*c*1850

Iain Macintyre

———

Here in the Uplands
The soil is ungrateful;
The fields, red with sorrel,
Are stony and bare.
A few trees, wind-twisted –
Or are they but bushes? –
Stand stubbornly guarding
A home here and there.

SIR ALEXANDER GRAY
(1882–1968)

———

It is from Scotland that we now receive the rules of
taste in all the arts from gardening to the epic poem.

VOLTAIRE
(1694–1778)

———

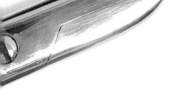

There is no European nation which, within the course
of half a century, or little more, has undergone so
complex a change as this kingdom of Scotland.

SIR WALTER SCOTT
(1771–1832)

INTRODUCTION

In the hundred years which followed the suppression of the 1745 Jacobite uprising, changes took place which transformed Scotland. Gray's poem paints a bleak picture of a country whose land and climate offered a harsh living. Yet during this period agricultural reform and industrialisation saw the population shift from predominantly rural living to predominantly urban, the greatest such migration in Europe at the time. The consequent expansion of Scotland's cities and burghs resulted in a doubling of the urban population. By the end of the eighteenth century, agricultural innovations such as draining and liming of soil and new crop rotations marked the transition, in lowland Scotland, from an inefficient, subsistence, agrarian economy dominated by the run-rig to one which was, by the mid-nineteenth century, highly productive and market oriented. These changes, and the introduction of crops such as potato and turnip, meant that the general nutrition of the population improved, so that the famines seen at the end of the seventeenth century now became more sporadic and largely confined to the Highlands and Islands. In the decade from 1846 the crofting communities were afflicted by the failure of the potato harvest through blight, but the resulting mortality was greatly mitigated by the distribution of food aid from the lowlands, in a co-ordinated initiative involving churches, charities and government. Yet potato famine triggered a mass migration from the western Highlands and the Hebrides, involving an estimated one-third of the population of the area.

The dogmas of the Presbyterian religion, which had so dominated Scottish life and politics since the Reformation, were increasingly questioned from the eighteenth century onwards, and the influence of the Church of Scotland began a slow decline from its position at the heart of every Scottish community. One of the central doctrines of Scottish Calvinism, predestination, which decreed that all events were predetermined by God, was now seriously questioned for the first time, enabling a new freedom of thought which allowed philosophers and scientists to think the previously unthinkable. The cities of Scotland witnessed an outburst of intellectual activity in arts, science and philosophy that was to make Edinburgh,

for a few remarkable decades, one of the intellectual hubs of Europe. Even Voltaire, that 'most celebrated man in Europe', observed that Scotland was the source of new ideas, from simple and practical to sophisticated and intellectual ones. The self-styled literati, men of genius of the Scottish Enlightenment, sought to improve their understanding of man, his mind, his body and his environment.

This led to a more rational approach to the understanding of the cause of disease. Enlightenment thinking brought about a progressive change from concepts of disease based on astrology, religious dogma or ancient aphorisms, to empirical ideas based on new observations and studies, which increasingly included experimental studies. This questioning of established principles, the scepticism promoted by the philosophy of David Hume and the new religious tolerance which emerged, all

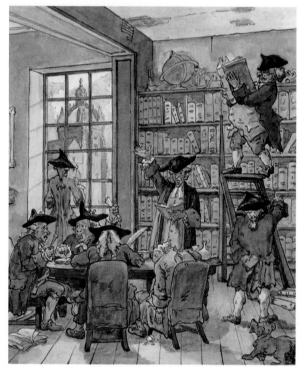

3.1 Aberdeen literati (Victor E. Davidson, 1986). The distinctive crown of King's College is in the background of this satirical view of Aberdeen literati, which demonstrates some of their characteristics – their love of reading, of scientific instruments, of writing, of holding forth in debate and of succumbing to excesses of claret (University of Aberdeen).

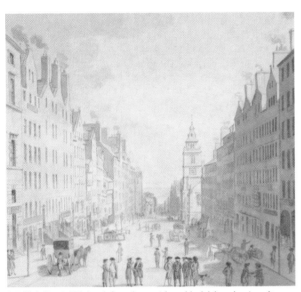

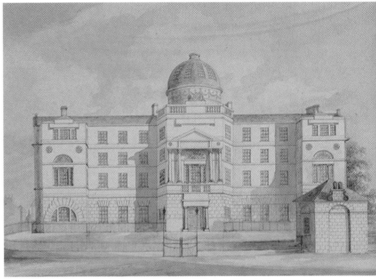

3.2 High Street, Edinburgh from the west (pen, black ink and watercolour over pencil on paper, David Allan, c1793). Tobias Smollett, who trained as a surgeon in Glasgow, described Enlightenment Edinburgh as a 'hotbed of genius'. Edinburgh's High Street was the hub of social and intellectual life in the city, where one English visitor reckoned he could 'in a few minutes take fifty men of genius and learning by the hand' (*National Gallery of Scotland*).

3.3 Glasgow Royal Infirmary (James Hopkirk, 1827). Glasgow Royal Infirmary was designed by Robert Adam and completed (under the supervision of his brother James) in 1794. The building was erected on the site of the old Bishop's Castle at the head of the medieval High Street and close to Glasgow Cathedral. Intended to convey an air of grandeur, it was built with an eye to teaching, with the lecture theatre under the dome holding around 200 students. This building was demolished in 1912. (*University of Glasgow*).

combined to make Scotland a fertile field for the growth and propagation of new and often radical ideas.

The Enlightenment produced talented individuals eager to explore philosophy and science, and their very presence in the clubs, societies, taverns and coffee houses stimulated innovative thinking by doctors. This included new ideas in medical education, particularly in Edinburgh, where the system of teaching imported from Leiden initially flourished, but was to be surpassed by other centres in continental Europe. The concept of a university medical school linked to a teaching hospital and offering systematic and clinical teaching attracted students from around the world, although Edinburgh did have other attractions. There were no religious barriers, there was freedom of movement between the classes of the University and extra-mural schools and the city had the advantage of two Royal Colleges. On a more practical level, both teaching and accommodation were inexpensive, students could select their own curriculum, could attend lectures at either university or extra-mural classes (or both) and many opted not to graduate. Glasgow had

a combined Faculty of Physicians and Surgeons, and educational co-operation between physicians and surgeons in Edinburgh led to Scotland producing doctors trained in both disciplines and so able to practise in the new genre of general practice, which they did in increasing numbers throughout Britain, her Empire and her armed forces. By the end of the eighteenth century, Glasgow offered a similar range of university and extra-mural teaching, while in Aberdeen, university-based clinical teaching was to replace the practice of awarding MD degrees by recommendation, a practice which persisted in St Andrews beyond the mid-nineteenth century. Nutton and Porter reckoned that 'between 1760 and 1826 17,000 medical students attended the Scottish universities to participate in a system that was in European terms remarkably open, flexible and free from state interference.' So successful was Scottish medical education that in the fifty years from 1800, more than 95% of British medical graduates had qualified from a Scottish university, although the practice of becoming a doctor through apprenticeship or by a college diploma was still recognised throughout Britain.

The Medical Act (1858) sought to impose a standardisation of curriculum and educational attainment on what had previously been a flexible market system where students frequently selected their own course topics and chose a university from which to graduate.

This meant more and better-educated doctors, but their services were largely used by the better-off, particularly in the cities. For many Scots, self-help for their ailments remained the norm, and wise women, clergymen, mountebanks, quacks and others were still commonly consulted and wells and spas increasingly frequented. The French revolution and the American Declaration of Independence had popularised the concept of rights of the individual, and an early manifestation of this in Scotland was the germ of the idea that this might include a right to health care. The sick poor could receive free treatment at the new dispensaries, and health provision was further improved with the building of new voluntary infirmaries. By the end of the eighteenth century there were infirmaries in Dundee, Dumfries and Montrose, and teaching had been established in the infirmaries of Edinburgh, Glasgow and Aberdeen.

Herman Boerhaave (1668–1738) and his followers in Scotland had taught the value of observation of the patient, and in the new hospitals these observations could be recorded, analysed and shared with others through publication. The printed word became the great engine that spread Enlightenment thought, and Edinburgh became a major publishing centre, producing important works which included *Encyclopaedia Britannica* and Buchan's *Domestic Medicine*, the latter destined to become the single most popular guide to health until the twentieth century.

The industrial revolution produced a further decline in general health associated with urban overcrowding and industrial diseases, and by 1850 serious public health efforts to combat these were under way, events which heralded the involvement of the state in disease prevention and public health. By the middle of the nineteenth century Scottish medicine and surgery were to have an influence out of all proportion to the size of the population.

POPULATION AND MORTALITY 1750–1850

The increase in Scotland's population during this period took place mainly in the towns and cities, and urban overcrowding was to bring a different pattern of disease, associated with a higher mortality.

Documenting the Population Rise

Webster's *Account of the Number of People in Scotland* (1755) is a good illustration of the Enlightenment quest for knowledge and the desire to see it published. It exemplifies the interest in numeracy and counting which was to become a hallmark of the period. The *Account* was one of the first censuses in Europe since Roman times, and the only population survey in Britain before 1801. It provides a valuable guide to the size and distribution of the Scottish population in the mid-eighteenth century. Rev. Alexander Webster (1707–84), minister of the Tolbooth Kirk in Edinburgh (Fig. 3.4), had studied under the gifted mathematician Colin MacLaurin (1698–1746), and with Rev. Robert Wallace had produced the world's first complete actuarial analysis of a pension fund for the widows and children of the ministers of the Church of Scotland and the teaching staff of the Scottish Universities. This gave him a popularity which, together with his standing as Moderator of the General Assembly, ensured full compliance (eventually), when he asked all Scottish church ministers to provide returns detailing the number of persons in their parish. His survey estimated the Scottish population at 1,265,380 (Edinburgh 31,122; Glasgow 23,546; Aberdeen 15,433; Dundee 12,477; Leith 9,405; Perth 9,019).

Almost half a century later *The First Statistical Account of Scotland* (1791–99) was compiled by Sir John Sinclair (1754–1835) in his capacity as a leading church elder. His questionnaire contained over 170 questions on a wide range of topics, and Church of Scotland ministers in all 936 parishes in Scotland provided returns between 1791 and 1799. The *Account* provides information about the detailed geography and history of each parish, about its population and its economy. It gives a detailed account at a personal level of, for example, the type of housing and the cost of food items and the wages received by different

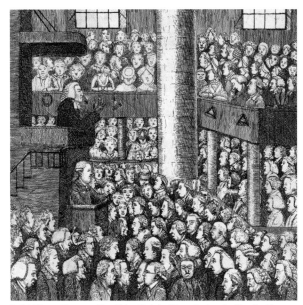

3.4 A Sleepy Congregation (John Kay). In this caricature by Kay, the Rev Alexander Webster, regarded as the most evangelical clergyman in the city, is preaching to a congregation composed, for purposes of the satire, of those not accustomed to churchgoing. His real congregation in the Tolbooth Kirk was noted for ultra-Presbyterianism and known as 'The Tolbooth Whigs'. John Kay (1742–1826) was an Edinburgh barber who sketched and caricatured the many celebrities who frequented the city. Biographical notes to accompany each of the sketches were later added by Hugh Paton, who published the work as *Kay's Portraits*.

groups of workers. Yet it is striking that so few of the questions are about health – one asks about epidemics in the locality, another about longevity.

Published some thirty years later, *The New Statistical Account of Scotland* (1834–1845) was modelled on the earlier *Account* and drew on its experience; on this occa-

sion informants included not only ministers but other local worthies considered credible, like doctors and schoolmasters. Comparison with the first *Account* demonstrates the improvements which had taken place in agriculture, in the economy, in education and in the daily lot of the Scottish people.

The population of Scotland more than doubled in the century to 1851 (table 1) with the growth of the major cities accounting for much of this. Edinburgh's population quadrupled and Glasgow's grew by a factor of fifteen, increases which were to have a damaging effect on the health of their citizens.

Mortality

The Bills of Mortality for Edinburgh for the year 1740 show that communicable diseases remained the commonest causes of death. In that year 1611 deaths were recorded with the causes listed as follows:

Consumption	349
Fever	304
Smallpox	206
Measles	112
Chincough	101
Flux	36
Convulsions	16

(Chincough was whooping cough and flux could include any diarrhoeal illness)

TABLE 2. Commonest causes of death in Edinburgh in 1740 as recorded in the Bills of Mortality

Population (000s) Date	Aberdeen	Edinburgh	Glasgow	Scotland
1755 (Webster)	15	47	23	1,265
1791–99 (1st Stat. Acct.)	24	71	61	1,700
1801 (Census)	27	83	77	1,608
1851 (Census)	71	202	357	2,888

TABLE 1. The growth in the population of Scotland and her three largest cities from 1755

Deficiencies in parish records make it difficult to establish trends of mortality in eighteenth-century Scotland. Flinn and colleagues (1977) attempted to do this by devising a mortality index which related the *total* burials in any one year to the *average* number of burials during the years 1615–1854. They demonstrated a fall from 90 in 1750 to 56 in 1800, followed by a progressive rise to 209 by 1849.

From this it can be presumed that there was an increase in life expectancy in the half century to 1800, probably due to improved nutrition and the disappearance of some infectious diseases like sibbens and ague (malaria). Malaria, prevalent in estuarine marshy areas of south-east Scotland from about 1700, died out through a combination of land drainage, increasing use of Peruvian bark and quinine, and improved general health. The rise in mortality from the start of the nineteenth century was caused to a large extent by progressive urbanisation, which not only increased the spread of infectious diseases but enhanced their virulence. The proportion of infected individuals who died (case mortality) increased as many of the immigrants to towns were poorly nourished and did not share the urban 'herd immunity', making them more susceptible to common infectious diseases. One exception to this was smallpox. Here, largely as a result of the widespread adoption of vaccination, the proportion of deaths fell from 15% to 5% of all deaths between 1801 and 1811 (see p. 148).

The population shift to towns in the first half of the nineteenth century resulted in urban overcrowding, poverty and squalor with their associated diseases, and the effects of these were duly reflected in the rise in urban mortality rates. Between 1835 and 1845 the average mortality rate in 331 *rural* parishes (total population 751,016) was 20.3 per 1000, while the average mortality rate in the 14 principal towns of Scotland, with almost exactly the same population, was 26.7 per 1000. In the latter half of the century it was to rise even higher. In adults, infectious diseases, convulsions and 'old age' were the commonest recorded causes of death in the mid-nineteenth century. Tuberculosis, the leading cause of death in adults, was not universally recognised as an infectious disease until several decades later.

ENLIGHTENMENT THINKING

In the latter half of the eighteenth century, as the Enlightenment swept through Europe, Scotland witnessed an extraordinary outburst of intellectual activity which took place in the midst of the rural poverty in the Highlands and urban squalor of the cities. The roots of the Scottish Enlightenment are complex, but a major factor in its genesis was the existence of a relatively well-educated population who had suffered a loss of national identity from 1707 and were loosening themselves from strict adherence to Calvinist dogma and faith, a change which was to allow greater freedom of thought. One feature of the Enlightenment which accelerated the spread of new ideas was the concept that acquired knowledge should be shared. At informal meetings in homes, taverns and coffee houses and at the more formal meetings of the societies which sprang up throughout the country, lectures, debates and discussions all encouraged exchange of new observations and development of new rational thought. So too did the writing of pamphlets, papers, books and journals. The literati and their students and followers aspired to the universal application of reason to improve the mental, physical and material condition of mankind. This led to new ideas about the causation of disease, the use of experiment in medicine, and the concept of evidence to prove or disprove hypotheses. This climate attracted doctors into Scotland, particularly from England, while conversely many Scottish doctors left to pursue and develop their ideas south of the Border and beyond.

Views on the Cause of Disease

The idea that disease could be explained by imbalance of humours had been questioned by Al-Razi (865–925) and by Paracelsus (1493–1541), yet the theory continued to appear in medical textbooks until the end of the nineteenth century. Fevers might be caused by *contagion* if acquired from the body of a sick person, or by *miasma* if acquired through the atmosphere from marsh water or rotting matter. The blossoming of science in the Renaissance had led to mechanistic theories on the working of the body and these gained popularity in the seventeenth century. Boerhaave's hydraulic theory of the working of

William Cullen

William Cullen (1710–90) had studied at Glasgow, serving an apprenticeship as a surgeon-apothecary before attending medical classes in Edinburgh, where he jointly founded the student society which would become the Royal Medical Society. After eight years of practice in his birthplace, Hamilton, as surgeon-apothecary, he moved to Glasgow in 1746 to teach chemistry, medicine and physiology, while continuing to practise as a physician. Here his innovative teaching methods and emphasis on critical analysis marked him out as a particularly gifted teacher. He was soon giving additional lectures in materia medica and botany before being appointed Professor of Medicine in 1751. Cullen returned to Edinburgh in 1755 as Professor of Chemistry. Within a year he was giving clinical lectures at the Royal Infirmary, was appointed Professor of the Institutes of Medicine and eventually, in 1766, became Professor of the Practice of Physic.

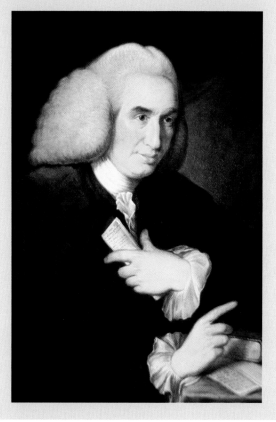

3.5 William Cullen (attributed to William Cochran, c1768). This copy of a painting by Allan Ramsay was presented to the RCPE by Cullen's great granddaughter. The letter in his left hand is a reminder that consultation and opinion by letter was the mainstay of his extensive consultative practice (*Royal College of Physicians of Edinburgh*).

the body was in tune with the thinking of an increasingly scientific age, while iatromechanical theory, which sought to explain body function through the laws of physics, was taught by the Edinburgh physician turned anatomist Archibald Pitcairne (1652–1713). In turn this was superseded by the idea promoted by George Stahl (1660–1734) that the soul was the driving force for all vital activity. Stahl's animist view was taken forward by Friedrich Hoffmann (1660–1742) who believed that a vital substance maintained the body in an equilibrium effected through the nervous system. This theory was further developed, elaborated and made popular throughout the medical world in the late eighteenth century by two rival Edinburgh physicians, William Cullen (1710–90) and John Brown (1735–88).

The concept of classification had become popular since the publication in 1735 of *Systema Naturae* by Carl Linnaeus (1707–78). William Cullen, who was to become one of the most influential medical teachers of his generation in the English-speaking world, first published his classification of disease as *Nosology* in 1769, and this had an immediate international influence. He described four classes of disease: pyrexiae, cachexias, neuroses (a word he introduced), and locales, subdividing these into nineteen orders and 132 genera. Introduced as a teaching aid and soon superseded by better, less contrived systems, this classification system led Cullen on to delve deeper into the cause of disease in each of his categories. This resulted in his major postulate, a development of Haller's hypothesis, that the cause of disease was governed by the nervous

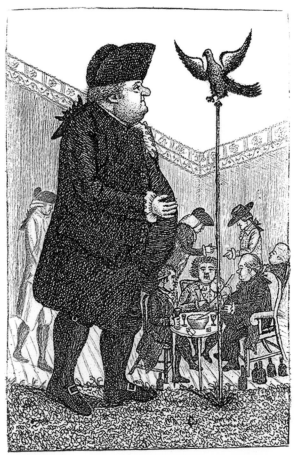

3.6 John Brown (John Kay). John Brown is depicted by Kay beside the ensign of the Roman Eagle Masonic Lodge, which he had founded, over which he presided and which, at his instigation, conducted all its business in Latin. The figures in the background include Dr William Cullen and Dr Alexander Hamilton, Professor of Midwifery, with a bowl of punch on the table (Kay's *Portraits*).

A rival theory was proposed by John Brown, a weaver's son from Duns in Berwickshire, a true lad o' pairts, endowed with great intellect, a prodigious memory and with a particular flair for Latin. Moving to Edinburgh he tutored Latin, became a 'grinder' or extramural coach, and was allowed to attend medical lectures free of charge. He tutored the children of William Cullen but, following a disagreement with his benefactor, Brown went on to devise a system for the diagnosis and treatment of disease which did away with mechanist and vitalist concepts and which directly challenged Cullen's. This became known as 'Brunonianism' and was published in his book *Elementa Medicinae* (1780). In it Brown proposed that bodily function and disease depended on 'excitability', mediated through the nervous system. Diseases were either 'asthenic', caused by lack of stimulation and treated by food or prescribed stimulants including opium and alcohol, or 'sthenic' caused by over-excitability and treated by mild 'stimulants' such as emetics and cathartics or by physical and mental rest. Bloodletting was used 'only in the most violent cases'. Brown aimed to lend credibility to his theory by the use of a 'Table of Excitement and Excitability' based on Newtonian quantification and mathematical formulae. Debates between Cullenians and Brunonians became heated and at times vitriolic, the former deriding Brunonian theory as simplistic, anti-establishment and a dangerous encouragement for quacks and self-help medicine. Its popularity with some doctors and the public at large perhaps owed more to Brown's advocacy of large doses of 'stimulant' alcohol and opium, stimulants which he himself used liberally.

Such public disputes were a common characteristic of Edinburgh medicine at the time, a failing observed by Benjamin Franklin who wrote in his *Autobiography* (1794): 'Persons of good Sense . . . seldom fall into [disputation], except Lawyers, University Men, and Men of all Sorts that have been bred at Edinburgh.'

Yet Brown was articulate and persuasive, and for a time Brunonianism enjoyed considerable popularity throughout Britain and Europe, particularly in Germany, Austria and Italy. In Germany, Brown's anti-authoritarian views and the simplicity of his excitability theory with its uncomplicated therapeutics, struck a chord with the

system, as opposed to the Newtonian mechanistic (iatro-mechanical) theory, which had been popularised by the teaching of Boerhaave.

Cullen's theory of nervous energy proposed that nerves needed stimulation to produce 'tonus' to maintain the flow of fluids into organs. Lack of such stimulus caused disease and was treated by 'tonics' such as blistering, quinine or camphor to stimulate the nervous system and thus maintain it in its normal state of 'excitability'. In contrast to Brown's system, Cullen's therapy was sparing in its use of alcohol or opium and made little use of powerful purgatives, the 'depletive' of humoral theory. Paradoxically Cullen made extensive use of bloodletting, the ultimate depletive.

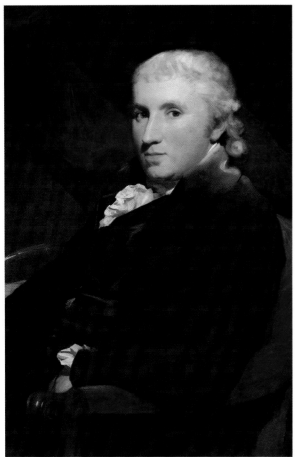

3.7 Benjamin Bell (oil on canvas, Sir Henry Raeburn c1790). Benjamin Bell was a major surgical figure of the Edinburgh School. His encyclopaedic textbook, *A System of Surgery*, published in six volumes between 1783 and 1788, went to seven English editions, was translated into Italian, French, Spanish and German, in addition to two American editions. He advocated the use of nerve compression and opiates for operative and post-operative pain relief. Bell's aphorism 'save skin' applied to amputation and mastectomy was to improve operative technique and wound-healing in both procedures (*Bourne Fine Art, Edinburgh*).

ADVANCES IN DIAGNOSIS

In contrast to this grand theorising about the cause of disease, the diagnosis of disease remained primitive, but increasing clinical observation of the patient became a feature of Enlightenment medicine. The emphasis on observation, documentation and experiment brought about improvements in the diagnosis of some diseases, none more so than sexually transmitted disease.

Syphilis and Gonorrhoea – Different Diseases?

Venereal disease was common, and attempts to treat it provided a major source of income for doctors. John Hunter (see p. 139) had gone from Lanarkshire to London where he became the most celebrated scientific surgeon of his day. Hunter, in common with most of his contemporaries, believed that syphilis (*lues venerea*) and gonorrhoea were different manifestations of the same disease, caused by the same agent. In his *Treatise on the Venereal Disease* (1786) he set out this view, supported by an experiment, characteristic of the new thinking, in which he had inoculated pus from a patient with gonorrhoea into a subject who had subsequently developed syphilis. Some believe that Hunter himself was the subject, although this is unlikely. Sadly for the subject and for Hunter's conclusions it seems likely in hindsight that the patient had both conditions. Hunter's view was authoritative and seemed to be the final word on one of the main medical dilemmas of the age. Benjamin Bell (1749–1806), an Edinburgh surgeon set out to demonstrate that these were two separate diseases in his *Treatise on Gonorrhoea Virulenta and Lues Venerea*. In this masterly monograph he argues clearly and logically that the two are different diseases, a conclusion based on clinical features, natural history, mode of transmission, geographical distribution and response to treatment with mercury.

As a riposte to Hunter's experimental evidence he describes another alarming and dangerous experiment in which 'two young gentlemen of this place failed to induce gonorrhoea in themselves by inoculating material from a chancre, or syphilis by inoculating gonorrhoeal pus'. In 1838 the French physician Philippe Ricord (1800–1889) was finally able to demonstrate beyond doubt that the two

doctors of the German Romantic movement.

It became popular too in America. Benjamin Rush, a young American who had come to Edinburgh to study under Cullen, took the theory even further, reducing Brown's two types of disease to one, a state of excessive excitability or spasm in the blood vessels, which he treated by depletion, usually in the form of massive bloodletting. Rush's pre-eminence as physician and teacher ensured the popularity, albeit transiently, of this variant of the theory in America.

Cullen, a sociable man and caring physician who embodied the spirit of the Enlightenment, made contributions as teacher, diagnostician and College president, all of which are considered later.

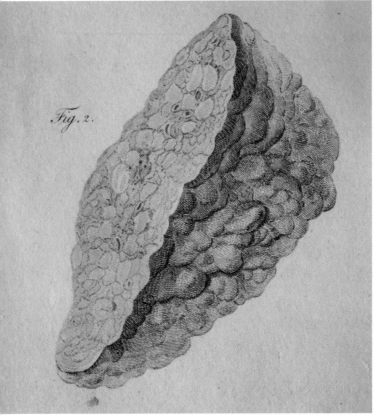

Fig. 2.

3.8a A scirrhous liver (William Clift). In this illustration showing what it now called cirrhosis of the liver, Baillie uses the term 'scirrhous', meaning 'hard', to describe one of the principal pathological features of the condition (*The Morbid Anatomy of Some of the Most Important Parts of the Human Body*).

PLATE II.

THIS Plate is intended to illustrate the most common kind of tubercles formed in the liver. The process by which they are formed is very slow, although it varies in this respect a good deal in different individuals, and it is commonly produced by a long habit of drinking spirituous liquors. When the liver has undergone this change, it is commonly said to be scirrhous, but the morbid appearance is very different from what is observed in the genuine scirrhus of other glands. It should rather be considered as a disease *sui generis*.

3.8b Baillie's description of the condition, which notes that it is commonly produced in those with 'a long habit of drinking spirituous liquors' (*Morbid Anatomy*).

were indeed different diseases and that Bell was correct. In doing so he quoted extensively from Bell's *Treatise*.

The Science of Morbid Anatomy

While postulating the cause of disease was largely an intellectual discipline and diagnosing it a clinical one, there were advances in medical science, notably in morbid anatomy, which saw develop the concept of disease arising within organs rather than resulting from humoural imbalance. Anatomy had been at the core of medical education even before Vesalius, and increasing anatomical knowledge paved the way for the growth of morbid anatomy, the study of disease in the dead body. The post mortem now increasingly became a means of understanding disease. Giovanni Morgagni (1682–1771) systemised and popularised the study of the relationship between pathological changes and symptoms of disease in *De Sedibus et Causis Morborum* (1761) and this concept was developed by Mathew Baillie (1761–1823) (see p. 138) a nephew of the brothers John and William Hunter. The immense contributions of the Hunters to science, anatomy, surgery and midwifery are discussed in detail later (see p. 139).

In *The Morbid Anatomy of Some of the Most Important Parts of the Human Body* (1793) Baillie presented pathology as an independent science and, crucially for the concept of organ-based disease, arranged his book organ by organ. In the first edition he aimed to describe 'our knowledge of the changes of structure produced by disease, which may be called the Morbid Anatomy' and went on to give remarkably clear and precise descriptions of changes to organs caused by disease. In the second (1797) edition, he noted correlations between symptoms and pathological change, including some which he regarded as of particular importance. Notably he recognised that liver cirrhosis could result from alcohol excess and his observation that 'ossification of the coronary arteries would seem to produce the symptoms of angina pectoris' was the first recognition of this association. The book became popular and influential around the world and was published in several English editions, but also in American, French, German, Italian and Russian editions.

This focus on organs as the seat of some diseases was a major advance in understanding of the cause of disease

Lind's Treatment of Scurvy

Twelve seamen with scurvy, 'as similar as I could have them', were given a common diet, and confined for two weeks within the ship. They were then grouped into pairs, and each pair prescribed a different potential remedy (cider; elixir of vitriol; vinegar; sea water; oranges and lemons; garlic and mustard seed). Only the pair prescribed the oranges and lemons recovered. Throughout the *Treatise*, published six years later, Lind presents the proof of the efficacy of both fruit and green vegetables in preventing scurvy, yet he believed that scurvy was caused by faulty digestion and excretion. Lind considered it impractical to take citrus fruits on long naval voyages, and neither in the conclusions in his *Treatise* nor in his subsequent practice did he clearly advocate citrus fruit to prevent scurvy.

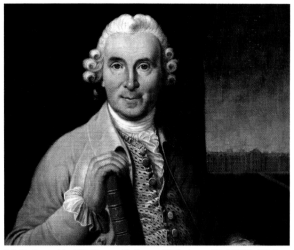

3.9 Dr James Lind (Sir George Chalmers, 1783). James Lind (1716–1794) served an apprenticeship to the Edinburgh surgeon George Langlands, and with no other qualification joined the Royal Navy in 1738 as surgeon's mate, going on to be promoted to surgeon. He returned to graduate MD from Edinburgh University in 1748 and set up in medical practice in the city before being appointed physician in charge at Royal Hospital Haslar. In this portrait the Royal Hospital, Haslar, is in the background, and his three-part *Treatise of the Scurvy* is in the foreground (*Hepner Family*).

and represented another step in the move away from theories based on imbalance of humours.

Ideas on Evidence-based Medicine

Until the eighteenth century evidence had not been a particular feature of medical diagnosis or treatment. The rational, empirical approach of the Enlightenment promoted the collecting, sharing and analysis of information about patients and their illnesses. The concepts of postulating hypotheses and of proving or disproving by experimentation were now gradually introduced into medical practice.

The natural philosopher Sir Francis Bacon (1561–1626) had set out the basis of logical enquiry with a system of observation and experience combined with inductive reasoning. John Gregory (1724–1773), Professor of Physic at Edinburgh University, advised his students to follow Bacon's model and adopt a systematic, scientific methodology for investigation into the cause of disease, the diagnosis of disease and the best ways to treat it.

This approach to evidence was developed further by George Fordyce (1736–1802), who had graduated in arts from Aberdeen University, then MD from the University of Edinburgh, where he was an early and favoured pupil of William Cullen. As a physician and teacher in London he lectured for some thirty years, on chemistry, materia medica and the practice of physic. Despite his Scottish

origins and qualification, he was elected a licentiate, then a fellow, of the Royal College of Physicians of London and appointed physician to St Thomas's Hospital. Throughout his life he conducted chemical analyses and a series of clinical experiments and observations on the nature of heat and bodily control of temperature. With the publication of his 1793 paper, *An Attempt to Improve the Evidence of Medicine*, Fordyce made the case for medical practice based on evidence, rather than on case studies.

Medical Experiment in Action – the First Prospective, Controlled Clinical Trial

One of the earliest examples of the use of experiment as evidence in clinical medicine was James Lind's 1753 *Treatise of the Scurvy*, which demonstrates his enquiring mind and his appreciation of the value of experiment. In the aims set out in the introduction he encapsulates the rational thought so characteristic of the Enlightenment.

'I shall propose nothing dictated merely from theory' he wrote 'but shall confirm all the experience and facts, the surest and most unerring guides'. He then went on to conduct what is widely regarded as the first controlled trial in medicine. This was at a time when scurvy was a major cause of morbidity and mortality in the Royal Navy, the force on which Britain's political and military supremacy depended. Lind's work may have been stimulated by Anson's disastrous voyage in 1740, when around 1000 of his 1400 sailors died of scurvy. Lind conducted his 'experiment' in 1747 when he was ship's surgeon on HMS *Salisbury*. Although the results would appear to show clearly that dietary oranges and lemons cure scurvy, Lind did not draw this conclusion, so that his advice was not 'the surest and most unerring guide' he had set out to produce.

Lind was appointed physician in charge of the Royal Hospital Haslar in 1758, but did not put into practice a preventative remedy for scurvy based on citrus fruit. It was not until 1795 that the Admiralty was persuaded to issue seamen with a regular ration of lime juice. Much of the credit for this policy belongs to two other Scottish naval surgeons, Thomas Trotter and Gilbert Blane, who freely acknowledged Lind's pioneering work (see p. 146). Lind's famous experiment exemplifies the opposition to medical innovation and the delay in introducing apparently proven ideas, both of which were to become all too common in medicine over the next two centuries.

Lind later engaged in 'comparative trials' of febrifuges (preparations used to lower temperature). In his time at Haslar he was among the first to publish outcomes of a single method of treatment of one disease entity, in one hospital over a given time period, and was an important figure in the movement towards a more objective evaluation of treatment methods. His important contribution to standards of hygiene in the Royal Navy is considered later.

Clinical Epidemiology – First Demonstration of the Contagious Nature of Puerperal Fever

One of the earliest examples of the use of patient observation and rational thought to establish the cause and spread of disease came from Aberdeen. Alexander Gordon (1752–1799) graduated MA from Marischal College in Aberdeen in 1775. He trained in medicine in Edinburgh and Leiden, then spent five years in the Royal Navy, first as surgeon's mate, then as surgeon. After studying midwifery in London, he was appointed physician to the Aberdeen Dispensary in 1785. Because of his midwifery training, Alexander Gordon was to play a major role in patient care during the epidemic of puerperal fever which struck Aberdeen and its environs in 1789. Puerperal fever has since been shown to be most commonly caused by a

streptococcal infection of the female genital tract after delivery. The prevailing explanation in Gordon's day was miasma theory, a belief that the disease was caused by a noxious constituent of the atmosphere.

Gordon meticulously recorded information about his patients. He compiled a table of mothers affected by puerperal fever and, crucially, noted the time of delivery and by whom they were delivered. From these data he concluded that the cause of puerperal fever was a 'specific contagion or infection' transmitted from one patient to another by a medical attendant. In this way he clearly identified the contagious nature of the infection, writing in his commentary on the table of those affected: 'The midwife who delivered [patient] No. 1 in the table carried the infection to No. 2, the next woman whom she delivered . . .' He goes on to describe in this way the disease transmission for all cases. With remarkable scientific objectivity Gordon implicated himself as an agent of transmission. He also recognised the relationship with erysipelas (a streptococcal infection of the skin): 'I will not venture positively to assert' he wrote, 'that the puerperal fever and erysipelas are precisely of the same specific

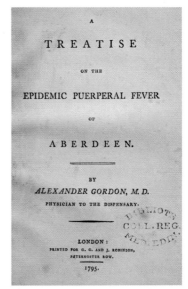

3.10 Frontispiece of *Treatise on the Epidemic Puerperal Fever of Aberdeen* by Alexander Gordon, 1795. Gordon proposed that puerperal fever was contagious, caused by 'putrid matter' introduced into the uterus by doctors and midwives, who in this way transmitted the disease. He suggested that it might be prevented by the medical attendants washing their hands and fumigating their clothes.

nature; but that they are connected, that there is an analogy between them, and that they are concomitant epidemics, I have unquestionable proofs.'

On the basis of these conclusions he went on to suggest methods of prevention of puerperal fever, citing James Lind's view that 'fire and smoke are the most powerful agents for annihilating infection; and, as he thinks, even the plague itself.' Gordon went on to suggest that 'The patient's apparel and bedclothes ought either to be burnt or thoroughly purified; and the nurses and physicians who have attended patients affected with puerperal fever ought carefully to wash themselves, and to get their apparel properly fumigated before it be put on again.'

So Alexander Gordon performed the first epidemiological study of puerperal fever and clearly and logically showed the contagious and transmissible nature of the condition and how it might be avoided. All this some forty years before the work of Oliver Wendell Holmes and Ignaz Semmelweis who are widely credited with demonstrating the mode of transmission of the condition and its prevention.

New Ideas on Medical Ethics

While some doctors of the period were concerned with the theory of disease and its scientific study, others developed ideas about the relationship between doctors and patients. John Gregory (1724–1773) believed that doctors' prime motivation must not be the pursuit of status, power and money, but rather concern for the welfare of the patient. His *Lectures on the Duties and Qualifications of a Physician* (1772) have been described by McCullough (1995) as 'the first secular, philosophical, clinical, and feminine medical ethics and bioethics in the English language'. In these lectures Gregory advocates the concept of a bedside manner demonstrating to the patient gentleness, compassion and tenderness, traits which had until then been regarded as essentially feminine. He promoted the concept of sympathy elaborated by David Hume who believed that sympathy could be developed by imagining the pain and suffering of others – an extension of his thinking on the senses. Sympathy was important as it helped gain the trust of the patient and was 'in many cases of the utmost consequence to his recovery.' Another quality, humanity 'that

sensibility of heart which makes us feel for the distresses of our fellow creatures' was, he believed, the single most important trait for the doctor to possess. In the spirit of the Enlightenment, Gregory taught that the physician should be honest and 'ready to acknowledge and rectify his mistakes'. He argued that the doctor must maintain intellectual rigour and standards and protect and promote the interests of patients. Gregory's influence was to prove powerful in shaping concepts which came to define Scottish medicine – a rejection of commercial motivation and a belief that rich and poor should be treated in exactly the same way. Gregory taught Thomas Percival (1740–1804), whose *Medical Ethics* (1803) became a classic throughout the English-speaking world. Benjamin Rush, another of his Edinburgh students, was to become a leading physician and statesman in America and as such had a major influence on medical ethics in that country. Gregory's ethical writings were also translated into French, German, Italian and Spanish.

Gregory was a member of a medical family which was to influence Scottish medicine over five generations (see p. 125).

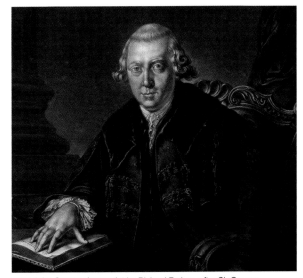

3.11 John Gregory (mezzotint by Richard Earlom, after Sir George Chalmers, 1774). John Gregory (1724–1773), son of James Gregory (1674–1733) the mediciner at King's College, Aberdeen, was appointed professor of philosophy there, and started to teach and write on philosophy. In 1764 he became a physician in Edinburgh and two years later was appointed professor of medicine in preference to William Cullen (*Wellcome Library, London*).

Dear Sir/
If it is agreeable for you to let me have 100 copies of the new Edition of your first Lines, I dare say many of them will be sold here. The Price I leave to yourself.
It is some months since I wrote for this Article to Mr Creech, but without success. He threw the blame of the delay upon Mr Smellie – & I was so disgusted at their dilatoriness that on the 10th march I cancelled the order.
I had the pleasure of seeing your Son this day in perfect health. I remain with great Respect Dr Sir/ Your very obedt Servant
London 23d April 1778. *J. Murray*
Dr Cullen. Edinburgh.

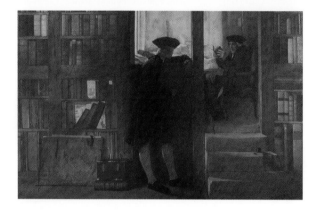

Publishing – Spreading Enlightenment Knowledge and Ideas

The doctors of the period were eager to spread their innovative ideas, theories and observations, not just by lecturing but by writing. Printers, publishers and booksellers played a major role in spreading the views of the Scottish Enlightenment throughout the world. In Glasgow the brothers Robert (1707–76) and Andrew (1712–75) Foulis established the Foulis Press, printing some 600 titles from 1740, which earned them a reputation for beautiful and accurate printings of Latin and Greek classics. John Murray (1737–1793) moved from Edinburgh to set up a bookselling business in London, which soon developed into a major publishing house, producing a wide literary output but with a particular interest in medical and scientific titles, which accounted for one-quarter of its output. He published, among others, William Cullen and Gilbert Blane. The business developed into John Murray publishing, which evolved under seven successive generations of the family, and whose imprint name survives into the twenty-first century. The John Murray Archive, comprising around 150,000 documents collected by the publish-

ing house over the centuries, was acquired by the National Library of Scotland in 2007.

It was characteristic of the Enlightenment ideal that knowledge should be shared that William Smellie (1740–95), a printer's apprentice in Edinburgh, should be allowed to attend the botany lectures given by John Hope and John Gregory. Smellie became the favoured printer of the publishers Charles Elliot, John Murray and William Creech among others, printing works by the Gregories, Andrew Duncan, William Cullen, Benjamin Bell and by virtually all the major figures of the Scottish Enlightenment. Smellie also founded *The Edinburgh Weekly Journal* (1765–70) and the radical and controversial *Edinburgh Magazine and Review* (1773–60). Having edited and printed the first edition of Buchan's *Domestic Medicine*, he wrote the first essays for and edited the first edition of *Encyclopaedia Britannica*. A sociable and learned man, his wide network of friends and contacts ensured a broad range of authoritative contributors from home and abroad to this massive and successful work.

Like Smellie, William Creech (1745–1815) was able to take advantage of the 'open' system of medical lectures at the University of Edinburgh, which he attended before setting up a successful bookshop in Edinburgh's High Street. He published work by Alexander Monro *secundus*, Cullen and James Gregory, but also poetry by Burns and Fergusson and Sir John Sinclair's *Statistical Account of Scotland* (1791–9).

An international dimension was provided by the Edinburgh bookseller and publisher Charles Elliot (1748–1790) who, from his bookshop in Parliament Square, traded with England, Ireland, Europe and America, specialising in medical books and translations of foreign works. He published James Lind, James Gregory, Alexander Monro *secundus*, John Brown, Alexander Hamilton and Andrew Duncan, but his most profitable works proved to be Benjamin Bell's *System of Surgery* and William Cullen's *First Lines of the Practice of Physic.* Elliot summarised his role in promoting the medical books of the period. 'I am,' he wrote, 'the principal Man Midwife (in the literary way) here, to Man Midwives, Physicians, Apothecaries etc.'

Origins and Development of Medical Journals

Important though they were, textbooks took time and effort to prepare and publish, and became dated as new knowledge emerged. The monograph was the conduit for more immediate announcement of new findings or opinions, but was traditionally confined to a single topic. The torrent of new observations and ideas generated by Enlightenment thinking created the need for a new type of publication to communicate these quickly and regularly to the increasing numbers of doctors eager to learn about innovations.

Between 1733 and 1744 the Society for the Improvement of Medical Knowledge had published *Edinburgh Medical Essays and Observations,* a journal which contained accounts of prevalent epidemic diseases, medical case reports and accounts of medical innovations. In 1773, Andrew Duncan founded *Medical and Philosophical Commentaries,* the first English-language medical journal with a wide readership (see p. 125), made possible by the distribution of each edition by John Murray in London. Its appeal to doctors was in part due to the reviews of what he regarded as 'the best new books' in medicine and a list of all recently published medical books. It became difficult to sustain quarterly publication because of Duncan's many other activities, so his son Andrew junior became joint editor and, renamed *Medical Commentaries,* the journal was published annually. In 1796 the periodical became *Annals of Medicine,* a name which lasted only until 1805 when it was again retitled, becoming the *Edinburgh Medical and Surgical Journal.* This journal, having dropped *Surgical* from the title in 1855, continued in publication until 1954, when a merger with the *Glasgow Medical Journal* resulted in the *Scottish Medical Journal,* which continues publication into the twenty-first century.

HEALERS

'The vulgar in most parts of this country, and particularly here, have an utter dislike to all regular physicians and surgeons, though in general their faith in drugs, quack medicines and old wives' nostrums is most implicit. In my attendance upon the sick, my first question has generally been, when I found the disorder dangerous, whether a physician had been called; and though I have always advised it, I do not remember that in any instance I have succeeded.'

Minister of Kilspindie, County of Perth, in *Statistical Account of Scotland* 1791–99

In late eighteenth and early nineteenth-century Scotland the choice of a healer still depended on what was available locally, on ability to travel and ability to pay. In this medical market-place the sick might seek the advice of a local wise woman or a minister, visit a clooty well or perhaps all three. For the better off there were options like a trip to a healing well or a spa, and if affordable and appropriate, a consultation with an itinerant quack, a surgeon-apothecary, or a physician. Physicians offered lifestyle advice, much of it wise and some of it seemingly in advance of its time. Benjamin Rush, for example, returning to America from Edinburgh, wrote 'Golf is an exercise which is much used by gentlemen in Scotland . . . A man would live 10 years the longer for using this exercise once or twice a week.'

Yet in the light of later knowledge, few of the cures in the array of herbal and other remedies on offer were effective, and excessive purging and bleeding could be positively dangerous. Robert Burns, in his satirical poem *Death and Dr Hornbrook* (1785), was scathing about lay healers (Hornbrook was the village schoolmaster), and by implication doctors who still relied on 'cures' which had their origins in folklore and were sprinkled with Latin names to imply credibility and learning.

Forbye some new, uncommon weapons,
Urinus spiritus of capons;
Or mite-horn shavings, filings, scrapings,

Distill'd *per se;*
Sal-alkali o' midge-tail clippings,
And mony mae.

He continues with a damning indictment of the harm
which the healer could inflict:

Thus goes he on from day to day,
Thus does he poison, kill, an' slay.

So, in the delivery of health care, ordinary people in the
eighteenth century did not seem to benefit immediately
from the grand theorising about the nature of disease
which was taking place in cities and universities.

Lay healers

As discussed in previous chapters, folk remedies were
commonly collected by a local wise woman who would
often remain the first port of call for advice, particularly
in country areas. The local blacksmith would often have
the expertise (and the strength) to draw teeth and set
broken bones. Schoolteachers, like Burns's Dr Hornbrook,
and clergymen could also offer help. The Rev George
Ridpath, minister in the Borders village of Stichel, exemplified the reach of the Enlightenment into a country
parish. He was 'a friend of the most celebrated Scots
literati of the time, and an earnest student in many
branches of science.' His diaries (1755–61) record that he
read Celsus, Mead and Boerhaave and was familiar with
Cleghorn's successful use of willow bark in fever. He would
provide what medical services he could free to parish-
ioners. The value of the clergy in this regard was recognised in the early nineteenth century when the committee
of the Edinburgh Royal Dispensary and Vaccine Institute
proposed to the general Assembly of the Church of Scotland that any minister willing to vaccinate against smallpox should have vaccine posted free of charge, and some
took up this offer.

Midwives

In his *Treatise on the Theory and Practise of Midwifery*
(1752), William Smellie (1697–1763) (the Lanarkshire-born
man-midwife, not to be confused with the Edinburgh

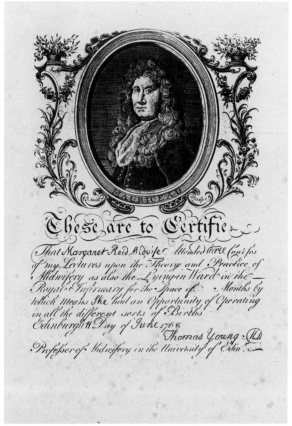

3.14 Certificate signed by Thomas Young in 1768. This certifies that
Margaret Reid, midwife, had attended his lectures on midwifery and
attended the lying-in ward of Edinburgh Royal Infirmary, where she had the
'opportunity of operating in all the different sorts of births'. The certificate
features an etching of the celebrated French obstetrician Francois
Mauriçeau (1637–1709) (*Lothian Heath Services Archive*).

publisher of the same name) gave his view of the attributes
of the ideal midwife:

A Midwife, though she can hardly be supposed
mistress of all these qualifications, ought to be a
decent, sensible woman, of a middle age, able to
bear fatigue; she ought to be perfectly well
instructed with regard to the bones of the Pelvis,
with all the contained parts, comprehending
those that are subservient to generation; . . . she
ought to live in friendship with other women of
the same profession, contending with them in
nothing but in knowledge, sobriety, diligence,
and patience.'

Licensing of midwives had been introduced by the Edinburgh Town Council as early as 1694. When John Gibson,
a Leith surgeon, was appointed the first City professor of

midwifery in 1726, the responsibility to test midwives for their licence fell to him. Gibson thus became the first professor of midwifery in Britain appointed to teach both student doctors and midwives. A register of licensed midwives was now kept by the town council. Thomas Young (c1730–83), the third professor, set up a lying-in ward in the Infirmary in 1756 where he offered practical instruction to midwives, who could also experience deliveries and attend his course of lectures. By advocating a policy of 'a midwife for every parish', he attracted pupil midwives from the length of Scotland. A further attraction for these pupils was the certificate they were awarded (Fig. 3.14), while the attraction for their parish was that they were cheaper than doctors and easier to attract to remote communities. Alexander Hamilton, the fourth professor, established the Edinburgh General Lying-in Hospital in Park House in 1793, and published a comprehensive textbook, *A Treatise of Midwifery* (1781). In keeping with Enlightenment thinking he required midwives to keep a record of all of their cases.

In Glasgow, the Faculty of Physicians and Surgeons issued licences for midwives from 1740, and from 1757, lectures were given to midwives, initially by James Muir and later by Thomas Hamilton. The Faculty's system of examination and licensing lasted until the early nineteenth century. A similar lecture course was delivered in Aberdeen by David Skene (c1731–70) and John Gregory. Skene had trained in Edinburgh and then in London where he attended the lectures of William Hunter and William Smellie. He went on to learn practical delivery from Smellie and, returning to Aberdeen, helped establish a lying-in ward and began to give courses of instruction 'particularly intended for the instruction of country midwives'.

As a result of these pioneering activities in its three main cities, the training of midwives flourished in Scotland, where between 1780 and 1818 over one thousand midwives qualified, compared to relatively small numbers south of the Border. The subsequent growth in the numbers of midwives has been documented by Mortimer (2002) who reckons that by 1851 there were 815 midwives in Scotland, of whom 52 were in Aberdeen, 41 in Glasgow, 40 in Edinburgh and 13 in Dundee.

Nurses

While lecture courses and certification were available for eighteenth-century midwives in Scotland, nurses did not at this stage have the benefit of formal training. They worked either as independent nurses who could attend the wealthy at home, or as institutional nurses in the new infirmaries. Independent nurses were familiar with medical practice and were able to carry out the instructions of the attending doctor. While 'wet nurses' were employed to breast-feed infants, 'dry nurses' cared for them. William Smellie in 1752 advised that a dry nurse should be 'an elderly woman properly qualified'. The 'sick' nurse, on the other hand, cared for adults. Some were able to bleed or to inoculate against smallpox, and all were expected to be able to lay out the dead. Infirmary nurses did not have the independence of their colleagues in the community and were paid less. They were employed by the hospital and, although they were required to live in, board and lodging were provided. Their nursing duties extended to ward cleaning, management of the domestic staff and preparing or supervising the preparation of meals.

When Mrs Wood was appointed matron of the Royal Infirmary of Edinburgh in 1840, she was required to be 'without dependants, so that she would be divested of every other care but that of the hospital, whose inmates she was to regard as her family'. She failed to live up to these criteria and was dismissed for dishonesty two years later, accused of stealing hospital crockery and furniture. Worse, her daughter and granddaughter were found to be living in her quarters, and her brothers had been removing 'unwanted' articles from the hospital workshop. By contrast her successor, Miss Peat, seems to have been an honest, reforming matron who began to impose standards of discipline not only on the nurses, but also on the resident house staff of doctors.

Mortimer has calculated that, by 1851, there were 53 nurses in Edinburgh's Royal Infirmary and 212 working independently in the city.

Dickens's caricature of the mid-nineteenth-century nurse as a gin-soaked Sarah Gamp, reeking of snuff, was a widely held perception. Dr James Burn Russell (1837–1904), medical superintendent of Glasgow's first munici-

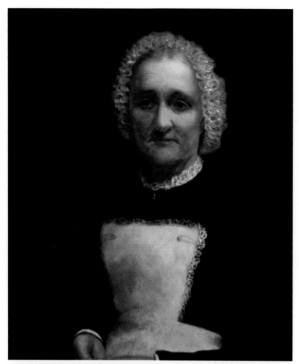

3.15 Janet Porter (painting by an unknown artist). Janet Porter, c1810–1890, nursed in the Edinburgh Royal Infirmary for 47 years, a career which spanned the introduction of Nightingale-based training. She cared for the patients of Syme, Lister and Joseph Bell, the latter describing her as a 'wonderful woman, of great natural ability and strong Scottish sense and capacity, of immense experience and great kindliness' (*Lothian Health Services Archive*).

pal hospital (and later Glasgow's MOH), gave this unflattering view: 'at present nursing is the last resource of female adversity. Slatternly widows, runaway wives, servants out of place, women bankrupt of fame or fortune from whatever cause, fall back on hospital nursing.' Russell was instrumental in improving nursing in Glasgow with careful selection of applicants, and the establishment of nursing training, which initially took the form of learning Florence Nightingale's *Notes on Nursing* (1859).

Thirty years later, the poet W E Henley, a long term patient under the care of Joseph Lister in Edinburgh Royal Infirmary, was able to give a much more appreciative account of Janet Porter, the ward sister.

> The broad Scots tongue that flatters, scolds, defies,
> The thick Scots wit that fells you like a mace.
> These thirty years has she been nursing here,
> Some of them under SYME, her hero still.
> Much is she worth, and even more is made of her.
> Patients and students hold her very dear.
> The doctors love her, tease her, use her skill.
> They say 'The Chief' himself is half-afraid of her.

Apothecaries and Surgeon-Apothecaries

While they retained an important function in the delivery of health care, apothecaries in Scotland were never to enjoy the power and autonomy of their London counterparts. This was partly because the apothecaries did not have sufficient numbers to be politically influential, and partly because the surgeons had always exercised their rights to practise pharmacy, often designating themselves as surgeon-apothecaries and effectively functioning as general practitioners. When some of these Scots with training and qualifications in both medicine and surgery began to emigrate to England to find work in the growing provincial towns, so the English apothecaries came to view them as unwelcome competition. Apothecaries could only charge for dispensing rather than consultation, while this Scottish breed could do both, representing a serious threat to their livelihoods. The English apothecaries lobbied Parliament for legislation that would define their role and enshrine in law their right to see patients. The College of Physicians in London did not regard the legislation as a threat, believing that the apothecary's role would always be subservient to that of the physician. When the Apothecaries Act (1815) was passed, however, it became clear that it applied to *all practitioners* who prescribed drugs in England and Wales, so that the Scottish surgeon-apothecary (or indeed any Scottish graduate) was now required to serve an apprenticeship under the aegis of the Society of Apothecaries if he wished to practise in England or Wales. A Royal Commission in 1831 concluded that 'The direct effect of the enactment is to vest the monopoly of practice in a person of very inferior education', by which was meant the apothecary. This power, whether given to the apothecaries unintentionally or by the design of the College of Physicians, resulted in a campaign, widely supported by factions within the medical establishment much more used to internecine squabbling, to protect their own vested interests. These included the London College of Physicians, the Scottish universities, the *Edinburgh Medical and Surgical Journal* and *The Lancet*. The eventual outcome was the Medical Act of 1858, which set up a General Medical Council to examine medical qualifications and established a register of those considered qualified to practise medicine in Britain.

Collegiate Surgeons

In the mid-eighteenth century, all Edinburgh and Glasgow surgeons were effectively surgeon-apothecaries, but over the next 100 years 'pure' surgeons began to emerge, and by the end of the period some surgeons would develop a special interest in an aspect of surgery such as dentistry or eye disease. In Edinburgh the Incorporation of Surgeons received a Royal Charter in 1778 to become the Royal College of Surgeons of the City of Edinburgh. Like the Faculty of Physicians and Surgeons in Glasgow, it continued to license local surgeons. From 1770 the Edinburgh College required country surgeons to sit a diploma examination, and, with the political help of Henry Dundas, Viscount Melville, the college diploma was recognised as a surgical qualification for prospective surgeons by the East India Company and subsequently for those wishing to serve in the Army and the Royal Navy.

From 1815 success in this diploma examination conferred the title of Licentiate, and the examination attracted medical students and candidates from around the world. The examination to become a Fellow (previously Master or Freeman) of the college tested knowledge at a higher level, but traditionally attracted only local candidates, so that by 1850 there had only been a total of 431 Masters or Freemen since 1505. This too was to change as the Fellowship developed into an international examination. Soon examination fees were to provide increasing income for the college, a situation which continued into the twentieth century. The new Surgeons' Hall building, designed by the leading Scottish architect William Playfair, opened in 1832. Housing one of the best medical museums in the world, the building attested to the increasing size, influence and confidence of the College. In Glasgow the Faculty diploma examination progressed along similar lines, albeit with smaller numbers of candidates involved. The Faculty, along with the two Edinburgh Colleges, became increasingly involved, in the early decades of the nineteenth century, in a struggle to maintain recognition of their basic medical qualifications. The 1858 Medical Act recognised the qualifications of all three establishments, and their Triple Qualification provided a registrable basic medical qualification until the start of the twenty-first century.

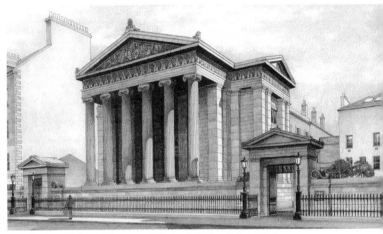

3.16 The Royal College of Surgeons of Edinburgh (William Fulton, 1991). The college building, opened in 1832, was designed by William Playfair, whose buildings had gained for Edinburgh the soubriquet 'Athens of the North'. The Ionic columns were a classical style favoured by Playfair, who designed the facade to convey the impression of a learned and prestigious organisation (*Royal College of Surgeons of Edinburgh*).

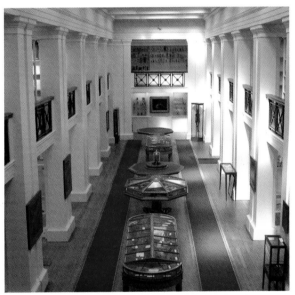

3.17 Surgeons' Hall Museum. The Playfair building was designed to house the recently acquired museum collections of Charles Bell and John Barclay. In the twenty-first century it remains open to the public and retains the original display cases designed by Playfair (*Royal College of Surgeons of Edinburgh*).

Collegiate Physicians

The role of Scottish Medical Royal Colleges differed in many respects from that of their English counterparts. All were to some extent elitist, but none more so than the London College of Physicians, which restricted its fellowship to graduates of the universities of Oxford and Cambridge. It functioned in many respects as a gentlemen's club, bent on maintaining standards among its members, and frowning on Scottish graduates who had been trained

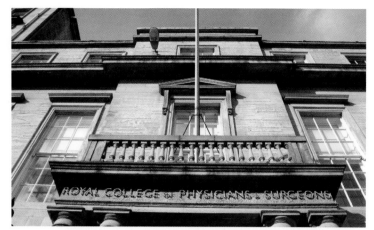

3.18 The Royal College of Physicians and Surgeons of Glasgow. The Faculty of Physicians and Surgeons of Glasgow moved from its original premises in the Trongate to this elegant terraced building in St Vincent Street (*RCPSG*).

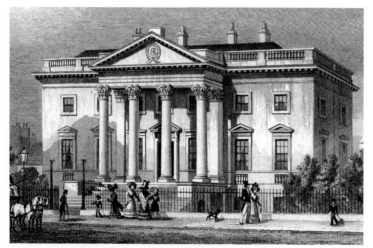

3.19 Physicians Hall, George Street, Edinburgh (drawing by Thomas H. Shepherd, engraving by J. Henshall, *c*1829). This was the hall of the Royal College of Physicians from 1781 to 1843. It was designed by James Craig, architect of Edinburgh's New Town, and was built to house the extensive library, the contents of which were deteriorating in the College's cramped quarters in Fountain's Close. In 1843 the building was sold to the Commercial Bank (which promptly demolished it to build its own headquarters) and the College moved to its current premises in Queen Street (*Royal College of Physicians of Edinburgh*).

in 'trades' like surgery and obstetrics. After the Union of 1707, ever more Scots doctors made their way to London, and, under increasing pressure to accommodate them, the London College, from 1761, admitted up to three licentiates per year. This was an inferior qualification, so much so that licentiates were not even allowed into the building, and in 1767 angry licentiates stormed into the College in protest. Yet it was not until 1835 that candidates from other universities were finally admitted to fellowship.

The Scottish colleges also adopted a licensing function, but in addition took on roles in education and in caring for the poor. The Faculty of Physicians and

Surgeons of Glasgow continued to license local practitioners in the west of Scotland, including midwives. So jealously did it guard its licensing powers that in 1815 the Faculty challenged graduates of Glasgow University who were practising as surgeons within its area of control. This resulted in litigation which lasted off and on until 1840. The Faculty won the case and, having resolved these differences with the University of Glasgow, now began to develop its aspiration to become a postgraduate teaching organisation rather than simply a licensing institution. The Faculty library was to produce the first major bibliography of books in the English language. Robert Watt (1774–1819), physician to Glasgow Royal Infirmary, compiled *Bibliotheca Britannica,* one of the largest works of bibliographical scholarship published to that time. It began as a bibliography for his medical students, which he expanded aiming to include every work published in English since printing began. He ended with a massive four-volume work containing over 200,000 books, pamphlets and periodicals printed from 1450 to the early nineteenth century. Having given up his career to complete this, sadly he did not live to see it published between 1819 and 1824.

The Glasgow Faculty members attended in rotation as physicians and surgeons to the Town's hospital and later to the Royal Infirmary, although, as in Edinburgh, these arrangements were the subject of bitter disputes. The Faculty opened the first vaccination station in Britain, offering vaccination from 1801, and within five years had vaccinated over 10,000 persons free of charge. By 1812 the practice was widespread throughout Glasgow and the west of Scotland.

In Edinburgh the Royal College of Physicians, in addition to licensing local physicians, continued to provide free medical care to the poor of the city. In 1781, during the presidency of William Cullen, the College moved to a new hall in George Street, largely in order to house its expanding medical library, perhaps the largest and one of the finest in Britain.

Yet within a few years, even this building was to prove too small for the expanding College, which next moved to its current premises in Queen Street. The College attempted to influence regulation of apothecaries and surgeon-apothecaries and to standardise medical prescribing by producing the *Edinburgh Pharmacopoeia* over many editions (see p. 117), until this was amalgamated with those of the London and Dublin Colleges to become the *British Pharmacopoeia* in 1864.

The Faculty in Glasgow and the Royal Colleges in Edinburgh became involved in the early nineteenth century in a struggle with the London College of Physicians and the universities over the right to grant qualifications to practise medicine. The universities regarded this as a necessary reform and standardisation of undergraduate medical education, but for the Colleges in Scotland it became a fight for the maintenance of privileges and patronage, and indeed for institutional survival. The Medical Act of 1858 brought about a standardisation of medical qualifications from universities and Colleges and this allowed the Colleges to continue to offer medical qualifications in the form of the Triple Qualification (the equivalent of Conjoint Boards in England) until the start of the twenty-first century.

The role of the Colleges in public health reforms is considered in the next chapter.

Medical Societies

Conviviality, the sharing of knowledge, argument and debate, were key elements of the Enlightenment, and so the founding of clubs and societies to promote these activities became a prominent feature of the period. 'The more these refined arts advance,' wrote David Hume, 'the more sociable men become.' Many of these societies were established by medical men, a further manifestation of the increasing number and organisation of doctors. Medical societies played an important part in the emergence of medicine as a profession, not only by enhancing social contact and friendship, but also by providing forums for the sharing of new ideas, knowledge and experience. Jenkinson (1993) has estimated that by 1830 some forty medical societies existed in Scotland, while in the next forty years a further forty-eight were founded.

Medical students were among the first to organise. The Medical Society of Edinburgh, founded in 1737 by ten students, met each week in a tavern for a discourse, a case study and questions on medical topics. From 1751 each

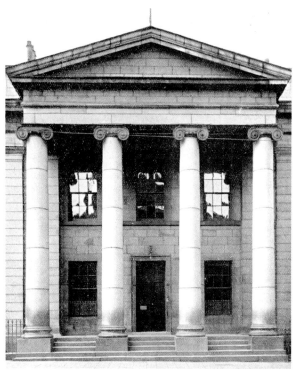

3.20 The hall of the Aberdeen Medico-Chirurgical Society in King Street, Aberdeen. This was designed by Archibald Simpson and opened in 1820. The Ionic pillars at the entrance show that even student buildings of this era were built to convey an impression of grandeur and learning. The Society met here until 1973, when it moved to the Foresterhill campus (*Aberdeen Medico-Chirurgical Society*).

member was expected to present a dissertation and defend it, providing ideal practice for the presentation which formed part of the MD degree. With support from prominent local doctors, the Society built its own hall in Surgeon Square in 1775 and three years later, with the award of a royal charter, became the Royal Medical Society (RMS). It was to be an important forum for medical students and young doctors to present research and new ideas.

In Aberdeen the Medico-Chirurgical Society was founded in 1789 by a group of students among whom James McGrigor was the driving force. He retained an interest in the 'Med-Chi' throughout his successful career as an army surgeon and 'watched its advancement and its success with the anxieties of a parent'.

Both societies were obliged to sell the bulk of their extensive libraries in the 1960s, but the demand for a student-led social and academic forum has ensured that both the RMS and the Med-Chi have survived over two centuries of change into the twenty-first century.

As the number of qualified practitioners increased, so medical societies sprang up in the cities and towns throughout the country as doctors felt the need for a forum where they could discuss cases and share experience. Not all of the societies were medical, political or scientific. 'Convivial' societies allowed doctors to socialise together, out of sight of their patients. The Aesculapians, a dining club established by Andrew Duncan in 1773 to cement relations between physicians and surgeons, thrives into the twenty-first century, as does the Harveian (founded 1782), which meets annually to commemorate the memory of William Harvey.

Specialist Interests Develop

The eighteenth century saw the emergence of physicians and surgeons developing a specialist interest, and the contribution of the Rae family to dentistry has been considered in the previous chapter. John Rae, William's younger brother, the first Fellow (as opposed to Master or Freeman) of the Royal College of Surgeons of Edinburgh, advertised in the *Edinburgh Advertiser* in 1784 that 'he continues to transplant teeth and to perform every other operation relative to natural teeth.' Dentists in the eighteenth century often practised as itinerants, moving, usually in a regular circuit, from town to town, their arrival advertised in the local press. These were not quacks, but usually able men who might continue such a practice for decades.

Midwifery had principally been the domain of the female midwife, but now doctors began to specialise in that branch of medicine, although not without the disapproval of some senior physicians, who considered it 'trade' and thus demeaning.

Eye surgery had seen 'specialists' in the form of the travelling couchers like the self-publicising oculist John 'Chevalier' Taylor (1703–72) who plied his trade throughout Europe. In Scotland, James Wardrop (1782–1869), surgical apprentice to Benjamin Bell, advanced knowledge of diseases of the eye by studying their pathology, particularly during his time as assistant to John Barclay at Surgeons' Hall Museum in Edinburgh. He recognised retinoblastoma as a malignant tumour, and recommended that it should be treated by removal of the eye. The operation of couching (dislocating) the lens for cataract had been performed for centuries, but Wardrop described, with great clarity, improvements in the technique of lens extrac-

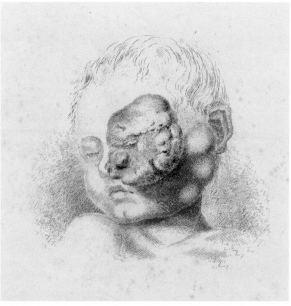

3.21 Illustration from *Observations on the Fungus Haematodes* by James Wardrop. This distressing picture depicts a child with what is now called retinoblastoma, a rare malignant tumour of childhood arising from the retina of the eye. In this case the tumour is advanced and the swellings behind the tumour suggest that it has already spread to lymph glands.

tion. His *Essays on the Morbid Anatomy of the Human Eye* contained a wealth of pathological description, including the first description of sympathetic ophthalmia, where injury to one eye can cause inflammation in the other, leading to blindness. Wardrop's friend John Wishart (1781–1834), in his probationary essay *Ophthalmia*, described the clinical and pathological features of various types of inflammation occurring in the eye. In 1822, with John Argyll Robertson (1798–1855), his apprentice, he founded the Edinburgh Eye Dispensary, the first specialist eye hospital in Scotland. When he retired, William Walker (1814–85) became surgeon to the Eye Dispensary, and in 1855 was the first surgeon appointed to the ophthalmic surgery department of the Royal Infirmary.

Like James Wardrop and John Wishart, William Mackenzie (1791–1868), a Glasgow physician, was inspired to a career interest in eye surgery by studying under the doyen of European eye surgery, Georg Josef Beer (1763–1821) of Vienna, who established ophthalmology as a scientific discipline. With George Moneta, Mackenzie founded the Glasgow Eye Infirmary in 1824, and was Glasgow University's first lecturer on diseases of the eye.

The moves toward increasing specialisation in hospital practice gained pace in the nineteenth century and progressively more so in the twentieth, when specialities further divided into sub-specialties.

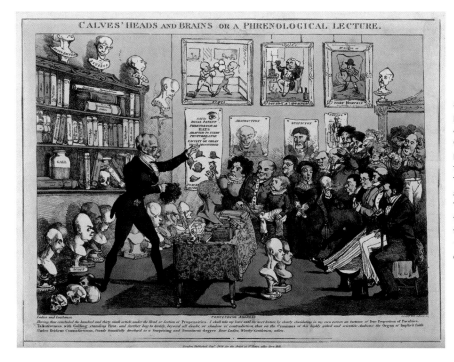

3.22 Calves' heads and brains or a phrenological lecture (L. Bump after J. Lump, 1826). This cartoon portrays George Combe, his head a mass of protuberances, lecturing on phrenology to an audience in his Edinburgh home. This satirical coloured lithograph is attributed to 'L. Bump, after J. Lump.' These names are presumed to be part of the satire and the print is thought to be the work of Henry Thomas Alken (1785–1851), a popular sporting illustrator and caricaturist (*Wellcome Library, London*).

ALTERNATIVE HEALERS

The medical establishment wished practitioners to be qualified, in order, it was argued, to maintain standards; and many of those who practised healing without such qualification were regarded by orthodoxy as quacks or mountebanks. Yet in the nineteenth century, many doctors advocated therapies which could be regarded as being on the fringes of mainstream medicine, because they seemed to have a quasi-scientific rationale – until they were found wanting. Phrenology and hydrotherapy are good examples.

Phrenology

The study of phrenology was espoused by some qualified doctors, and while it flourished in Edinburgh in the early nineteenth century, by the second half of the century it had come to be regarded as quackery. The Viennese physician Franz Joseph Gall (1758–1828) is regarded as the originator of the study of relating the size and shape of the skull to personal characteristics and brain function. His theories were popularised in Britain by Johann Spurzheim (1776–1832) who visited Edinburgh in 1815 to promote the theory and face up to the scathing criticism by the Surgeon Square anatomy lecturer John Gordon (1786–1818), which had been published in the influential *Edinburgh Review*. Spurzheim's impressive and persuasive lecture included a dissection of the brain. Among those he convinced were the brothers Andrew Combe (1797–1847) and George

Combe (1788–1858). Andrew, an Edinburgh physician, who studied with Spurzheim in Paris, and George, a lawyer, were to become the major advocates of the theory in Britain. In 1820, with others, they founded the Edinburgh Phrenological Society. Andrew wrote extensively on phrenology, making claims about its value in clinical practice which came to be regarded with increasing scepticism by medical orthodoxy. Latterly, in publications on mental illness and on physiology, he adopted a more mainstream approach, but it was his advocacy of phrenology that was to be his legacy. His brother George devoted himself to the promotion of the theory, in his textbook *A System of Phrenology*, in a series of essays and in his seminal work *The Constitution of Man* (1828). Claiming that phrenology was 'the greatest and most important discovery ever communicated to mankind', he developed the hypothesis that phrenology could predict character in individuals and determine their characteristics and moral code. His advocacy of moral retraining and discipline found a resonance in nineteenth-century society, not only in Britain, but also in Europe and America where *The Constitution of Man* became a bestseller. His theories influenced philosophers, educationalists, writers and politicians. By the end of his life, however, his theories had been denounced by the religious and medical establishments and even by factions within the phrenology movement.

Hydrotherapy

Hydrotherapy was to become fashionable in the late eighteenth and nineteenth centuries. One of its leading advocates was James Currie (1756–1805), who was born in Kirkpatrick Fleming, Dumfriesshire, and graduated MD from Glasgow University. As a physician in Liverpool he advocated cold sea-bathing for fevers. In *Medical Reports on the Effects of Water, Cold and Hot as a Remedy for Fever and Other Diseases* (1797), he claimed cures for techniques variously using hot or cold immersion with douches and copious drinks, claims supported by observations on the pulse rates and temperatures of febrile patients. His therapy was also promoted by influential practitioners like William Buchan and Andrew Duncan. In the late eighteenth and early nineteenth centuries, Scotland, like England and coastal Europe, enjoyed a boom in sea-water bathing to promote health, but Currie did not live to see the heyday of the water cure in the late nineteenth century. He is perhaps better known as the first biographer and editor of the works of the poet Robert Burns.

Healing wells which had been used for centuries were now subjected to chemical analysis and given medical endorsement, like Dr Taylor's *Medical Treatise on the Virtues of St Bernard's Well* (1790).

While spiritual healing wells were visited less often, spas like those at Moffat, Innerleithen and Strathpeffer became more popular, a trend which lasted until the early twentieth century. Typically a chemical analysis, still crude by later standards, would demonstrate the presence of iron or sulphur in the water (although the therapeutic benefits were still not understood), and a doctor would write a laudatory report. Many doctors were happy to act as medical promoters of spas, often because there was a pecuniary benefit for them. The water could usually be guaranteed to induce diarrhoea, vomiting or diuresis, which seemed to attest to its potency and contribute to its popularity. Yet even Strathpeffer, the most frequented Scottish spa, was never to enjoy anything like the popularity of those in England.

DISEASES

Diagnosis of disease improved throughout the period 1750–1850 largely as a result of the increasing emphasis on history-taking and accurate observation, and the recording and publishing of these. It is striking that even in the mid-nineteenth century the diseases which could be diagnosed in life and which were judged to have caused death were largely communicable diseases (tables 1 and 2), whose pattern in Scotland was similar to that seen in other European countries.

Some infectious diseases like smallpox and measles could be diagnosed relatively easily, but discriminating between febrile diseases, particularly those associated with diarrhoea, still taxed early-nineteenth-century physicians who lacked any form of corroborative test.

Fever

While fever remained a diagnosis as well as a symptom, it is now recognised that many cases described as fever were typhus. Fever was variously classified as miliary or intermitting (perhaps malaria), nervous, remitting or continuous. Bloodletting remained a mainstay of treatment, particularly for the 'continuous' form. Yet as knowledge increased, Buchan was able to differentiate the different forms of ague (malaria), although he still adhered to miasma theory, believing that it was caused by 'effluvia from putrid, stagnant water'. In an age when few effective medicines were available he considered the only reliable treatment to be Peruvian bark (from which quinine was isolated in 1820).

Communicable Diseases

Epidemic typhus was variously known as jail fever, hospital fever, ship fever, camp fever, war fever, famine fever, putrid fever, brain fever, bilious fever, spotted fever or petechial fever. The many descriptive terms describe both the locations in which it would commonly strike and some of the clinical features. For centuries epidemics had been common in crowded conditions and during times of privation and war, although it was to be the latter half of the nineteenth century before it could be clearly differentiated from typhoid. Because of its prevalence in over-

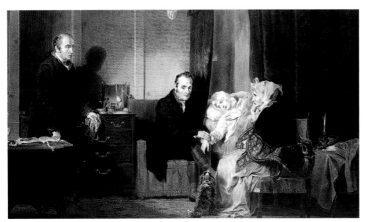

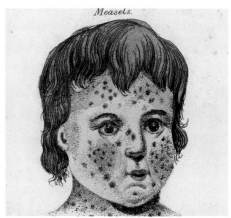

3.23 A bedridden, sick, young woman being examined by a doctor, accompanied by her anxious parents (engraving by F. Engleheart, after Sir David Wilkie, 1838). Wilkie, a minister's son from Fife, became one of the foremost British painters of his generation. Here, in a well-to-do household, he has captured the gloomy resignation of a doctor, evidently aware of the little he can do for his seriously ill young patient. The concern and anxiety of her parents seem to be shared even by the family dog (*Wellcome Library, London*).

3.24 Measles. The characteristic facial rash of measels [*sic*] as portrayed in Buchan's *Domestic Medicine*.

crowded army barracks and naval vessels, it was naval and military doctors who first took steps to try to reduce its spread (see pp. 144–146).

Measles epidemics were sporadic and mortality varied, increasing for example during periods of famine. Robert Watt's inquiry into child mortality reckoned that in Glasgow between 1803–13 measles accounted for some 15% of all child deaths. Measles epidemics with a high mortality spread throughout Scotland in 1808 and again in 1818.

A major epidemic which swept Scotland in 1758 was described by Robert Whytt as characterised by fever, coryza (nasal mucus), muscle pains and frequently complicated by pneumonia. From his description this was, almost certainly, influenza. Observing subsequent regular epidemics, James Gregory concluded that it was seasonal, episodic, probably infectious, and that some epidemics carried a higher mortality than others.

Epidemics of puerperal fever had been recognised for centuries, appearing in Graunt's Bills of Mortality for seventeenth-century London. It remained a common cause of maternal mortality in Scotland until the twentieth century. As described earlier, Alexander Gordon of Aberdeen played an important role in our understanding of its mode of transmission and prevention (see p. 102).

As the cholera pandemic of 1831 and 1832 spread east across Europe, local authorities in Britain were given some time to prepare means to combat it. Many local Boards of Health were set up in Scottish burghs well before the Privy Council established a Central Board of Health in London to coordinate prevention and treatment and

investigate outbreaks. The local boards tried to limit spread by methods which included the enforcing of quarantine and the cleaning and limewashing of passageways and houses thought to be at greatest risk (Fig. 3.25). Many boards, however, expressed their frustration at their lack of effective means to counter the outbreak. The first Scottish case was in Haddington, from where it spread throughout Scotland, sparing only the Highlands and Islands and a few fortunate lowland burghs like Linlithgow and Montrose. The industrialised towns and fishing ports were worst affected and, with about half of those who caught the disease dying from it, death rates increased towards seventeenth-century levels. Scotland accounted for some 10,000 of the 23,000 British deaths.

One notable event in this epidemic was the use of intravenous infusion as therapy for the first time. Thomas Latta (d. 1833), a Leith physician, put into practice the suggestion made by William O'Shaughnessy (1808–1889), a young Edinburgh medical graduate, that infusion into a vein of salt-containing fluid should be used to treat 'blue cholera' (the late stage of the illness where gross fluid loss through diarrhoea results in cold, clammy and blue extremities). Latta used a silver cannula to inject saline solution intravenously and, in a series of letters to the *Lancet*, gave a detailed account of his successes and failures, clearly describing the classical clinical features of the resolution of shock following fluid replacement. His colleague Dr Lewins prophetically wrote that 'this astonishing method of medication will lead to wondrous changes and improvements in the practice of medicine'.

CHOLERA.

The **BOARD** of **HEALTH** considering that **CHOLERA** has renewed its ravages in this Town and Neighbourhood, deem it to be their indispensable duty to urge upon all classes the necessity of strict attention to the directions formerly issued by the Board in regard to **CLEANLINESS**, **VENTILATION**, and **REGIMEN**.

The Board also request the Visitors to renew their inspection of the Lanes and Closes in their several districts, and to report every instance of inattention to Public Cleanliness, that the offenders may be proceeded against according to Law.

PAISLEY, 28th JUNE, 1832.   ALEX. GARDNER, PRINTER, PAISLEY.

3.25 Cholera poster. This poster, drawn up by the local Boards of Health, in this case for Paisley in 1832, recommend cleanliness, fresh air and sobriety to avoid the disease (*Renfrewshire Libraries*).

Yet it was to be almost 50 years before the technique was accepted into routine clinical practice.

A second epidemic spread from Leith in 1848 and resulted in over 6,000 deaths in Scotland over the next two years, fewer than in the earlier epidemic, and on this occasion relatively fewer than in England.

In the early years of the nineteenth century it is likely that tuberculosis was the single greatest killer in Western Europe, flourishing and spreading in the overcrowded, squalid conditions of the newly industrialised cities. Even allowing for the possibility of over-diagnosis, about a quarter of the Scottish population was affected by the disease. Manifestations of the disease which erupted onto the skin (scrofula or King's Evil) had long been recognised, and the advent of the stethoscope in the 1820s was to improve the diagnosis of the pulmonary manifestations. This condition was commonly described as phthisis or consumption, where wasting was a prominent feature.

HEALING

Medical Therapy Evolves

While ideas about the cause of disease abounded in the late eighteenth century, as we have seen earlier, this was not accompanied by equivalent advances in effective treatment. For all the grand theorising there was little in the way of practical benefit for the patient. Mathew Baillie summarised the paradox. 'I know better, perhaps than any other man, from my knowledge of anatomy how to discover disease but when I have done so I don't know better how to cure it.' In the busy medical market place, where a variety of healers could be consulted, the special contribution of the physician was advice about lifestyle, diet, fresh air, spas and sea bathing. Yet, even by the mid-nineteenth century, much of the medicine practised by doctors was of doubtful benefit to the patient, and some medication, such as mercury, was potentially dangerous. Infirmary records from Edinburgh and Glasgow record the regular use of cupping (usually with prior scarification) and leeching, which increasingly aimed to remove blood from as close as possible to the site of the perceived problem. The use of blistering and poultices was common, as was the use of cautery with a hot iron and galvanism, in which an electric current was applied to the skin, in the hope that this might induce a 'life force'. Other therapies, like copious bloodletting and violent purging, could be positively harmful and, despite the array of herbal remedies, it is now appreciated that there was little in the way of effective drug treatment. The fifth edition of the *Edinburgh Pharmacopoeia* (1756) was the first one to banish many medicines that had been previously included through 'superstition' or 'credulity' or 'established custom'. (Surprisingly, digitalis was also removed, reappearing later in the 1783 edition.)

Although Paracelsus had postulated a 'quinta essentia' (which boiled down to a specific cure for a specific illness), the first line of medical treatment in the eighteenth century and into the nineteenth was usually depletive, based either on *humoralism*, the idea of balancing the humours, or on *solidism*, the Cullenian and Brunonian concepts of regulating tone in the nervous system (pp. 96–99). The main depletives were bloodletting, emetics,

A Selection of Drugs from Domestic Medicine *1782*

A selection from the list of 'Simples' (drugs which were single preparations) in the 1782 edition of Buchan's *Domestic Medicine* (see p. 126) gives some insight into the therapeutic armamentarium of the Enlightenment period, and many of the names remain familiar in the twenty-first century.

Ipecacuana – a widely used emetic.

Castor oil, senna and Epsom salts – cathartics.

Antimony powerfully combined both these functions. (Antimony compounds subsequently found a role in the twentieth century in effectively treating the parasitic infection Leishmaniasis.)

Mercury – treatment of fevers, especially syphilis and gonorrhoea (although for the latter Buchan thought it seldom necessary, and Benjamin Bell thought it ineffective).

Hemlock, extract of poppies and gum opium – sedatives and analgesics.

Sal ammoniac and sal volatile – to treat hysteria or fainting.

Opiates and hemlock – cough suppressants.

Liquorice – expectorant.

Herbs include garlic, gentian, ginger, ginseng and St John's wort.

Peruvian bark – to treat fevers. (It was regarded as a 'tonic' and in the dose recommended the quinine it contained would have had little therapeutic effect.)

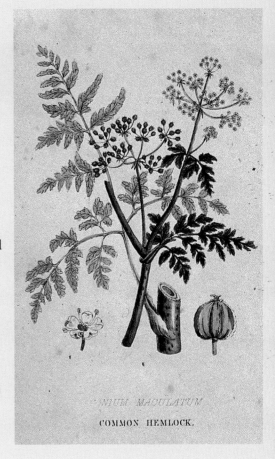

3.26 Hemlock (*Conium maculatum*) (coloured reproduction of a wood engraving by J. Johnstone). Hemlock has been recognized as a herbal medicine and as a poison for centuries. Buchan recommended it for 'hooping-cough', for scrophula and King's evil (tuberculosis) and as a poultice on the eye after cataract extraction. He is sceptical about its widely recommended use in cancer. (*Wellcome Library, London*).

CONIUM MACULATUM

COMMON HEMLOCK.

cathartics, narcotics, and diuretics. Solidism also required the use of stimulants or tonics, which included fresh air, meat, ale and wine. Camphor, musk and aether were among the most common drugs used as tonics. While Brown advocated opiates, especially laudanum, as stimulants, Buchan did not, advising caution in their use. Buchan had claimed good results using musk in such disparate conditions as epilepsy, nervous fever, hiccup and epilepsy. Aether (nitrous or sulphuric ether) was recommended as a useful 'bracer' in nervous asthma, and indeed diethyl ether was subsequently shown to be effective in reducing bronchospasm, the constriction of the airways occurring in asthma.

Cullen's *Treatise on Materia Medica* (1789) attempted to place therapeutics on a rational basis. In true Cullenian fashion the *materia medica* were systematically classified according to their action, i.e. as astringents, tonics, stimulants, sedatives, antispasmodics, emetics, cathartics, diuretics, antiseptics and diaphoretics (perspiration promoters). Yet this classification and the contents of the 1790 *Edinburgh Pharmacopoeia* clearly demonstrate that therapeutics was still firmly embedded in humoralism and solidism. But by the last decade of the eighteenth century a third major treatment concept began to emerge – chemical therapy – although it was to be more than half a century before the new understanding of chemistry was to be translated into everyday therapeutics.

The Edinburgh Pharmacopoeia and Dispensatories

By the mid-nineteenth century, therapeutics was still largely based on herbal remedies. Despite the progressive deletion from the *Edinburgh Pharmacopoeia* of agents originally included because of superstition or common usage, such preparations still formed the bulk of the reme-

Growing knowledge about the nature and composition of chemical agents was reflected in the pharmacopoeias and dispensatories. The 1819 edition of the *Edinburgh New Dispensatory* now listed elements including oxygen, chlorine, iodine, fluorine, nitrogen, hydrogen, carbon, sulphur and phosphorus. Knowledge of chemical reactions was also apparent by the use of terms like 'metallic oxides', 'alkanisable metals' and 'oxydisable metals'. By the 1842 edition there were chemical formulae and descriptions of chemical processes like distillation and percolation. Yet this increasing knowledge had not led to the introduction of new chemical agents by the mid-nineteenth century, and of over 2,000 preparations in the 1842 *Dispensatory*, few were subsequently found to be effective as intended.

Surgical Treatment before Antisepsis and Anaesthesia

In the late eighteenth century, routine treatment offered by surgeons was still largely confined to bloodletting and to surgery of superficial, visible problems such as minor skin lesions, abscesses, ulcers, burns and wounds, including gunshot wounds. Limb amputation, the immobilisation of fractures and the aspiration of hydrocoeles and pleural effusions all fell within the surgeon's domain. By the mid-nineteenth century, more major procedures had been added to the repertoire.

Charles Bell's *Illustrations of the Great Operations of Surgery* (1821) describes, with clear illustrations, ligation for aneurysm (ballooning of an artery) at various sites, repair of groin hernia, limb amputation, trepanning and cutting for bladder stone – previously the domain of the travelling lithotomist. In this pre-anaesthetic era some formidable procedures were successful, a tribute to the fortitude of the patient and the dexterity and anatomical knowledge of the surgeon. Excisions of the maxilla (upper jawbone) for huge facial tumours performed by Robert Liston and James Syme are good examples.

There are isolated examples before this period of abdominal operations where the patient survived. The surgical procedure which heralded the era of successful abdominal surgery was ovariotomy – the removal of large ovarian cysts. Ephraim McDowell (1771–1830), a surgical apprentice from Kentucky, went in 1793 to Edinburgh

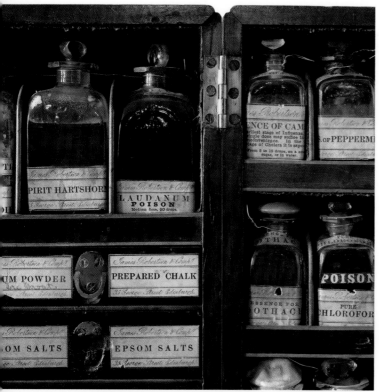

3.27 Domestic medicine chest, Georgian House, Edinburgh. In the heart of Edinburgh in the mid-nineteenth century, pharmacy was a mixture of traditional, herbal and a few chemical preparations. The chest contains laudanum, a tincture of opium, used for a wide variety of ailments including pain relief; Epsom salts was used for constipation and chalk for diarrhoea; spirit of hartshorn (prepared from powdered staghorn) was used as a smelling salt. As chloroform came into medicinal use as an anaesthetic agent after 1847, the preparations date from after that year (*National Trust for Scotland*).

dies in the 1841 edition. This was to prove the last edition before the merger with the pharmacopoeias of London and Dublin.

Yet the Edinburgh influence was continued by the *Dispensatories*, commentaries on the pharmacopoeias of Edinburgh, London and Dublin. The 1819 edition of the *Edinburgh New Dispensatory*, edited by Andrew Duncan junior, aimed to explain the 'language and principles of modern chemistry'. Despite this, even the 1842 edition, edited by Duncan's successor in the Edinburgh chair of Materia Medica, Robert Christison, still consisted mainly of herbal remedies and many remedies described as 'tonics'.

Peruvian bark had been widely used to treat fevers since the seventeenth century. Francis Home (1719–1813), the Professor of Materia Medica at Edinburgh University, carried out trials of bark on patients with intermittent fever in the Edinburgh Royal Infirmary, demonstrating that its efficacy could be improved by the timing of administration. The naval surgeon Robert Robertson (1742–1829), who graduated MD from Aberdeen University in 1779, showed that mortality could be reduced four-fold when fever was treated with bark. Yet, by the mid-nineteenth century, there were no cinchona trees in Europe, Africa, India or the Far East, and there were fears that the South American trees might become extinct through massive exploitation. The successful transfer of cinchona trees to India was largely accomplished by two Scottish botanists, William McIvor (c1820–76) and Robert Cross (1836–1911), working under the aegis of Sir Clements Markham. Sir William Osler described the introduction of cinchona into the eastern hemisphere as 'one of the greatest events in the history of medicine'.

Opium, derived from the poppy *Papaver somniferum*, had long been known to have narcotic properties, and had been advocated by such influential figures as Paracelsus and Thomas Sydenham. By the early eighteenth century it was widely used in Europe. What might be regarded as the first pharmacological research was carried out on it by Charles Alston (1683–1760), Professor of Botany and Materia Medica at Edinburgh University. In a series of experiments in which he administered opium to animals and to himself, he recorded many of its properties. He observed microscopically the slowing of capillary blood flow in frogs given the drug and the analgesic effect when the drug was given orally to humans. Robert Whytt and Alexander Monro *secundus* added further experimental observations. An Edinburgh medical graduate, William Gregory (1803–58), son of James Gregory, Professor of Physic at Edinburgh University (see Gregory family tree, p. 125), became Professor of Chemistry at the university, and in 1831 isolated pure morphine hydrochloride. John Macfarlan, an Edinburgh pharmacist who founded the pharmaceutical firm bearing his name, was a major supplier of laudanum, and seeing the potential of Gregory's work began commercial production of morphine.

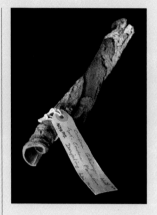
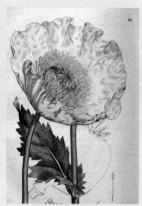
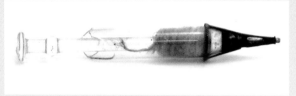

3.28 *Top left*. Cinchona bark prepared as a roll for ease of shipment. This specimen originated from a cinchona plantation in Darjeeling, India (*Science Museum, London*).

3.29 *Top right*. Opium poppy (*Papaver somniferum*) (print by M. A. Burnett after Gilbert T. Burnett, 1853). The principal source of all natural opiates (*Wellcome Library, London*).

3.30 *Above*. Syringe used by Dr Andrew Wood. The syringe was made by Daniel Fergusson, London. Wood was the first to use it for subcutaneous injection of morphine (*Royal College of Surgeons of Edinburgh*).

In 1853 the Edinburgh physician Alexander Wood (1817–84), first used a syringe to inject morphine subcutaneously, around a painful joint. He observed the beneficial local and systemic effects, and his publication led to its widespread use in clinical practice as a powerful analgesic.

The first successful attempt to correlate the chemical structure of salts of opium alkaloids with their biological activity was performed in Edinburgh in 1868 by Alexander Crum Brown and Thomas Fraser, later to be knighted for his contributions to pharmacology. At St Andrews University, the correct chemical structure of morphine was first established by John Masson Gulland and Robert Robinson, who was to win the Nobel Prize for chemistry for his work on plant products of biological importance, especially the alkaloids. Macfarlan Smith became major suppliers of the drug, and remain a world leader in the manufacture of opium alkaloids into the twenty-first century.

A Selection of Drugs from the 1842 Dispensatory, *edited by Professor Robert Christison*

Of over 2000 preparations listed, the following are amongst the small number which have subsequently been shown to produce the intended effect. The comments are from the original.

Belladonna – drops for ophthalmic surgery; antispasmodic for anal spasm

Bismuth – for dyspepsia

Cinchona bark – febrifuge; arrests ague

Colchicum – for gout

Digitalis – diuretic in dropsy especially those caused by heart disease

Ergota – stimulate labour pains; promote uterine contraction for retained placenta; overdose may cause gangrene of digits

Henbane – sedative

Iron preparations – a tonic. The iron of the blood is increased and the blood becomes 'florid'

Opium – multiple preparations

Salix (willow bark) – febrifuge

Strychnia – causes muscle twitching; used in paraplegia and hemiplegia

Tin preparations – anthelminthic effective against ascaris and lumbrici worms

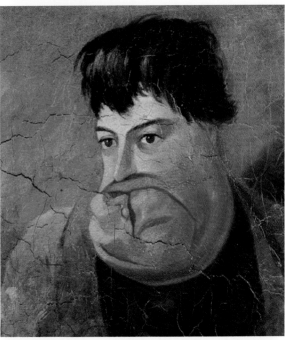

3.31 Robert Penman (painting, unknown artist, *c*1828. This portrait shows the large facial tumour which was excised by James Syme in 1828, without anaesthetic and in 24 minutes. This rapidly growing tumour of the lower jaw measured about 15 inches in circumference. The fact that it was successfully removed says much for the skill of the surgeon and the fortitude of the patient (*Royal College of Surgeons of Edinburgh*).

3.32 Robert Penman (photograph, *c*1855). This photograph was taken some 27 years after the procedure. Robert Penman survived the procedure, emigrated to the United States and was able to partly disguise his residual facial deformity with a beard. These two portraits were donated to the museum of the RCSEd by Syme's son-in-law, Joseph Lister (*Royal College of Surgeons of Edinburgh*).

1793, where he attended the lectures of John Bell, who is thought to have suggested how the operation might be performed. In 1809 McDowell performed the first successful ovariotomy, his patient surviving for 32 years. These and the other cases he reported effectively mark the start of abdominal surgery. McDowell wrote of this success to John Lizars in Edinburgh, who performed the first successful ovariotomy in Britain in 1823.

For patients, the pain associated with such procedures was intense, and at times barely tolerable. A harrowing and moving account of the courage shown by patients in the face of such pain is given in *Rab and His Friends,* a novel by Dr John Brown (1810–82), based on his experience working as a surgical dresser to James Syme in Minto

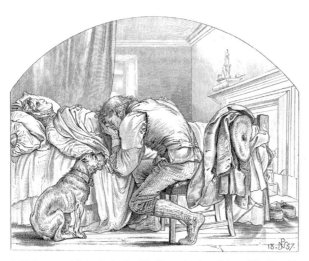

3.33 James and Rab grieving for Ailie (illustration from *Rab and His Friends*). After the operation Ailie dies from infection, and her husband James and dog Rab grieve at her bedside.

House Hospital in Edinburgh. Here the patient, Ailie, has a mastectomy without anaesthesia, watched by a group of students.

> The operating theatre is crowded; much talk and fun, and all the cordiality and stir of youth. The surgeon with his staff of assistants is there. In comes Ailie: one look at her quiets and abates the eager students. That beautiful old woman is too much for them; they sit down, and are dumb, and gaze at her . . . The operation was at once begun; it was necessarily slow; and chloroform – one of God's best gifts to his suffering children – was then unknown. The surgeon did his work. The pale face showed its pain, but was still and silent . . .
>
> It is over: she is dressed, steps gently and decently down from the table, looks for James; then, turning to the surgeon and the students, she courtesies, and in a low, clear voice begs their pardon if she has behaved ill. The students – all of us – wept like children.
>
> From *Rab and His Friends*, John Brown.

Anaesthesia and antisepsis, the great innovations which would allow surgery to become more humane, more successful and more complex, were yet to come.

'THE GREAT DOCTORS' – THE NEXT GENERATION

In this period a generation of remarkable doctors ensured that Scotland's contribution to medicine was, yet again, out of all proportion to the size of the country.

Surgeons

In the later years of the eighteenth century in Edinburgh, Benjamin Bell gained a worldwide reputation as a surgical writer; John Bell (no relation) became a leading surgical anatomist, while his younger brother, Charles Bell, was to make lasting contributions to surgery and physiology.

The early 1830s marked the beginning of a memorable era for Edinburgh surgery with the appointment of important figures to the three surgical chairs. In 1833, James Syme (1799–1870) was appointed to the University chair of Clinical Surgery in succession to James Russell. On the death of J. W. Turner in 1836, the College of Surgeons appointed John Lizars (1787–1860) to its chair of Surgery. In the same year Sir Charles Bell returned to Edinburgh from London to take up the University chair of Systematic Surgery.

Benjamin Bell (1749–1806) had emerged as an influential surgical thinker (see p. 99). His *System of Surgery* (1796) was widely read throughout the world, and his advocacy of the routine use of opium for the relief of post-operative pain did much to introduce this into surgical practice.

Despite his international reputation, he and his works were subjected to local ridicule by John Bell, another successful local surgeon. The school of anatomy, which John Bell set up in Surgeon Square in 1788, was an immediate success because of his emphasis on surgical anatomy, in contrast to the more theoretical approach of Monro *secundus*, a physician. Yet for all John Bell's brilliance as a teacher, his artistic gifts and his surgical skills have tended to be overshadowed by his perennial arguments with and criticism of other colleagues.

John Bell's younger brother, Charles Bell (1774–1842), showed artistic talent from an early age, a skill enhanced by tutoring from the painter David Allan (1744–96). Bell was to put these artistic gifts to great use throughout his

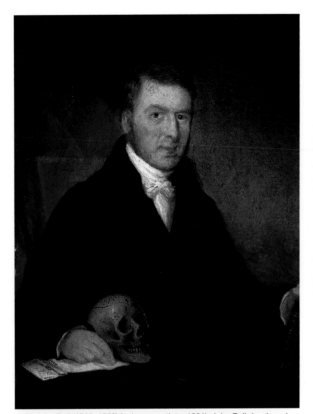

3.34 John Bell (1763–1820) (unknown artist, c1801). John Bell developed a large surgical practice in Edinburgh and his *Principles of Surgery* (3 volumes between 1801 and 1806) proved an influential textbook. Yet because of rivalry and jealousy, particularly involving James Gregory, the Professor of Physic at the University, he was excluded from the Royal Infirmary in 1800. Much of his career was dominated by bitter quarrels, conducted through pamphlet wars, and even derogatory remarks in his textbooks about his enemies, particularly Gregory and Benjamin Bell (*National Portrait Gallery, London*).

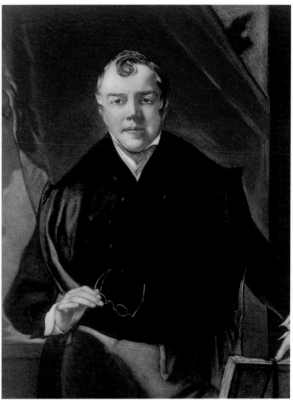

3.35 Sir Charles Bell (painting, John Stevens, c1821). Born in Fountain-bridge, Edinburgh, the son of a clergyman, Bell achieved success as a teacher, anatomist, physiologist, surgeon, author and artist. He developed his collection of anatomical and surgical specimens during his time in London and sold it to the Royal College of Surgeons of Edinburgh, where much of it remains on display. In addition to anatomy and pathology speci-mens showing disease, it includes skeletons showing bony abnormalities, wax and plaster models and his Corunna oil paintings (*National Portrait Gallery, London*).

life. While still a student at the Edinburgh medical school, he taught anatomy in his brother's anatomy school in Surgeon Square, and published his illustrated *System of Dissections* in 1798. Having failed to obtain the post of surgeon-in-ordinary to the Royal Infirmary, Bell moved to the Middlesex Hospital in London, and soon published *Anatomy of Expression*, another superbly illustrated classic of its kind. Having taught at the London College of Surgeons and the Hunterian Great Windmill Street School, Bell became professor at the new London Univer-sity Medical School and gave the inaugural address at its opening in 1828. Internal political conflict caused him to resign and return to Edinburgh to take up the University chair of Systematic Surgery in 1836. His discovery, brought to fruition by the French physiologist François Magendie, that the anterior nerve roots carried motor nerves and the dorsal ones sensory nerves, was his greatest contribution to physiology. Bell's other legacy is his art, notably his illus-

trations in his *Illustrations of the Great Operations of Surgery* (1824), his Corunna oil paintings and his Waterloo water-colours, the latter two depicting battle injuries in the Napoleonic Wars. The Corunna oils (Fig. 3.36) are on display in the Royal College of Surgeons of Edinburgh.

John Lizars (1787–1860) was surgical apprentice to John Bell, and after service as a naval surgeon, joined him in what was one of the most renowned surgical practices in Scotland. He taught anatomy and surgery at the extra–mural school, his classes enhanced by his beautifully illus-trated books on anatomy and surgery. *A System of Anatomical Plates of the Human Body* (1822–26) and *A System of Practical Surgery* (1838) were both superbly illus-trated by his brother William Lizars, regarded as one of the best engravers of his day. In marked contrast to Monro *tertius* in the University chair, Lizars was a gifted and popular teacher, who continued his surgical practice while teaching anatomy. An innovative surgeon, he performed

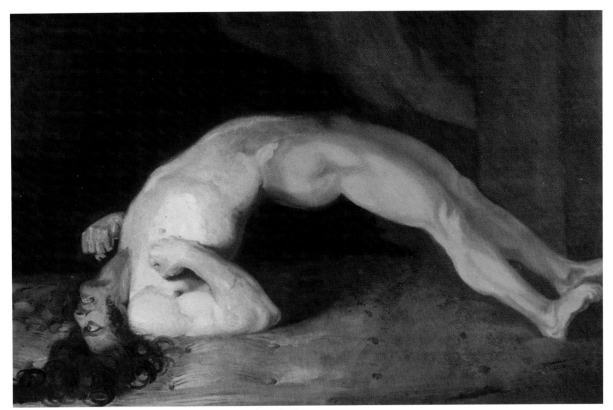

3.36 Opisthotonos (Charles Bell, 1809). This, perhaps the most dramatic of Bell's Corunna oils, shows the terrible effects of tetanus, a bacterial infection which results in muscle spasm, usually starting with mild spasm of the jaw muscles (lockjaw). Here, in the final agonal stages of the condition the large muscles of the back have gone into spasm, causing a grotesque arching of the spine. Bell's commentary indicates that the subject is a composite from three victims, and indeed the joins between these can be made out below the neck and at the waist (*Royal College of Surgeons of Edinburgh*).

the first ovariotomy in Britain, and was one of the first to ligate the innominate artery, a major vessel in the root of the neck, for aneurysm. In his appointment as professor of surgery at the College of Surgeons of Edinburgh in 1831, Lizars had defeated James Syme, and the latter harboured a continuing grudge, a source of bitter enmity between the two which eventually cost Lizars his career. As a result of pressure from Syme the college did not renew Lizar's professorship in 1838, and his practice progressively declined.

Robert Liston (1794–1847), a minister's son from West Lothian, learned anatomy as assistant to John Barclay in the extra-mural medical school. Here his uncompromising personality resulted in friction and the quarrels which were to characterise his professional life. After surgical training in Edinburgh Royal Infirmary and the London Hospital, he returned to teaching anatomy in the extra-mural school in competition to Barclay, having recruited a distant rela-

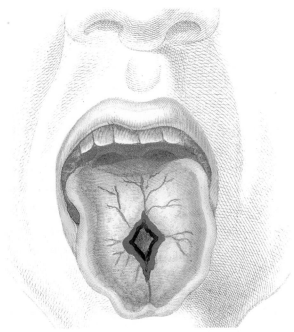

3.37 Malignant ulcer on the tongue (John Lizars, 1859). This ulcer was ascribed by Lizars to excessive use of tobacco. In 1859, the year before he died, Lizars published the eighth Edinburgh edition of *Practical Observations on the Uses and Abuses of Tobacco in* which he suggested that tobacco use might cause a number of health problems. With remarkable foresight he predicted that tobacco-induced 'injury to the constitution of the young may not appear immediately, but cannot fail ultimately to become a great national calamity'. The book continued to be published well after his death (*Royal College of Surgeons of Edinburgh*).

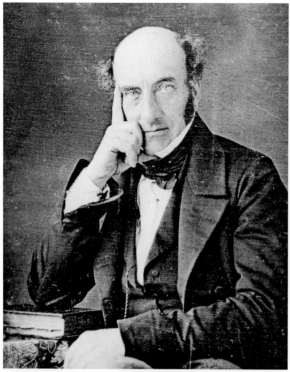

3.38 Robert Liston (calotype, David Octavius Hill and Robert Adamson, c1847). A portrait taken before 1847 by the Edinburgh photographic pioneers David Octavius Hill and Robert Adamson. It may have been taken in their studio in Rock House, Carlton Hill, Edinburgh, where calotype photography flourished from 1843, free of Fox Talbot's patent of the process which applied only in England (*Wellcome Library, London*).

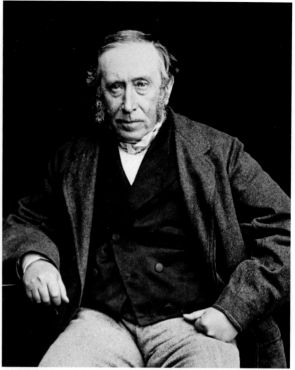

3.39 James Syme (albumen print, John Adamson c1855). This studio portrait was taken by John Adamson when Syme was at the height of his fame. It probably dates from 1855, the year before his daughter Agnes married Joseph Lister (*Scottish National Portrait Gallery*).

tive, the young James Syme, as his partner. At first the two were close colleagues in surgical partnership, assisting at each other's operations. Liston's time as a surgeon in the Royal Infirmary was a turbulent one, marked both by the brilliance, boldness and success of his surgery and by expulsion from the staff for constant quarrelling. He quarrelled even with Syme, and when the latter was preferred as professor of surgery in the University, Liston moved to London where he became professor of clinical surgery at London University (University College). Liston's legacy was as a skilled, dextrous, innovative technical surgeon.

While a medical student at Edinburgh, James Syme (1799–1870) published an account of waterproofing cloth using a rubber solution, but the idea was patented by Charles Macintosh who thus achieved eponymous fame. After his partnership with Liston, first as anatomy teachers and then in surgical practice, had ended through professional jealousies, Syme established himself as a successful surgeon in his own private hospital, Minto House. In the pre-anaesthetic era, he successfully performed surgical operations which required courage, precise anatomical knowledge and dexterity on the part of the surgeon, and

courage and forbearance on the part of the patient. Foremost among these procedures were major excisions for tumours of the face (Figs. 3.31–32) and the tongue, and amputation through the hip joint. Yet for all that he was a conservative, and not particularly fast surgeon, who, according to one of his apprentices Alexander Peddie, 'never unnecessarily wasted a word, a drop of ink or of blood'. As professor of clinical surgery at Edinburgh University he established a reputation as a leading surgical teacher, a reputation which attracted young surgeons, like Joseph Lister, to Edinburgh. Antiseptic practice and anaesthesia were introduced during his tenure of the chair, and it is a mark of his vision that he embraced both.

Physicians

Scottish physicians of the period made contributions which were directly to benefit patients everywhere. Foremost among these were Andrew Duncan, James Gregory, Francis Home and William Buchan (Fig. 3.80).

Andrew Duncan senior (1744–1828) was to become one of the most important medical reformers and innovators of his day, a position he attained without the family

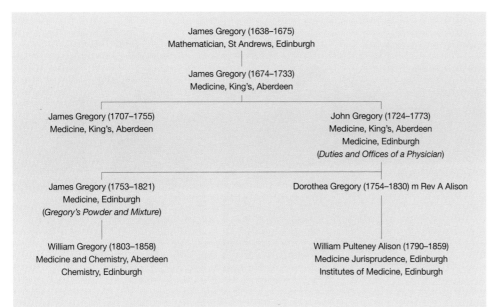

3.40 Gregory family tree. While the progenitor, James Gregory, was a mathematician, his descendants held chairs of Medicine in the Universities of Aberdeen and Edinburgh over four generations.

wealth or patronage enjoyed by most of his medical contemporaries. As a medical student at Edinburgh he befriended great figures of the Enlightenment like David Hume, Adam Smith and William Robertson, and his career was furthered by presidency of the Royal Medical Society, an office which he held for an unprecedented six times. Duncan was instrumental in obtaining the Society's Royal Charter (which remains the only one held by a medical undergraduate society), and in establishing a hall in Surgeon Square in which the society could meet (Fig. 3.49). Disappointed at his failure to be appointed to the chair of the Institutes of Medicine, but with his ambition undiminished, he delivered a successful lecture course in the extra-mural school and founded *Medical and Philosophical Commentaries,* essentially the first English-language medical journal in the world, a quarterly which printed 1000 copies simultaneously in London, Dublin and Edinburgh. By the end of the decade it was read in France, Denmark, Russia and America.

Duncan demonstrated his concern for the welfare of the poor by inviting the sick poor to attend his lectures, which, although primarily for student instruction, 'will be also the means of furnishing the indigent with advice and medicines gratis, when subjected to chronical diseases.' The Royal Infirmary did not offer outpatient facilities, so Duncan raised the funds to open the first public dispensary in Edinburgh in Richmond Street.

His innovation continued with his proposal for the lunatic asylum, his ideas on medical policy, the foundation of the Gymnastic Society and the Aesculapians, all of which are described later. Duncan, originally regarded as an outsider by the medical establishment, became a pillar of that establishment with his election as President of the Royal College of Physicians of Edinburgh, and appointments as Professor of the Institutes of Medicine and as Physician to the King in Scotland.

James Gregory (1753–1821) was fortunate in being well prepared by his father John (see p. 103) for a career in medicine. Educated at Aberdeen, Edinburgh, Oxford, Paris and Leiden, he was appointed professor of the Institutes of Medicine at Edinburgh University in succession to William Cullen in 1776. His textbook of medicine, *Conspectus Medicinae Theoreticae*, became a standard work and he was an outstanding lecturer. Yet much of his time and energy was taken up with vitriolic and sarcastic attacks on colleagues, both verbal and in the form of pamphlets. His physical assault on James Hamilton, professor of midwifery, resulted in a fine, and he was expelled by the College of Physicians for publicly divulging their proceedings. Gregory's powder, a mixture which included rhubarb, ginger and magnesium oxide, became a popular cathartic and antacid in the nineteenth century and remained in use well into the twentieth.

Francis Home (1719–1813) was a polymath who embodied the spirit of the Enlightenment with observation and experiment, not only in medicine but in chemistry and agriculture.

He was apprenticed to John Rattray (the Edinburgh surgeon who signed the first rules of golf in 1744 and survived service as surgeon to the Jacobite army from the

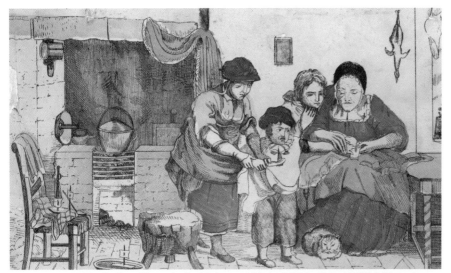

3.41 'The Cut Finger' (engraving by Joly from an original painting by Sir David Wilkie). Many minor ailments (and some not so minor) would be treated by a mother or grandmother with their own experience and knowledge, often supplemented by reference to Buchan's *Domestic Medicine* (*Wellcome Library, London*).

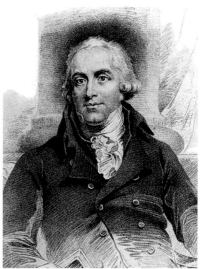

3.42 William Buchan (1729–1805) (unknown artist). Buchan was born in Roxburghshire and studied medicine in Edinburgh under Rutherford, Whytt and Cullen, graduating MD in 1761. After practice in England he returned to Edinburgh, where he was an unsuccessful candidate for the chair of the Institutes of Medicine vacated by the death of John Gregory (*Wellcome Library, London*).

battle of Prestonpans to Culloden). After medical studies in Edinburgh and Leiden Universities and military service, Home became a physician in Edinburgh where he suggested the possibility of inoculation against measles. 'I should do no small service to mankind,' he wrote in 1759, 'if I could render this disease more mild and safe in the same way as the Turks have taught us to mitigate the small-pox.' Taking blood from the vicinity of the spots of the most febrile patients, he inoculated other children, concluding that it resulted in milder cases of the illness. His detailed description of the laryngeal oedema or swelling in diphtheria in *A Treatise on Croup* (1765) included a recommendation that tracheostomy should be used when the condition threatened life. His writing introduced the word 'croup' into medicine.

Home's textbook *Principia Medicinae* (1758), which was popular for decades in Britain, Europe and America, was first published in Latin and subsequently in English and several European language editions. His interest in chemistry led him to publish recommendations, based on experiment, that bleachers should use specified chemicals and that farmers should add chemical nutrients like potassium nitrate to the soil. In 1768 Home became the first professor of Materia Medica in the University of Edinburgh, a position in which, in the nepotistic way of eigh-

teenth-century Edinburgh medicine, he was succeeded by his son.

For many Scots, who could not afford the luxury of a qualified practitioner or even an unqualified one, medical treatment was delivered in the home, often by a female family member or a local 'wise woman' (Fig. 3.41).

Medical texts aimed at the lay public had been available from the sixteenth century, but in the late eighteenth century the movement toward self-help in medicine, combined with the boom in printing, saw their numbers increase substantially. *Avis au Peuple sur Sa Santé* by the French physician Samuel Tissot (1728–97) had proved popular in France but a poor translation into English had hindered its dissemination. It was, however, to inspire a Scottish doctor motivated by the same ideals as Tissot to write a similar book. *Domestic Medicine or a Treatise on the Prevention and Cure of Diseases by Regimen and Simple Medicines* by William Buchan, first published in 1769, was based on *Avis au peuple* but was to prove one of the most widely read medical books for the laity ever written.

Buchan was a populist who regarded the medical profession as monopolistic. Through *Domestic Medicine* he wished to demystify medicine and to remove, as he put it 'the veil of mystery, which still hangs over Medicine.' His wish to give lay people the knowledge and means to

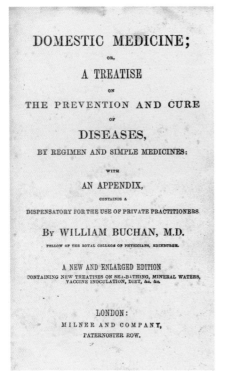

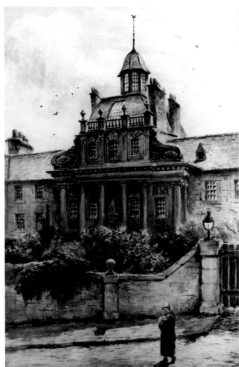

3.43 *Far left*. Frontispiece of *Domestic Medicine* by William Buchan. *Domestic Medicine* enjoyed a lasting and worldwide popularity, running to no fewer than 142 English language editions alone between 1769 and the final American edition in 1913. It was also translated into French, German, Italian, Portuguese, Russian, Swedish and Spanish (*Wellcome Library, London*).

3.44 *Left*. Edinburgh Royal Infirmary 1741–1889 (print of watercolour painting by J. Sanderson, 1885). This, the second Edinburgh Infirmary, was designed by William Adam. It was funded by organisations and individuals from all over Scotland, and indeed by the Scottish diaspora throughout the Empire. The building is an imposing one, with Doric columns and ornate masonry. In the foreground a woman and child in arms are perhaps hoping to be admitted to the Infirmary. If treated she would be expected to show her gratitude for the charity of the founders and supporters (*Lothian Health Services Archive*).

diagnose and treat their own illnesses proved hugely popular with increasingly literate populations. The emphasis which he placed on simple remedies and the health benefits of improved lifestyle – better diet, temperance and improved hygiene proved both popular and influential. He set out basic rules of hygiene – hand washing when dealing with patients, frequent change of linen in the sick bed and keeping rooms well ventilated. This populist and philanthropic approach incurred the wrath of fellow doctors which he shrugged off, writing in the foreword to the second edition that neither 'interest, nor prejudice, [would] ever deter him [Buchan] from exerting his best endeavours to render the Medical art more extensively beneficial to mankind.'

Domestic Medicine was still being used in Scotland in the mid 1920s, a reflection of its popularity, its lasting authority and the inability of many poor people to pay for treatment by doctors.

The concept of self-help was further stimulated by the Edinburgh medical graduate Samuel Smiles (1812–1904) whose book '*Self-Help*' (1859) sold a quarter of a million copies, was translated into fourteen languages and was the basis of some of the political philosophy of the British Conservative governments of the late twentieth century.

ORGANISATION OF HEALTH CARE

The early eighteenth century had witnessed the establishment of infirmaries in Scotland, part of the voluntary hospital movement which developed rapidly throughout Britain and Ireland. These infirmaries were financed by public subscription, the subscribers motivated, on the surface at least, by philanthropic ideals. As explained in the previous chapter, these voluntary hospitals became important by attracting celebrated physicians and surgeons to work, but also to teach, in them. The students contributed their services free, gained experience 'walking the wards' and, with the clerks and residents, helped to make the observations and write the casenotes and records which generated much of the knowledge contributed by these hospitals.

Glasgow Royal Infirmary (Fig 3.3), designed by Robert and James Adam, was built at the head of the medieval High Street next to Glasgow Cathedral and opened in 1794. Initially it housed 136 patients, which increased to 208 when an extension was added in 1815. A separate 220-bed Fever House was added in 1828–34.

Aberdeen Infirmary at Woolmanhill (opened 1742) appointed James Gordon as first physician to visit daily and to keep 'proper books on the Edinburgh plan'. Here too, continued expansion was required to meet increasing demand. By the turn of the nineteenth century, infirmaries had been opened in Dumfries (1776), Montrose (1782) and Dundee (1798), and more followed in the early years of the century.

Dispensaries

Inspired by the success of the Aldersgate Dispensary in London, Andrew Duncan senior opened the Edinburgh Public Dispensary in 1776 in West Richmond Street. This provided advice and medicines to the sick poor, the doctors providing their services free and the students, who attended to learn, paying towards the cost of this practical education. The enterprise was largely funded by charitable donations, and its success was endorsed by the award of a Royal Charter in 1818, when it became the Royal Public and Vaccine Dispensary. Vaccination, obstetric care and domiciliary visits were usually provided by Scottish dispensaries.

Dispensaries were often promoted by local philanthropists, as was the case in Kelso, where the dispensary founded by the Earl of Haddington in 1777 was free by letter, and in Montrose where the dispensary was part of the hospital and asylum established by Susan Carnegie.

In Aberdeen the Public Dispensary founded in 1781 was staffed by Alexander Gordon, whose pioneering work on puerperal fever was centred here and is described earlier (see p. 102). The early years of the nineteenth century saw the development of insurance schemes, but few dispensaries in Scotland attempted a contributory scheme. One which did was the provident scheme adopted by the Perth dispensary in 1834, but this proved to be a failure, and charitable status resumed until the opening of Perth Royal Infirmary in 1838.

In 1815 the New Town Dispensary of Edinburgh was founded, one of many established in the city. In Glasgow the life of the public dispensaries tended to be short, like the Glasgow Dispensary (1801–15) and the Celtic Dispensary (1837–47). By contrast the dispensary work of the Medical Missionary Societies in Edinburgh (established 1841) and Glasgow (established 1867) continued into the twentieth century.

MEDICAL EDUCATION

As emphasised in the previous chapter, education had been a prominent feature of Scottish life from the sixteenth century, when King James IV required the sons of landowners to learn Latin, and John Knox and the Reformers codified in the *Books of Discipline* their ambition to found a school in every parish. The establishment of five universities by the mid-sixteenth century meant that Scotland was well placed to promote medical education within these universities. This position was further enhanced by the presence of two medical royal colleges in Edinburgh and the Faculty of Physicians and Surgeons in Glasgow. From the mid-eighteenth century, medical training was based on a free trade principle with students electing to study at one or more centres and perhaps presenting themselves for examination at yet another, but with many choosing the cheaper option of not graduating at all. Some Scottish medical degrees went through a phase when their award was abused, but by the late nineteenth century, over 95% of British medical graduates had graduated from a Scottish university. This virtual monopoly of medical graduates was in part the result of the policies of the Universities of Oxford and Cambridge, whose long medical courses, even in the late eighteenth century, offered 'no patients and no clinical lectures' and who restricted admission to members of the established church. While medical apprenticeships were available throughout England, it was not until the foundation of the medical school at University College, London in 1828 that the number of medical graduates from England began to increase.

Edinburgh University and Extra-Mural Schools

The founding of the Edinburgh Medical School in 1726 had provided, for the first time in Britain, a system of university-based teaching linked to a teaching hospital, the students submitting and defending a thesis before graduating MD. The century from 1750 was to see the Edinburgh Medical School become one of the most successful in the English-speaking world, its graduates practising in the armed forces and in cities, towns and villages throughout Britain and the Empire. Edinburgh

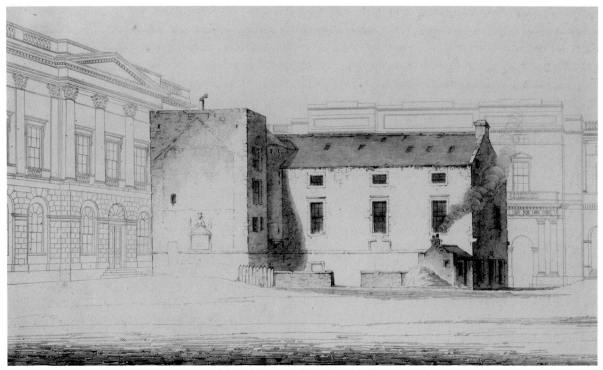

3.45 Edinburgh University Old Quadrangle by William Playfair (etching by W. H. Lizars, 1823). This view, looking east, shows the elegant new Adam/Playfair building in the background, contrasting with the 1617 building in the centre, which housed the University Library behind the three large windows on the first floor. The Anatomy department, where Professors Monro primus and secundus taught, had previously occupied the lower floor. This building was demolished and anatomy teaching moved into the north-west corner of the new building (*National Museum of Scotland*).

had widespread appeal to aspiring doctors for a number of reasons. There were no religious barriers, the teaching was largely in English and both teaching and accommodation were less expensive than in London. Indeed in the latter half of the eighteenth century there were more English and Irish graduates than Scots, who barely outnumbered the students from the Americas. In 1790 over 500 students matriculated in medicine at the university and a similar number were 'auditors', who attended lectures without intending to graduate from Edinburgh University. The remarkable rate of growth of the medical school can be gauged by the progressive increase in size of the anatomy classes from 83 in 1730 to 158 in 1750 to over 436 by 1783.

Anatomy Teaching in Edinburgh

This flourishing of anatomy teaching while Alexander Monro *secundus* occupied the chair of anatomy between 1756 and 1804 was due in no small part to his intellect and ability to teach. Monro *secundus* had been educated with the intention that he would succeed his father to the chair.

He was appointed joint professor with his father while only 21 years old. The tribute from his American pupil Benjamin Rush was typical. 'In anatomy he is superior perhaps to most men in Europe. He is a gentleman of great politeness and humanity and much admired by everyone who knows him.' From a twentieth-century perspective Comrie thought that his achievements were greater than those of his father. 'The second Monro showed himself the greater man, both as a teacher and investigator. Among more brilliant colleagues than those with whom his father had to compete, he maintained an easy equality and was the acknowledged head of the developing medical school.' The genius of the Monro dynasty finally faltered, however, with Alexander Monro *tertius*, who succeeded his father to the anatomy chair in 1804. Monro *tertius*, old-fashioned and unpopular with students, made 'his lectures on human anatomy as dull as he was himself', according to Charles Darwin, who attended his lectures between 1825 and 1827. A rival anatomy teacher, the surgeon John Bell, described other deficiencies in Monro's teaching. 'Not three subjects are

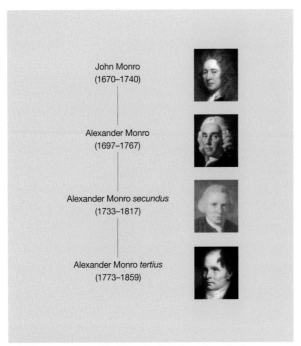

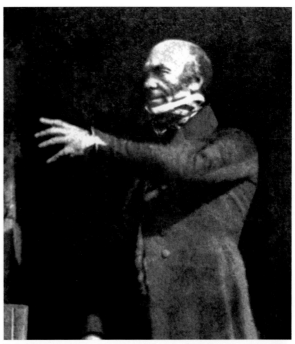

3.46 Four generations of the Monro family. Between them the three Alexanders Monro held the chair of anatomy at the University of Edinburgh for 126 years (*Royal College of Surgeons of Edinburgh*).

John Monro
(1670–1740)

Alexander Monro
(1697–1767)

Alexander Monro *secundus*
(1733–1817)

Alexander Monro *tertius*
(1773–1859)

3.47 Robert Knox (from an original calotype by David Octavius Hill (*c*1843)). This portrait with Knox posed as though lecturing was taken at Hill's Rock House studio, Calton Hill, Edinburgh (*Wellcome Library, London*).

dissected in a year. On the remains of a subject fished up from a tub of spirits are demonstrated those delicate arteries and nerves which are to be avoided or divided in our patients; and these are demonstrated once at a distance of 100 feet.' Monro's unpopularity resulted in students moving, in increasing numbers, to anatomy lectures in the extra-mural schools.

John Bell seized the opportunity and built an anatomy school in Surgeon Square, where he taught until 1799. While the Monros *secundus* and *tertius* were physicians, Bell was a surgeon, perhaps the foremost in Scotland of his day, and was able to relate anatomy teaching to surgical practice. His book *Anatomy of the Bones, Muscles and Joints* (1794), written as a student teaching aid, was a beautifully illustrated volume and was to form the basis for the magnificent anatomical texts that he was to produce with his younger brother Charles. Charles Bell had begun to assist his brother in dissection and lecturing in Surgeon Square in 1794 and, by 1804 when he departed for London to teach at the Great Windmill Street anatomy school, he had become an accomplished lecturer.

In that year John Barclay's anatomy lectures were recognised by the College of Surgeons, and his classes too grew in size. Barclay had set up a school of anatomy in 1800 in his house in 10 Surgeon Square. By devoting

himself to anatomy teaching, research and the collection of anatomy specimens, he was able to attract up to 300 students to his classes. His anatomical collection was donated (while that of Charles Bell was sold) to the museum of the Royal College of Surgeons of Edinburgh.

After Barclay's death in 1826, his anatomy teaching was taken on by Robert Knox, whose anatomy classes became the largest to date, exceeding 500 students in some years, making them almost certainly the largest anatomy classes ever taught in Britain. This increase exacerbated the problem of the shortage of bodies for dissection. When one of the victims of the Burke and Hare murders was identified in Knox's dissecting room, Knox was caught up in the public outrage which followed. This association with the Burke and Hare scandal saw his student numbers decline, and he stopped teaching at Surgeon Square in 1833. The new Surgeons' Hall was opened in 1832, but the original Surgeons' Hall was retained for teaching, and Knox continued to teach there and then at the Argyle Square School of Medicine, but without the success or popularity he had previously enjoyed.

Public outrage at grave robbing, and now murder, to obtain bodies for dissection led to the Anatomy Act (1832), which allowed the bodies of the unclaimed poor to be used for this purpose (see also p. 150).

Teaching of Surgery in Edinburgh

Surgical teaching in Edinburgh University had been included in the anatomy course by Monro *primus* and his son *secundus*, despite the fact that *secundus* was a physician whose knowledge of surgery was theoretical rather than practical. James Rae (1716–91), a local surgeon, began in 1769 to give lectures on surgery at Surgeons' Hall with the support of the Incorporation of Surgeons, which was 'desirous to promote . . . the advancement of the knowledge of surgery'. His course included 'practical discourses' on surgical cases in the Royal Infirmary. The success of this venture prompted the Surgeons to propose that a chair of surgery be established in the University. This was blocked by Monro *secundus*, who successfully petitioned the Town Council in 1777 to be styled 'Professor of Medicine, Anatomy and Surgery'. Such was the influence of the Monro dynasty that a physician, without surgical experience, was the University's professor of surgery. The anomaly was perpetuated when Monro *tertius*, also a physician, succeeded to his father's chair. It was not until 1803 that the University founded a Regius Chair of Clinical Surgery, spurred by Monro's unpopularity. This demise in the Monro influence prompted the Royal College of Surgeons (as it had now become) to establish in 1804 its own chair of surgery to which John Thomson (1765–1846) was appointed. Thomson also practised as a physician, and was involved with others in the founding of the New Town Dispensary. His lectures on ophthalmology paved the way for the opening of the first eye dispensary in Edinburgh in 1822. Thomson remained College professor, and from 1806 occupied in addition the University Chair of Military Surgery. When Thomson resigned from the college chair in 1821 he was succeeded by J. W. Turner (1790–1836). Dogged by chronic ill health, Turner proved to be 'a most uninteresting lecturer, a timid shy man who could not look his class in the face.' Yet after such a modest start, surgical teaching in Edinburgh was about to embark on a period of remarkable success.

Teaching of Physic (Medicine) in Edinburgh

The founding of the medical school had gained Edinburgh a reputation for medical teaching which increasingly attracted teachers and students from all over Britain

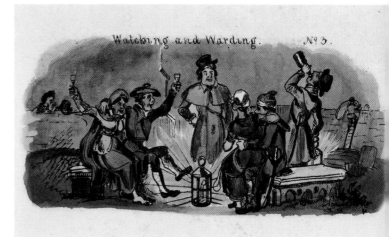

3.48 Watching and warding (*Northern Looking Glass*, August 1825). Graveyards would be guarded against resurrectionists by groups of relatives or concerned citizens. Here those on watch have enlivened their cold, lonely vigil by drinking and merrymaking, enabling the graverobbers in the background to escape with a body in a sack (*University of Glasgow*).

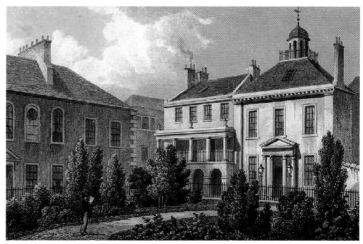

3.49 Surgeon Square (Thomas Shepherd, *c*1829). This painting shows the south west corner of Surgeon Square. The building on the left is the 1697 Surgeons' Hall (still in use by Edinburgh University in the twenty-first century). Next to it and set back is No 9, where John Gordon and then John Thomson taught anatomy, while No 10, with the colonnaded balcony, was used for medical teaching by Andrew Duncan senior and for anatomy teaching by John Barclay and then Robert Knox. The Royal Medical Society Hall, number 11, is on the right (*Royal College of Surgeons of Edinburgh*).

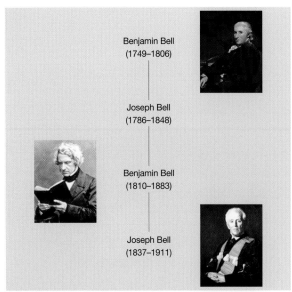

3.50 Bell family tree. Four generations of the Bell family produced presidents of the Royal College of Surgeons of Edinburgh. While some regarded this as a gifted family, from others it drew accusations of nepotism. (*Royal College of Surgeons of Edinburgh*).

and later from around the Empire. In the latter half of the eighteenth-century Enlightenment Edinburgh provided a rich milieu in which new medical ideas flourished.

The appointment by the University of Edinburgh of John Gregory (1724–73) as Professor of the Practice of Medicine in 1766 and that of William Cullen (1710–1790) as Professor of the Theory of Medicine two years later placed two of the most influential physicians of their day at the heart of Edinburgh medicine. In his lectures and writing Gregory promoted concepts of a doctor-patient relationship which were to form the foundation of modern medical ethics (see p. 103). Cullen taught that medicine must be based on a coherent, unified 'system' into which all observations about the patient and his illness must fit. With his roots in chemistry and in experiment, Cullen had no time for the empiricism which had dominated conventional medical thought. Perhaps influenced by his friend David Hume, he emphasised scepticism, and his concept of 'sceptical dogmatism' was to become one of the hallmarks of Scottish medical education, discernible well into the twentieth century. His nosology, or disease classification, was published in American and British editions as late as 1823, yet by then was largely discredited. His theory of nervous energy as the cause of disease barely survived after his death. Yet his consultation practice, both personal and postal, was immense.

Patronage and Privilege

Patronage had been a prominent feature of mainstream medicine for centuries. The appointment to chairs in Scottish universities involved a system governed by patronage and mired in corruption. Henry Dundas (later Viscount Melville), the Lord Advocate, was a shrewd and effective political operator, who controlled many professorial appointments. Nepotism too was endemic in appointments – witness the Monro dynasty. The Gregory family too filled chairs of medicine in Aberdeen and Edinburgh over four generations (see p. 125).

Benjamin Bell ensured that his son Joseph inherited his appointments as surgeon to George Watson's Hospital; in turn this passed to his other son George, and to his grandson Benjamin and to his great grandson Joseph. These Bells, spanning four generations, were all presidents of the Edinburgh College of Surgeons. In this climate it was all the more difficult for anyone from humble origins (the 'lad o'pairts'), to obtain the most sought-after appointments. Some who did were John Brown (see p. 98), John Thomson (see p. 131) and Andrew Duncan (see p. 124).

Medical Teaching in Glasgow

The origins of the medical school date from 1704, with the appointment of John Marshall, botanist and surgeon of Glasgow, as keeper of the physic garden. The establishment of chairs of medicine (1713) and anatomy (1720) allowed the University to start examining for the degree of MD, although at this stage there appeared to be little in the way of systematic teaching.

In the eighteenth century the city of Glasgow flourished, the population increased and the city's merchants grew wealthy through a flourishing sea trade in tobacco, linen and sugar. This sea trade also brought interchange of ideas with Europe, and, as Enlightenment values combined with the Scottish hunger for education and acceptance of new ideas, the West of Scotland was to produce three medical figures of world importance – John and William Hunter and William Cullen. While the Hunter brothers made their careers in London, Cullen began a tradition of excellence in chemistry research and teaching in Glasgow.

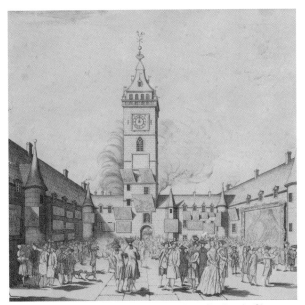

3.51 Foulis Academy of Arts exhibition, 1761. Inner Quadrangle, Glasgow University (from engraving by David Allan). The Inner Quadrangle of the Old College of the University of Glasgow, sited on the High Street, was completed by 1661. Robert Foulis established his bookshop here in 1741. The Foulis Academy of Arts exhibition depicted in this engraving was held to mark the coronation of King George III in 1761. Teaching took place here until the University moved to a new campus at Gilmorehill in the west end of the city (*University of Glasgow*).

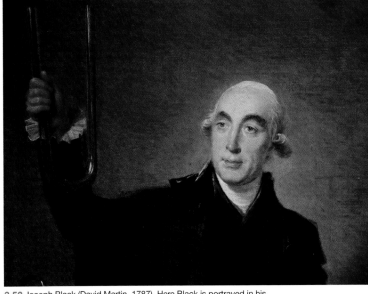

3.52 Joseph Black (David Martin, 1787). Here Black is portrayed in his laboratory, holding up a piece of laboratory glassware, probably used in his experiments on heat. Black graduated MD from Edinburgh University in 1754, with a thesis describing the formation of a gas produced by heating magnesia alba, the first chemical identification of a gas, which he called fixed air, now recognised as carbon dioxide. He succeeded William Cullen in the chair of the Practice of Medicine at Glasgow University (*Royal Medical Society and National Galleries of Scotland*).

Although there had been medical chairs in Glasgow University since 1713, William Cullen's lecture course which began in 1746 effectively marked the start of systematic teaching. His lectures at first were on physic, botany and material medica, but it was chemistry that was to become his main scientific interest during his time in Glasgow, and here began his research on heat, although his legacy was as a teacher rather than researcher. The University provided a laboratory, and Cullen's flair for teaching involving practical demonstration and experiment made his lectures famous throughout Britain. By the time he left for Edinburgh in 1755, Cullen had established and popularised medical teaching in Glasgow.

One student attracted to his teaching was Joseph Black, later to become a friend and colleague. In his Glasgow laboratory Black investigated the properties of heat, particularly the *transfer* of heat which occurred on liquefaction or solidification of a substance, work which led to his discovery of the phenomenon of latent heat. He went on to show that different bodies have different heat capacities, a characteristic which he was the first to describe and for which he coined the term 'specific heat'. His ideas were developed by a number of students and associates, including James Watt (1736–1819), instrument maker to the university, who used Black's theory of latent heat to modify the steam engine. Watt's brilliant contribution was to build a separate condensation chamber, making his engine so efficient that it became the industry standard and powered the industrial revolution, which, as a result, came early to Scotland. Black's lectures attracted large numbers of students to Glasgow and he was persuaded to accept the chair of chemistry at Edinburgh University. He produced no further research work, but with Thomas Charles Hope (1766–1844) was one of the most influential teachers of chemistry of his generation. Hope had graduated MD from Edinburgh in 1787, and that year was appointed lecturer in chemistry in Glasgow University. Working on a mineral mined near and named for the Argyll village of Strontian, he prepared pure strontium oxide and hydroxide, and described the preparation of thirteen other compounds of strontium. This led to the isolation of the element strontium by Humphry Davy, and Hope was to assert modestly that 'the greatest service which it has been in my power to render to Chemistry is the recommendation of Davy to the Royal Institution'. Like Cullen and Black before him he moved to the Chair of Chemistry at Edinburgh University, where his lectures attracted unprecedented numbers of students.

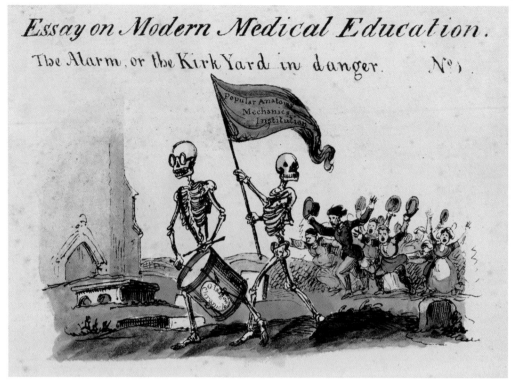

3.53 'The Alarm, or the Kirk Yard in Danger' (*Northern Looking Glass*, 1825). This satirical view of graver-obbing in Glasgow shows two skeletons in a graveyard, carrying the flag of the 'Popular Anatomy Mechanics' Institution', and being followed by an angry mob. As in Edinburgh there were not enough fresh cadavers to meet the need of anatomy students, who often resorted to becoming resurrection-ists themselves. This caused a public outcry, and in 1803 Glasgow University had to call in the army to protect the college buildings from a mob (*University of Glasgow*).

Midwifery Teaching in Glasgow

The eighteenth century witnessed the rise of the man-midwife, a reflection of the 'medicalisation' of childbirth. Two of the most prominent man-midwives in England, William Smellie (1697–1763) (see pp. 137–139) and William Hunter (1718–83), were Scots from Lanarkshire, yet the man-midwife genre was never popular in Scotland, largely because influential physicians like James Gregory and Andrew Duncan regarded midwifery as a demeaning profession for men.

Formal midwifery teaching in Glasgow began with Thomas Hamilton, who gave midwifery lectures at Glasgow University from 1768. His son, William Hamilton, professor of anatomy and botany, practised as a man-midwife, having trained under William Hunter in London. He introduced Hunterian obstetric techniques into Glasgow, and when he died in 1790, the midwifery lectures were continued by James Towers, who founded a lying-in hospital largely to facilitate student teaching at the University. His son, John Towers, was appointed to the first chair of midwifery at Glasgow University in 1820. The most notable contributions to midwifery teaching were made by John Burns (1774–1850) who lectured in anatomy and surgery, initially in his own private school in College Street and, from 1800, at Anderson's Institution, where he also lectured in midwifery. Burns was an effective lecturer and a prolific writer, his *Principles of Midwifery* (1809) being published in German, French, Dutch and American editions, in addition to ten English editions.

The Extra-Mural Schools in Glasgow

The extra-mural schools in Glasgow and Edinburgh became important features of medical education in both centres. The universities were unable to cope with the demand, and young, energetic doctors, eager to establish a reputation and supplement an often meagre income, taught private classes.

Extra-mural teaching in Glasgow was started by John Burns, who began to lecture on anatomy in 1797 in his private medical school in College Street, but his association with grave-robbing temporarily impeded his career. In 1815 he was appointed to the newly created chair of surgery at Glasgow University. His younger brother, Allan Burns (1781–1813), showed a natural aptitude for anatomy, so much so that he was able to take charge of dissection at the College Street School at the age of 16 and continued to teach anatomy in the extra-mural school until about 1830. Allan Burns is remembered for another innovation. In his classic work *Observations on Some of the Most Frequent and Important Diseases of the Heart* (1809) he clearly recommends the use of electric shock stimulation

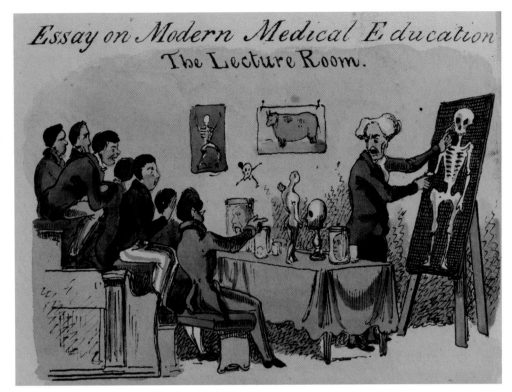

3.54 The Lecture Room (*Northern Looking Glass*, 1825). This cartoon shows Professor Jaffray lecturing on anatomy. With a reputation as a showman, he performed a notorious experiment in 1818 to demonstrate the effects of 'galvanism' (electricity) on the corpse. He passed electrical current through various parts of the body of the hanged murderer, Mathew Clydesdale. The grimaces produced by the contracting facial muscles resulted in apparent return of life, to the obvious alarm of the spectators. As a result the exercise became known as 'galvanic raising of the dead'. Jaffray held the Chair of Anatomy and Physiology at Glasgow University for 58 years (*University of Glasgow*).

in cases of sudden death. He wrote 'where, however, the cessation of vital action is very complete, and continues long, we ought to inflate the lungs, and pass electric shocks through the chest'. It was a technique that was to be taken on by the burgeoning Humane Societies around the country, but fell into disuse until the rationale was better understood in the twentieth century.

Anderson's Institution had been founded as a result of a bequest by John Anderson (1726–96) professor of natural philosophy at Glasgow University. He intended that it should be a large university with faculties of law, medicine, arts and philosophy, each granting degrees. These ambitions were thwarted by inadequate funding and political opposition, but teaching of various trades at Anderson's Institution was popular and it became the prototype for what would later become the Mechanics' Institute movement in Britain and beyond. Medical teaching did not start until 1815. By 1831 chairs had been established in Midwifery, Materia Medica, Practice of Medicine and Medical Jurisprudence. Anderson's never achieved the status to which its founder aspired, but it became the centre of extra-mural teaching in Glasgow, and as such it flourished. It opened the study of medicine to many who would not otherwise have been able to afford it by providing a cheaper medical education than Glasgow University. In 1828 it became Anderson's University, and in 1877

Anderson's College. (A fuller account of Anderson's is given on p. 190, chapter 4.)

By the end of the eighteenth century, Glasgow was well placed to provide medical education. Its attributes included University teaching in a range of pre-clinical and

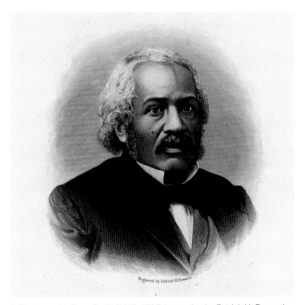

3.55 James McCune Smith (1813–1865) (engraving by Patrick H. Reason). McCune Smith was the first African-American to obtain a medical degree, graduating MD from Glasgow University in 1837. He became active in the Glasgow Emancipation Society, before returning to New York to become a successful doctor and leading abolitionist (*New York Historical Society*).

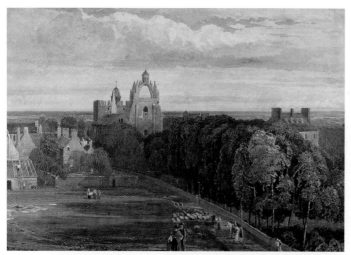

3.56 King's College and Old Aberdeen (Francis Oliver Finch, c1820). King's was built in the rural setting of the village of Old Aberdeen and dates from the turn of the sixteenth century. This painting shows that its rural surround-ings continued into the early nineteenth century (*University of Aberdeen*).

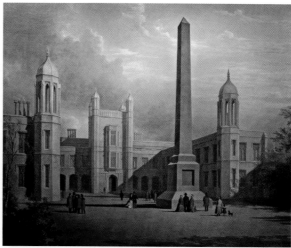

3.57 Marischal College, Aberdeen (James Giles, 1840). This iconic building, which dates from the mid-nineteenth century, has undergone extensive expansion and modernisation. Said to be the second largest granite building in the world, it now houses the Mitchell Hall and Marischal Museum and the headquarters of Aberdeen City Council. The obelisk in the foreground, a monument to Sir James McGrigor, was moved to Duthie Park, Aberdeen (*University of Aberdeen*).

clinical subjects, extra-mural schools, a large teaching hospital and a Faculty of Physicians and Surgeons. At this stage, however only about one third of the students grad-uating MD had actually studied in Glasgow. The impro-prieties previously associated with the Glasgow MD were long gone, and potential graduates now had a robust process of assessment. They were examined on Hippo-cratic aphorisms, on a medical case and submitted a Latin thesis which they publicly defended. Student numbers continued to increase throughout the first half of the nine-teenth century in both Glasgow University and the Ander-son University Medical School. While the Portland Street and College Street schools had disappeared, the medical school of the Anderson University attracted up to 150 students per year by the mid-nineteenth century.

Aberdeen

Aberdeen had long enjoyed the privilege, unusual for a city of its size, of housing two Universities, King's College in Old Aberdeen and Marischal College. Yet rivalry between them was to delay the local progress of medical education.

There had been a 'mediciner' on the staff of King's since its foundation in 1495, making it the oldest chair for the teaching of medicine in Britain. The role of the medi-ciner was to impart some knowledge of medicine as part of the traditional Scottish rounded education, rather than to produce graduates in medicine. John Gregory (1724–

1773), who had studied at Leiden, succeeded his brother James as mediciner in 1755. He gave lectures in medicine and, as one of the early physicians at the Aberdeen Infir-mary, published *Lectures on the Duties and Qualifications of a Physician* in 1772 (see p. 103). His attempt to found a medical school was frustrated by lack of funds and he transferred to the Chair of Physic in Edinburgh in 1766. The position of mediciner fell into disrepute during the tenures of Dr Alexander Bannerman and his son James, who between them held the post from 1793 to 1838. During those 45 years neither was to give a single lecture!

Repeated attempts over the years to unite the two colleges had always been thwarted, with the result that most students who attended classes in Aberdeen went on to qualify elsewhere. It was the students themselves, organ-ised as the Medical Society, who brought about a joint medical school from 1818. This seemed to work well until in 1836, when Marischal College was awarded a govern-ment grant to improve the existing teaching facilities and build new ones. The old enmities re-emerged and the medical union was dissolved in 1839.

Throughout this time MD degrees continued to be awarded by both colleges. In the eighteenth century these could be obtained by recommendation alone, but by the time of the union the regulations were more stringent, requiring proof of attendance at university medical classes or a recognised medical diploma before entry to a degree examination. Between 1826 and 1839 King's awarded four medical degrees and Marischal twenty-five.

It was not until the Universities (Scotland) Act of 1858 that the two colleges were finally united, four new chairs were endowed and an undergraduate medical school was formed.

St Andrews

The Chandos Chair of medicine and anatomy had been in place since 1721, but without funding, clinical beds or colleagues, the first incumbent, Thomas Simson (1696–1764), failed to establish a medical school. The practice of awarding the degree of MD *in absentia* on the recommendation of two referees, which had begun at the end of the seventeenth century, now began to expand and was to become notorious. The St Andrew's MD proved attractive to those from around Britain who had served an apprenticeship, gained a diploma, or had failed to gain a medical degree elsewhere by reason of cost or religious bar. Possession of an MD enhanced professional status, allowed a doctor to charge higher fees and was a valuable source of income for the university. There was justifiable resentment, particularly in England, at what were regarded as 'worthless Scotch degrees', and no less an authority than William Cullen described their award as 'a shameful traffic in degrees in physic at some of the universities in Scotland'. Yet the practice continued for more than a century. In 1826, anticipating government legislation, the awarding of degrees *in absentia* ceased. Despite the recommendations of the Universities Commission of 1826–30 that no further medical degrees should be awarded until St Andrew's had medical classes taught by professors for one academic year the 'shameful traffic' continued with degrees awarded if the individuals attended to receive them. The regulations were further tightened as a result of the Medical Act of 1858 and a subsequent visit by the newly constituted General Medical Council. Yet despite all this, although undergraduate medical teaching was still rudimentary, in 1862 alone no fewer than 530 individuals applied for medical degrees from St Andrew's University and 466 were conferred. The founding of University College, Dundee in the late nineteenth century allowed a conjoined medical school to be established with the Bute medical buildings in St Andrews.

THE INFLUENCE OF SCOTTISH MEDICINE OUTWITH SCOTLAND

Throughout the period under consideration, people, it has been argued, were Scotland's greatest export. Large medical schools in a small country meant that many Scots medical graduates had to travel to find gainful employment. Yet this was certainly a time of opportunity for those prepared to do so. The expanding worldwide Empire, the armed forces which defended it and the trading companies which it supported, all required doctors. One Scottish character trait to emerge was a curiosity about the world, whether fired by the quest for knowledge or the desire for a life better than the croft or urban deprivation could offer. The result was that Scottish doctors were to be found throughout the world – and were to prove influential.

Scots Exiles in London

Many Scottish doctors made their way to London after the Union of the Crowns in 1603, yet 'Scotch medical degrees' were not recognised by the Royal College of Physicians of London. The Scots graduates were young, had studied for three to five years as opposed to the ten to twelve years demanded by the Universities of Oxford and Cambridge, and with their broad training in medicine, surgery and obstetrics, they could effectively practise as general practitioners. Furthermore many had received degrees from St Andrews or Aberdeen regarded by the London Physicians as 'worthless' for reasons described earlier.

Yet many of these émigré Scots were men of talent. They included James Douglas (1675–1742), anatomist and man-midwife; Sir David Hamilton (1663–1721) from Lanarkshire, who became physician and confidant to Queen Anne; John Arbuthnot (c1667–1735), Royal physician, satirist and man of letters; and John Clephane (1701/2–1758), Physician to St George's Hospital and an activist in the fight between the College of Physicians and its licentiates.

However, the best known were a remarkable quartet of doctors: William Smellie, William Cullen and the

SONS OF LANARKSHIRE WHO BECAME LEADERS IN WORLD MEDICINE

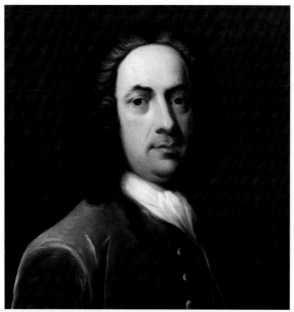

3.58 William Smellie (self-portrait, oil on canvas). William Smellie served apprenticeships as an apothecary and as a surgeon, then practised in Lanark for some 15 years, gaining further experience in midwifery in Paris, before moving to London, where he lectured in anatomy and midwifery. His success was such that he came to be described as the 'master of British midwifery' (*Royal College of Surgeons Edinburgh*).

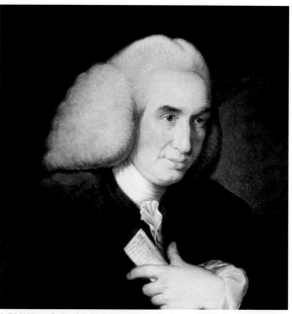

3.59 William Cullen (attributed to William Cochran, *c*1768). Born in Hamilton, Cullen set up his first practice near Shotts, also in Lanarkshire. In Edinburgh he established a large consulting and corresponding practice and became famous throughout the medical world as a teacher and author (*Royal College of Physicians of Edinburgh*).

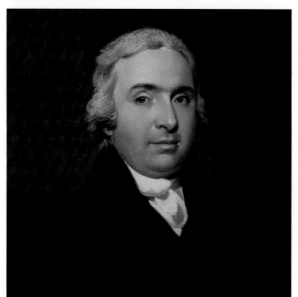

3.60 Mathew Baillie (portrait attributed to Thomas Barber). Born in Shotts and educated in Hamilton, at Glasgow University and at Balliol College, Oxford, Baillie moved to London to live with his uncle, William Hunter. He attended lectures and demonstrations at the Windmill Street School of Anatomy which had been founded by another uncle, John Hunter. Eventually he took charge of the school and was appointed physician to St George's Hospital. The success of his large private practice culminated in his appointment as physician to King George III, and he latterly abandoned anatomy and pathology for a career as a royal and society physician (*Royal College of Physicians of London*).

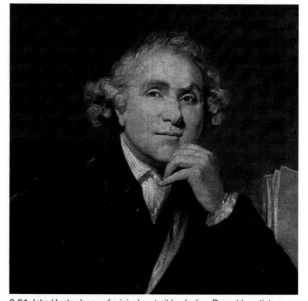

3.61 John Hunter (copy of original portrait by Joshua Reynolds, artist unknown). Hunter left Scotland aged 20 and, despite his lack of formal qualifications and distaste for books, he became, in London, the most celebrated surgeon of his generation. He embodied many core values of the Enlightenment, none more so than in his continued quest for knowledge. Hunter excelled as surgeon, anatomist, naturalist and collector. Much of his collection remains on display in the Royal College of Surgeons of England (*Royal College of Surgeons of Edinburgh*).

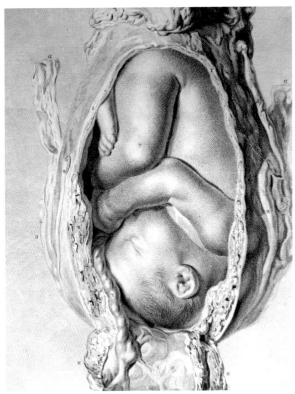

3.62 Gravid uterus from a dissection by William Hunter (Jan van Rymsdyk, 1774). This drawing of the foetus in late pregnancy is one of a series from *The Anatomy of the Human Gravid Uterus Exhibited in Figures*, in which Hunter's dissections, illustrated by van Rymsdyk's superb etchings, helped the understanding of growth, development and anatomical changes in late pregnancy.

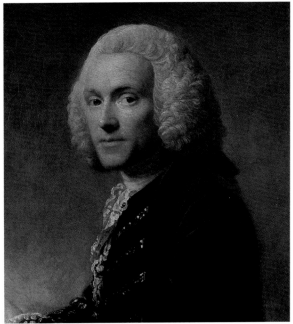

3.63 William Hunter (Allan Ramsay, *c*1764–65). William Hunter (1718–83) from Long Calderwood, near East Kilbride in Lanarkshire, served an apprenticeship under William Cullen in Hamilton, studied anatomy under Alexander Monro primus in Edinburgh, then set off for London, aged 22, to learn midwifery from William Smellie. He served as anatomy assistant to James Douglas, where his interest in the anatomy of pregnancy began. Hunter came to enjoy success as an anatomy teacher, surgeon and man-midwife (eventually becoming *accoucheur* to Queen Charlotte), but it was his anatomical discoveries and their presentation in books and lectures and his collection that brought him lasting fame (*Hunterian Museum and Art Gallery, University of Glasgow*).

brothers John and William Hunter, all born within 30 miles of each other in Lanarkshire, and all destined to become major figures in world medicine.

Smellie became the foremost obstetrician of his day, often described as 'the master of British midwifery'. His *Treatise of the Theory and Practice of Midwifery* (1752) described the physiology of pregnancy and the mechanisms of both normal and abnormal labour more comprehensively than any previous work. It was translated into several languages and became the classic obstetric work of its time. Writing and measurement were Enlightenment traits which Smellie used to great effect. His meticulous case notes were models of clarity (he was, after all, a lifelong friend of Tobias Smollett, doctor turned author), and his emphasis on pelvic measurement in obstetrics introduced much needed science into the emerging speciality. Smellie also modified the obstetric forceps to include a pelvic curve and devised the 'English lock', which enabled

the blades to be inserted separately. The guidelines which he developed for the use of obstetric forceps still form the basis of practice today.

The surgeon who, more than any other medical figure, exemplified the core values of the Enlightenment in England, was John Hunter (1728–1793). Despite leaving formal education at the age of 13 and declaring a distaste for books which was to last a lifetime, Hunter, through meticulous observation, repeated questioning and experiment, became the most important surgeon-scientist of his generation. Indeed it was his scepticism of the views of others expressed in books and treatises that drove the young Hunter to rely on his own observations to satisfy his intense hunger for knowledge. Leaving Scotland at the age of 20 without qualifications, he became assistant at the anatomy school in London founded by his brother William, where he was tasked with procuring bodies for dissection. Such was his natural flair for dissection that he

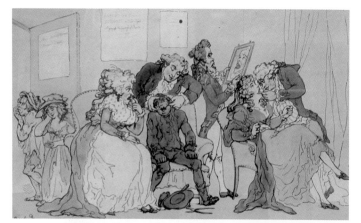

3.64 *Above*. The transplanting of teeth (Thomas Rowlandson, 1787). John Hunter popularised the transplantation of teeth, and in this satirical view Rowlandson highlights some of the ethical problems associated with the practice. The dentist appears to be removing a tooth from a chimney sweep before transplanting it into one of his wealthy patients. The wealthy had access to sugar and were more prone to caries. The results of his efforts are being admired in a mirror by the character on his left (*Royal College of Surgeons of Edinburgh*).

3.65 *Right*. Thomas Garvine (attributed to William Mosman, *c*1738). This portrait may have been painted by the Scottish artist William Mosman on the occasion of Garvine becoming a fellow of the Glasgow Faculty of Physicians and Surgeons in 1738. Garvine is depicted in an elegant silk coat, while on the table is a box of surgical instruments and documents in Chinese and Latin. Garvine, from Ayrshire, worked as a physician in St Petersburg, from where he was summoned to Peking to give an opinion on the health of the Chinese emperor in 1716. The coat in the portrait may have been a present from the grateful emperor (*Wellcome Library, London*).

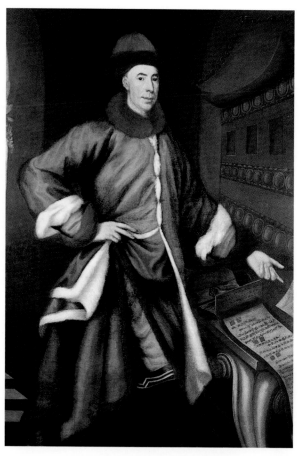

was soon teaching anatomy and, having learned his skills from William Cheselden and Percival Pott, before long was practising as a surgeon, destined to become the most sought-after surgeon of his day. It was the remarkable and innovative biological experiments which he performed that marked him as a hugely influential medical thinker and innovator. Hunter shared David Hume's scepticism about the widely held view that ideas took precedence over experience.

Having studied the growth and development of human teeth, and recognised *inter alia* the destructive nature of plaque, Hunter transplanted a human tooth into a cock's comb, with apparent success, and went on to popularise the practice of tooth transplantation in man (Fig. 3.64). He was, however, dismissive of the possibility that the procedure might cause disease transmission, and several recipients in his experiments went on to develop syphilis.

By tying off or ligating arteries in experimental animals, he confirmed his theory that collateral circulation developed rapidly around a blockage in an artery, which led him to develop ligation of arteries in man to treat aneurysm, a dangerous ballooning and weakening of the artery. This bold, innovative technique has been known ever since as Hunterian ligation. Hunter's tangible legacy is his magnificent collection of comparative anatomy, displayed to this day as part of the Hunterian collection at the Royal College of Surgeons of England.

Scottish influence was also disseminated by the many students from England who came to study at Scottish universities before returning, some to distinguished careers. Notable among these were the 'three men of Guy's', Richard Bright (1789–1838), Thomas Addison and Thomas Hodgkin.

Bright graduated MD in 1813 before returning to England where, as physician at Guy's Hospital, he was the first to describe the correlation between the pathology and the clinical features of the kidney disease which came to bear his name. A contemporary of Bright at Edinburgh was Thomas Addison (1793–1860) from Newcastle, who graduated MD in 1815, and was appointed physician at Guy's Hospital. He is best remembered for his description of the condition which bears his name, caused by the failure of the function of the adrenal cortex, and also for

Addisonian pernicious anaemia (although the Edinburgh physician James Scarth Combe had previously published a clear account of the condition). Thomas Hodgkin (1798–1866) graduated MD from Edinburgh in 1823 and, returning to practice in Guy's Hospital, gained eponymous fame through his description of the neoplastic condition of the lymphatic system.

The tradition of students from England studying medicine in Scotland continues into the twenty-first century.

Emigrés to Russia

From the sixteenth century, British doctors played a key role in shaping and developing medicine in Russia. Peter the Great was the driving force behind the radical reforms of the Russian medical system which took place during his reign. The implementation of these reforms was carried out by Robert Erskine (1677–1718), a pioneering genius endowed with outstanding organisational and executive ability, which was applied not only to medicine but to botany and natural history. Erskine, from Alva, was apprentice to an Edinburgh surgeon-apothecary before studying in Paris and eventually becoming physician to the Tsar and 'archiater', effectively the first director of the Russian Medical Services. Among his many achievements was the reorganisation and centralisation of medical herbalism in Russia in his capacity as head of the Apothecaries' Chancery.

The Scottish influence continued under James Mounsey (1710–73) from Dumfriesshire, who became Physician-in-Chief to the army of Catherine the Great, and then director of the medical chancery of the Russian Empire. It is likely that he paved the way for his nephew John Rogerson (1741–1823) from Lochmaben in Dumfriesshire, an Edinburgh medical graduate who, in 1746, became physician to Catherine the Great as well as her confidant. In 1816, after some fifty years of medical service at the Russian court, he returned to Scotland, a wealthy man.

The Scot credited with establishing military medicine in Russia was Dr (later Sir) James Wylie (1768–1854) from Kincardine, who studied medicine in Edinburgh before graduating from Aberdeen University. Through Roger-son's influence he became a court physician in Russia and personal surgeon to the Emperor Paul I. Wylie was essentially a military surgeon who claimed in his lifetime to have treated 600,000 sick or wounded Russian soldiers. He was first director of the Academy of Military Medicine and President of the Medical Academy of St Petersburg and Warsaw. In 1814 Wylie was made physician to the Emperor Alexander I.

His contemporary Sir Alexander Crichton (1763–1856) was born in Edinburgh and served as surgical apprentice to Alexander ('Lang Sandy') Wood. He matriculated in medicine in Edinburgh before graduating MD from Leiden. After being appointed physician to the Westminster Hospital in London, Crichton became physician to the emperor of Russia in 1803, and the following year became personal physician to Tsar Alexander I of Russia and to Maria Feodorovna, the Dowager Empress. Following his departure from Russia in 1819 he continued to be consulted by members of the Imperial family. His nephew, Sir William Crichton (1791–1865), graduated MD from Edinburgh University in 1810 and became physician to Tsar Nicholas I.

American Students/Graduates

Scottish doctors had been prominent in the American colonies from their earliest days. Yet the greatest impact on American medicine was made by the young Americans who crossed the Atlantic to study in Edinburgh and Glasgow before returning home with a medical degree. In the 100 years from 1750, no fewer than 650 North Americans graduated MD from Edinburgh University, together with an unknown number who simply attended lectures (the so-called 'occasional auditors'). In Glasgow about 60 Americans graduated MD over the same period. Americans were drawn particularly to Edinburgh by the increasing reputation of its teaching, by its tuition in English and by the efforts of Benjamin Franklin (1706–90), polymath, scientist, statesman and supreme patriot.

The advantages of the Edinburgh model of a university medical school linked to a teaching hospital were clear to Franklin, and in 1760 he was able to write 'We have imitated the Edinburgh institution of an Infirmary [in Philadelphia].' The Pennsylvania Hospital had been made

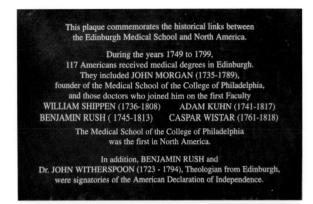

This plaque commemorates the historical links between
the Edinburgh Medical School and North America.

During the years 1749 to 1799,
117 Americans received medical degrees in Edinburgh.
They included JOHN MORGAN (1735-1789),
founder of the Medical School of the College of Philadelphia,
and those doctors who joined him on the first Faculty
WILLIAM SHIPPEN (1736-1808)   ADAM KUHN (1741-1817)
BENJAMIN RUSH (1745-1813)   CASPAR WISTAR (1761-1818)
The Medical School of the College of Philadelphia
was the first in North America.

In addition, BENJAMIN RUSH and
Dr. JOHN WITHERSPOON (1723 - 1794), Theologian from Edinburgh,
were signatories of the American Declaration of Independence.

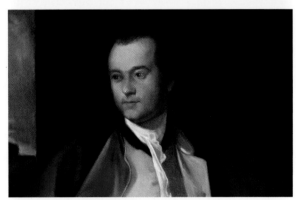

3.66 *Top*. Plaque in the Edinburgh Medical School commemorating links
with North America (*Iain Macintyre*).

3.67 *Above*. John Morgan (1735–1789) (Vincent Desiderio, 1981. Copy from
the original by Angelica Kauffman). Morgan graduated in Arts from the
College of Philadelphia in 1757, and after studying in Edinburgh graduated
MD from Edinburgh University six years later. After a tour of Europe, where
he met Morgagni and Voltaire, he returned to Edinburgh and was elected
MRCP in 1765. He was instrumental in establishing the Medical School of
the College of Philadelphia (*Royal College of Physicians of Edinburgh*).

possible through the benefaction of another Edinburgh
graduate, John Fothergill. Franklin, based largely in
London during his time in Britain, used his influence and
contacts to direct American students to Edinburgh, often
by letters of introduction to figures like William Cullen.
Notable among these were the students who were to return
to establish the first medical school in North America, a
school unashamedly based on the Edinburgh model.

Among the first of these was William Shippen, whom
Franklin recommended to the Edinburgh physician Sir
Alexander Dick 'to obtain the sanction of a degree if found
to merit it.' One of Franklin's other protégés, John
Morgan (1735–89), had academic and organisational qual-
ities that were to be crucial in establishing a medical school
in Philadelphia. 'Mr Morgan is a young gentleman of
Philadelphia whom I have long known and greatly esteem
. . . I wish him the advantage of your conversation and

instruction. I wish it also for the sake of my country where
he is to reside,' wrote Benjamin Franklin to William
Cullen.

On his return home with an Edinburgh MD, Morgan
persuaded the trustees of the College of Philadelphia to
establish the Medical School of the College of Philadelphia,
recommending himself as Professor of Physic and William
Shippen as Professor of Anatomy. He went on to become
Director-General of American Hospitals and Physician-in-
Chief to the Army. Morgan's career, however, was blighted
by a subsequent longstanding feud with Shippen.

These first five faculty members of America's first
medical school were all Edinburgh graduates (see p. 143),
who took to Philadelphia not only the view that medical
teaching should be university-based; they also took,
initially with minimal modification, the Edinburgh
medical curriculum. The textbooks, specimens and
student tests were all transplanted to Pennsylvania, but
soon the new medical school adapted these to the new
environment.

In New York too Edinburgh graduates were influential in establishing a medical school. Samuel Bard (1742–
1821), MD Edinburgh 1765, was a joint founder in 1767
of the country's third medical school, King's College, New
York (later Columbia). In Edinburgh the ideas of David
Hume, Francis Hutcheson and John Gregory on medical
ethics (see p. 103) had influenced both Bard and Benjamin
Rush, and Bard was to write the first American publication on medical ethics.

Morgan and his American peers held the Edinburgh
school in the highest regard. 'Its reputation' he wrote in
1765 'already rivals if not surpasses that of every other
school of Physic in Europe.' The influence of the University of Pennsylvania medical school formed in Edinburgh's
image was substantial.

Scottish influence was prominent in establishing the
first Canadian medical school, the Montreal Medical
Institution, whose founders had all studied at Edinburgh.
It became the medical faculty of McGill University, where,
as in Pennsylvania, the Edinburgh curriculum was adopted. Later in the century the Edinburgh influence would
again be to the fore, when medical schools were established in Sydney, Australia and Dunedin, New Zealand.

FOUR EDINBURGH GRADUATES WHO WERE MEMBERS OF FACULTY OF THE FIRST MEDICAL SCHOOL IN NORTH AMERICA, IN THE COLLEGE OF PHILADELPHIA

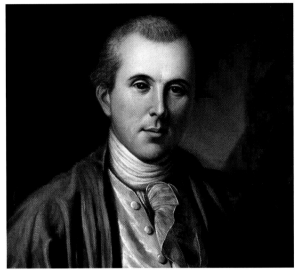

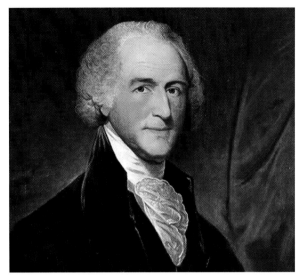

3.68 Benjamin Rush (oil on canvas, Charles Willson Peale, 1783). Benjamin Rush (1745–1813) attended the first lectures of John Morgan and William Shippen at the newly founded Medical School of the College of Philadelphia. Of his time in Edinburgh, where he attended the lectures of Joseph Black and William Cullen before graduating MD, he would later write, 'The years I spent in Edinburgh I consider as the most important in their influence upon my character and conduct'. He became Professor of Medicine at Philadelphia, wrote the first American textbook on psychiatry, and advocated, on health grounds, restrictions on the use of alcohol and tobacco. Rush supported better education for women and free schooling, and was an active campaigner against slavery and capital punishment. He was the only medical signatory of the American Declaration of Independence (*Winterthur Museum*).

3.69 William Shippen (1736–1808). Having graduated in arts from the College of New Jersey (later Princeton University) and served as medical apprentice to his father in Philadelphia, Shippen came to London, where he learned anatomy and surgery under John Hunter and midwifery under William Hunter. After graduating MD from Edinburgh University in 1761, he became the first Professor of Anatomy and Surgery in the new Medical School of the College of Philadelphia, controversially giving lectures in midwifery (*Clendening Library, Kansas University Medical Centre*).

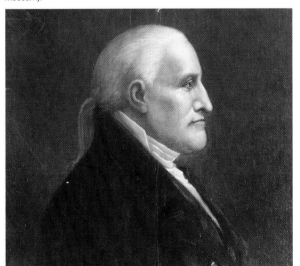

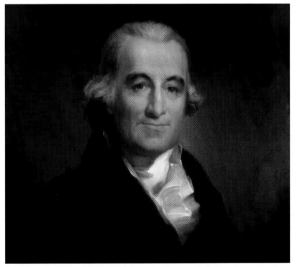

3.70 Adam Kuhn (1741–1817) (copy by Louis Hasselbusch in 1912 from original painting by unknown artist). Kuhn studied botany and medicine with Carl Linnaeus in Sweden, graduated MD from Edinburgh in 1767 and the following year became Professor of Materia Medica and Botany at the Medical School of the College of Philadelphia, and then Professor of the Theory and Practice of Medicine. (*University of Pennsylvania Archives*).

3.71 Caspar Wistar (1761–1818) (copy by Thomas Sully from the original painting by Bass Otis, oil on canvas, 1830). Wistar graduated MD from Edinburgh in 1786 and succeeded Benjamin Rush as Professor of Chemistry at Philadelphia, going on to become Professor of Anatomy and Midwifery. Noted for his innovative teaching methods, his collection of comparative anatomy was housed in the Wistar Institute, which is largely concerned with cancer research. His name also lives on in the plant genus Wisteria (*American Philosophical Society*).

MILITARY MEDICINE AND SURGERY

From the mid-eighteenth century the continuing growth of the Royal Navy and the British Army stimulated by the wars against France and the growth of Empire resulted in a concomitant increase in the number of doctors entering military service.

Army Medical Reforms

This was a time when armies lost more men from illness than from battle wounds. The causes of those illnesses were not understood, but there was a dawning realisation that the appalling standards of hygiene and sanitation endured by soldiers played a part. As physician-general to the Army in Flanders, Sir John Pringle (Fig. 3.72) campaigned to have military hospitals regarded as neutral territory, an innovation implemented for the first time by both sides at the battle of Dettingen in 1743. Yet his greatest contribution was in improving military hygiene and sanitation. He published *Observations on the Nature and Cure of Hospital and Jayl Fevers* in 1750 in which he proposed that these were the same disease – typhus. In his seminal work *Observations on the Diseases of the Army in Camp and Garrison* (1752) he suggested that, 'in the camp, the contagion [of dysentery] passes from one who is ill to his companion in the same tent, and from them perhaps to the next.' In later editions he speculated that the contagion might be spread by the 'animalicula' discovered by Antoni van Leeuwenhoek's microscope. He went on to anticipate antiseptic theory, as the first physician to use the word 'antiseptic' in 1752. 'The faeces,' he wrote, 'are rendered less, if at all infectious, by means of a strong acid combined with the parts that are really septic – especially, in the dysentery, where the faeces are highly corrupted and contagious . . .' Thus Pringle gave the first scientific account of the epidemiology, pathogenesis and prevention of hospital cross-infection, and was one of the first to suggest antiseptics to prevent the spread of disease. He returned to a thriving practice in London, and such was his reputation that, when the philosopher David Hume wished the best medical opinion, he travelled to London to consult Pringle.

The theme of military reform to improve the welfare of the fighting soldier was continued by Sir James McGrigor (1771–1858) (Fig. 3.73), whom the Duke of Wellington considered 'one of the most industrious, able, and successful public servants I have ever met with'. In 1815 he was appointed Director-General of the Army Medical Department, and brought about improvements in the techniques and speed with which wounded soldiers could be evacuated from the battlefield. This 'chain of battlefield evacuation' has formed the basis for the staged evacuation of battlefield casualties ever since. His concern for the welfare of his troops and their dependants resulted in his founding the Army Friendly Society (1816) and the Army Benevolent Society (1820) which supported soldiers' widows, orphans and dependants. He established a system of statistical returns of the health of the army by requiring all military stations to submit reports on the health of their men, and this later formed the basis of the *Statistical Returns of the Health of the Army*.

Preventative Medicine in the Army

The concept that doctors might prevent disease rather than simply attempting to cure it was a novel one in the eighteenth century. Sir George Ballingall (1780–1855) (Fig. 3.74) believed that most diseases and illnesses could be avoided or at least ameliorated through preventative measures, and the conditions which he found in India confirmed this view. He published the first description of Madura foot, initially known as Ballingall's disease, and later published *Practical Observations on Fever, Dysentery and Liver Complaints, as They Occur amongst the European Troops in India* (1818), which was influential in improving living conditions for British troops serving overseas. In 1822, on appointment to the chair of Military Surgery at Edinburgh University, the only such chair in the British Isles, he delivered a lecture course. This was published as *Outlines of Military Surgery* in 1833, and became the most authoritative textbook of its day on the subject, eventually running to five editions. His teaching was highly regarded, and both Sir James McGrigor and the Physician-general of the Royal Navy, another Scot, Sir William Burnett, recommended his course to their medical officers. The

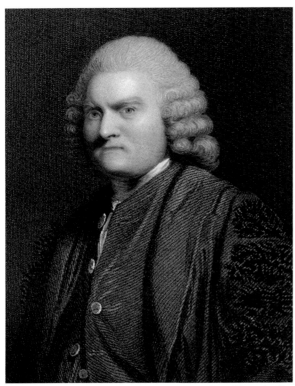

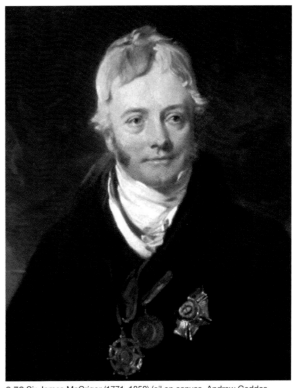

3.72 Sir John Pringle (1707–82) (engraving by William Henry Mote, after Sir Joshua Reynolds). Pringle studied at the universities of St Andrews and Edinburgh before graduating MD from the University of Leiden in 1730. He set up in practice in Edinburgh and was appointed Professor of Pneumatics (Metaphysics) and Moral Philosophy at Edinburgh University. In 1742 he joined the army as physician (*Royal College of Physicians of Edinburgh*).

3.73 Sir James McGrigor (1771–1858) (oil on canvas, Andrew Geddes, *c*1840). As a medical student in Aberdeen, James McGrigor was one of the founders of the student society which became the Medico-Chirurgical Society. He graduated MA from Marischal College in 1788, then studied medicine there and in Edinburgh, but, as was common at the time, did not graduate. After various postings as an army surgeon, he obtained the MD degree from Aberdeen in 1804 (*Aberdeen Medico-Chirurgical Society*).

East India Company, at that time the biggest and most important commercial arm of Empire, required candidates for their service to attend his course in military surgery. Ballingall was influential in persuading the Army to improve what he called military hygiene and to adopt preventive medicine. This included improved design of military camps and barracks and greater attention to diet and leisure activities.

Reforms in the Royal Navy

The conditions of squalor, deprivation and disease which prevailed in the ships of the Royal Navy were graphically described by Tobias Smollett (1721–71) in his tale *The Adventures of Roderick Random* (1748). Smollett had been

a surgical apprentice in Glasgow and served as a surgeon's mate in the Royal Navy. Having set up in medical practice in London he began to write satirical verse and plays. His first novel about the adventurous and unprincipled Roderick Random was an instant success, establishing him as a writer. In describing how Random leaves Scotland for London and serves as a ship's surgeon's mate, Smollett was clearly drawing on his own experiences. Random undergoes a series of misfortunes, is the victim of fraud and oppression, suffers extreme privation and develops contempt for authority. The work vividly depicts the misery of life below decks in the navy of the day, while surgeons and apothecaries are variously depicted as cruel, insensitive and untrustworthy. The resentment shown

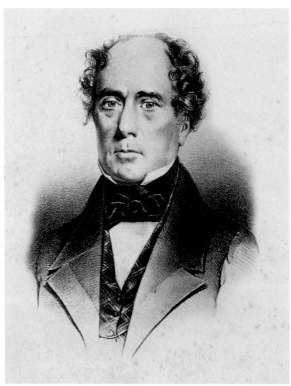

3.74 Sir George Ballingall (engraving by W. Stewart after original painting by T. Lawrence). Ballingall supplemented his medical studies at Edinburgh University by attending John Barclay's anatomy lectures in the extra-mural school. He qualified with a diploma from the RCSEd in 1805, before joining the Army Medical Department and becoming Assistant Surgeon to the 2nd Battalion of the Royal Scots, with whom he served in India (*Wellcome Library, London*).

bays, regular changing of patients' linen and frequent washing of the surgeon's hands.

Lind left Edinburgh in 1758 to become Physician-in-charge at the Royal Hospital, Haslar, in Portsmouth. He continued to promote reforms to improve the health of sailors (and other travellers) in his final work *Essay on Diseases Incidental to Europeans in Hot Climates* (1768). This contained a painstaking review of the literature on tropical disease, and public health recommendations such as avoiding building settlements on marshy ground. Lind's works were influential in Britain and overseas, being published in several European languages and in America.

Sir Gilbert Blane (1749–1834) had studied in Edinburgh, where he had learned from Cullen the value of nosological tables and of statistics, which he used to good effect in persuading the Admiralty of the need for reform. His publication in 1780 on the 'most effectual means of preserving the health of seamen' was to presage a series of reforms. Principal among these was his recommendation that sailors' diets should include fresh fruit, and the following year he was able to demonstrate its efficacy in preventing disease. With a growing reputation, Blane went on to become physician to King George IV, and, unusually for a Scottish graduate, was appointed physician to St Thomas's Hospital in London. On return to naval service Blane was promoted Physician to the Fleet and a Commissioner to the Board for Sick and Hurt Sailors, advising on health problems in British armed forces throughout the world.

At much the same time, a slave-ship surgeon, Thomas Trotter (*c*1760–1832) from Melrose in the Scottish borders, had witnessed at first hand a devastating outbreak of scurvy among the slaves, which was, he was convinced, the result of their inadequate diet. As a result he became an ardent abolitionist and became devoted to the prevention of scurvy. His *Observations on the Scurvy* (1786 and 1792) was influential in the lead up to Blane's 1795 diktat that lime juice become a routine part of naval diet. In 1825 Blane was able to report that the Navy was free from scurvy.

The emphasis on the value of recording clinical data, which was such a feature of Enlightenment medicine, can be seen in Blane's other contribution. He introduced the use of data collection by naval surgeons and began the

toward the young Scot in London in the aftermath of Culloden almost certainly reflected Smollet's own experience.

In many ways eighteenth-century naval surgeons were the true pioneers of preventative medicine, improving diet, hygiene and sanitation before their colleagues ashore. The theme of improved hygiene in the Royal Navy was championed by Dr James Lind (see p. 101). In his *Essay on the Most Effectual Means of Preserving the Health of Seamen in the Royal Navy* (1757), Lind argued for better standards of sanitation on ships and for more humane treatment of seamen at much the same time as Pringle was proposing similar changes for the army. He proposed measures such as increased space between patients in sick

The enigma of Dr James Barry

One of the most unusual tales to emerge from nine-teenth-century medicine is that of Dr James Miranda Steuart Barry, who graduated MD from Edinburgh University in 1812 with a thesis on femoral hernia. He went on to a successful career as a military surgeon, serving in Cape Town, where in 1826 he successfully performed a caesarean section, believed to be the first such successful procedure in Africa. Over the next twenty years he served in postings throughout the Empire, from the Caribbean to the Mediterranean and from the Crimea to Canada, eventually becoming senior Inspector General of Military Hospitals. Shortly after his death in London in 1865, his maid alleged that Barry had been a woman, and the story was widely reported in the national and medical press. Recent evidence appears to show that Barry was born Margaret Ann Bulkley in Cork and emigrated to London with her mother as a child. The plot to change her identity was made possible with the help of her maternal uncle, the painter James Barry RA, and some of his influential friends, including General Miranda, a Venezuelan exile in London. Under the name James Miranda Steuart Barry the new medical student arrived in Edinburgh, where studies and early career were facilitated by the patronage of David Steuart Erskine, Earl of Buchan.

It was to be 82 years after Barry's graduation before women were allowed to graduate in medicine from a Scottish University.

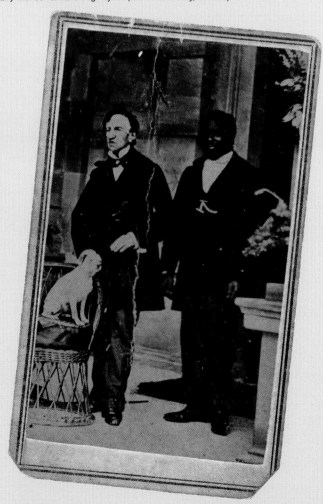

3.76 James Barry (photograph by Adolphe Duperly, 1862). This photograph, taken in the studios of Duperly in Kingston, Jamaica, depicts the 72-year-old Barry with servant and dog Psyche (*Wellcome Library, London*).

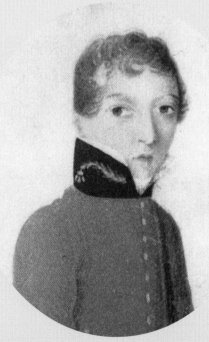

3.75 James Barry as a young military surgeon (artist unknown, *c*1813–1816). This miniature of Barry was painted before his first posting abroad. It was given to Thomas Munnick, father of the boy whom Barry in 1826 delivered by what is thought to be the first Caesarean section in Africa in which both mother and child survived. Barry subsequently kept in touch with the boy, who was named James Barry Munnick, and the painting still remains in the possession of the Munnick family (*Dr James Barry Munnick*).

system of subjecting these to statistical analysis. All naval surgeons were encouraged to report on the health of their seamen using standard forms and log books.

Largely as a result of Blane's reforms, the proportion of sailors on the sick list had by 1793 dropped from 1 in 3 to 1 in 10, greatly enhancing the fighting strength of the Navy.

The Regius Chair of Military Surgery at Edinburgh

For a nation so dependent on its armed forces, it is remarkable that Great Britain did not have a school of military surgery in the eighteenth century. Colleges of military surgery were well established in France, Russia, Prussia, Austria and Holland. Gilbert Blane and Thomas Trotter had recognised the need to train naval surgeons in the particular skills that they would need on active service. The Edinburgh surgeon John Bell wrote to the Government in 1798 proposing, as a matter of urgency, the setting up of 'one great school of military surgery' for naval and army surgeons. In 1806 the University of Edinburgh appointed John Thomson (1765–1846) as foundation professor to the Regius Chair of Military Surgery, the first such appointment in the British Isles. Two Scots, Sir James McGrigor, Director General of the Army Medical Department, and Sir William Burnett, Head of the Naval Medical Department, recommended his lecture course to their officers and in 1826 both reported to the Royal Commissioners their satisfaction with the results of his teaching. Many of the Edinburgh medical students who attended these lectures felt inspired to join the medical arm of the Army, Navy or East India Company. In 1822 Thomson was succeeded in the chair by Mr (later Sir) George Ballingall (see p. 144), whose lecture course was to enjoy the approval of the Medical departments of the Army, Navy, Ordnance and East India Company. Ballingall campaigned in the medical press and lobbied government to establish chairs of military surgery in London and Dublin. A chair was established in Dublin between 1844 and 1860, and in that year an Army medical school was established at Fort Pitt, Chatham, Kent. James Syme, professor of surgery at the University of Edinburgh, persuaded the University to abolish the chair of Military Surgery in 1856, a year after Ballingall's death.

DISEASE PREVENTION

Until the eighteenth century, disease prevention took the form of containment or isolation. Smallpox was the target of the first efforts to prevent a disease by active intervention, efforts eventually so successful as to lead to its eradication in the twentieth century.

Prevention of smallpox

In 1715, Peter Kennedy, a Scottish surgeon working in London, published *An Essay of Internal Remedies*, which contained an account of the 'engrafting' of fluid from smallpox vesicles by scarification of the skin, to confer immunity, a technique which he had seen in Turkey. He compared this practice with that in his native Scotland, where in 'some parts of the highlands of Scotland they infect their children by rubbing them with a kindly pock'. This technique, inoculation or variolation, was well known in China and India. The first written account of it in Scotland was from Aberdeen in 1726, but because of the death of a child following the procedure, it fell into disrepute. When Alexander Monro *primus* surveyed Scottish doctors in 1765, only 88 appeared to use the technique, representing about one third of all doctors. He found that there was resistance to its introduction by the young. 'Young people,' he wrote, 'are not much inclined toward inoculation'. There was further opposition on religious grounds. 'The notions of absolute predestination which are still deeply rooted in the minds of country people, lead the generality of them to look upon inoculation as implying an impious trust of Divine providence.'

William Cullen gave a detailed description of inoculation technique in 1771, and in 1781 Andrew Duncan, an early advocate of public health measures, suggested 'general inoculation' of the Scottish population. This endorsement by such a leading thinker may have contributed to increasing popularity of the technique. It had also become cheaper, but was not available in Scotland under the Poor Law as it was in England. By the end of the century, Sinclair's *Statistical Account* shows marked variation in practice throughout Scotland. There were apparent successes like those of Dr Lindsay, in Jedburgh, who inoculated one thousand patients, of whom only two

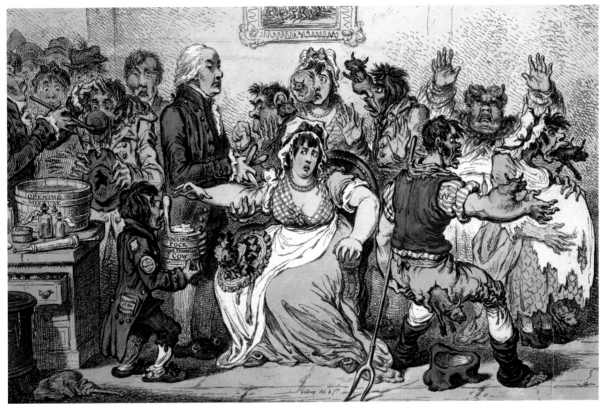

3.77 The Cow Pock (James Gillray, 1802). Gillray, the son of a Scottish soldier, was a leading satirical caricaturist of his day. Here he depicts some of the popular misapprehensions about the technique. A serene Edward Jenner is vaccinating an apprehensive patient, while those already vaccinated have cow parts growing out of their bodies (*Wellcome Library, London*).

died from smallpox. In Shetland the *Account* described the success of the technique of John Williamson (c1730–96): 'Formerly the small-pox occasioned the most dreadfull ravages, in these islands; frequently carrying off the fifth part of the inhabitants. Now, hardly any suffer from this disorder. Inoculation is successfully practised, even by the common people; but in particular by a person, whose name is John Williamson. Several thousands have been inoculated by him, and he has not lost a single patient.' But inoculation remained sporadic, and Brunton's review in 1992 concluded that inoculation probably had little effect on smallpox mortality.

Jennerian vaccination, on the other hand, was enthusiastically taken up after its introduction in 1796. This involved taking fluid from cowpox vesicles and introducing it under the skin by scarification. This time the Church of Scotland approved of the practice, and indeed, according to the 1811 census, it was frequently performed by ministers themselves. This remarkable *volte face* may be attributed to the Edinburgh Public Dispensary and

Vaccine Committee, who in 1803 wrote to the Church advocating vaccination, offering 'proper' vaccine and urging the clergy that they themselves should 'disseminate the blessings of vaccine inoculation'. With remarkable foresight they even suggested that smallpox might be 'completely exterminated' by vaccination. The General Assembly approved, casting aside previous doctrinal objections that disease prevention contravened preordination, and the letter was circulated to every minister in Scotland.

Vaccination was also provided free to the children of the poor by the Faculty of Physicians and Surgeons of Glasgow from 1801. The success of the practice can be seen from Watt's analysis of Glasgow burial registers, which show a progressive fall in the proportion of deaths from smallpox from 18.7% in 1795–1800 to 1.07% in 1813–19.

The Vaccination Act (1840) in England enabled free vaccination for all, chargeable under the poor rates, but it was not until the Vaccination (Scotland) Act (1863) that vaccination became compulsory in Scotland.

Evolving Attitudes to Anatomical Dissection

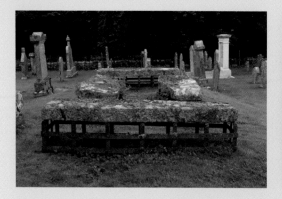

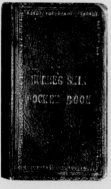

3.78 *Far left.* Mortsafes. These mortsafes, at Cluny in Aberdeenshire, demonstrate how the graves could be protected by a wrought-iron cage, on top of which was placed a mortstone, a heavy, coffin-shaped block of granite (*Allan Shedlock*).

3.79 *Left.* Pocket book made from Burke's skin. As was customary after the execution of a murderer, William Burke's body was dissected by Alexander Monro tertius. Ironically, as Professor of Anatomy in the University of Edinburgh, he had been the great rival of Robert Knox, the likely recipient of Burke's victims, but a much less popular teacher. This gruesome memento is on display in Surgeons' Hall Museum (*Royal College of Surgeons of Edinburgh*).

The growth of formal medical teaching in the eighteenth and early nineteenth centuries led to one gruesome consequence – grave-robbing, the practice of stealing fresh bodies from cemeteries for anatomical dissection. Although this was widespread throughout the British Isles, Edinburgh gained a particular notoriety as a result of the activities of Burke and Hare, who resorted to mass murder, selling on the bodies of their victims to anatomy teachers.

Anatomy dissection had been a core part of medical learning since the Renaissance. In Scotland the 1505 Seal of Cause (or charter) had granted the Edinburgh surgeons the right to dissect the body of one condemned man each year. Yet by the seventeenth century this was insufficient to meet the need for subjects; when a body was taken from Greyfriars Kirkyard in 1678, suspicion fell on 'some chirurgeon or his servant'. Anatomists and their students seemed to have started the practice, but as the demand increased they were joined by organized criminals, who came to be known as resurrectionists or 'sack-em-up-men', from their practice, usually nocturnal, of breaking open a recently buried coffin and removing the body in a sack.

Dr Robert Knox's extramural anatomy classes in Edinburgh exceeded 500 students, the largest ever seen in these islands. His popularity was due in no small measure to his advertising 'fresh anatomical subjects' for each course, with the chilling addendum that 'arrangements have been made to secure as usual an ample supply of anatomical subjects.' Even the supply of bodies from as far afield as London, Manchester, Leeds and Dublin failed to satisfy the unprecedented need. William Burke and William Hare, two Irishmen living in Edinburgh, took procurement to a new low, murdering their victims by suffocation, so introducing the macabre term 'Burking' into the language. When one of their victims was identified in Knox's dissecting-room, Burke and Hare were arrested and Knox was caught up in the public outrage which followed.

Hare turned King's evidence and fled; Burke was found guilty and hanged in January 1829. The Edinburgh mob, furious at these revelations, burned an effigy of Dr Knox and attacked his house. Although he was exonerated by a committee of inquiry, his student numbers declined and he stopped teaching at Surgeon Square in 1833, subsequently leaving Edinburgh under a cloud of suspicion, and ending his career in relative obscurity in the south of England.

Such public outrage helped shape the nation's response, and the 1832 Anatomy Act brought about a progressive decline in grave robbing. Yet bodies were still required, and the Act allowed unclaimed bodies from infirmaries, poorhouses, work-houses, asylums and jails to be given (or sold) for anatomical teaching. Public anger over grave-robbing came to be replaced in the public mind by a fear that institutionalised poverty, chronic illness or insanity was a condemnation to be dissected after death. In the 20th century voluntary bequest became the accepted source of bodies for anatomical dissection. In the 21st century medical students' exposure to dissection has been greatly reduced, as sophisticated imaging and plastinated models are used increasingly to teach anatomy. At least one UK medical school does not use cadavers at all to teach anatomy. Societal and medical attitudes to human remains continue to evolve.

ORIGINS OF PUBLIC HEALTH

This period saw the beginnings of the entry of the state into the regulation of medicine. The health of the populace, as opposed to individuals, became a matter of increasing concern, if only because of the perceived need to maintain fit and healthy workers and armed forces. The concept was developed in continental Europe and described by Johann Peter Frank, Professor of Medicine at Pavia and later at Vienna, in his book *System Einer Vollständigen Medizinischen Polizey* (*A Complete System of Medical Policy*). ('Polizey' became 'Police' in English translations). Frank put forward the view that the state should be responsible for virtually every aspect of medical care and preventative medicine. Andrew Duncan drew on this experience and promoted the idea that doctors' care should encompass the health of the entire population in addition to that of the individual. He advocated these views in his lecture course from 1792 but, unlike Frank, envisaged that this would be achieved through private acts of philanthropy rather than by state intervention. In 1801 he published his *Heads of Lectures on Medical Jurisprudence and Medical Police* to promote his views more widely.

Police Acts, giving local authorities powers over sanitary matters like street-cleaning, were passed earlier in Scotland than elsewhere, in Glasgow in 1800 and in Edinburgh in 1805. These might be regarded as the first legislative steps in the regulation of health, as the state became increasingly involved in legislating for the health and welfare of its citizens and those who sought to provide their health care.

SUMMARY

This was a period dominated, at one level, by the intellectual brilliance of the Enlightenment, a phenomenon whose influence in Scotland was out of all proportion to the size of the country and its population. The Enlightenment produced in and attracted to Scotland men of genius and creativity, free to express new, often radical and iconoclastic ideas, in a new age of tolerance. There were benefits from this new age of discovery for ordinary Scots;

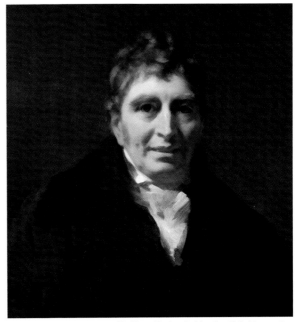

3.80 Andrew Duncan senior (Sir Henry Raeburn). A leading Enlightenment physician, Andrew Duncan senior left a rich and varied legacy. He founded the first English language medical journal, a dispensary for the sick poor, a chair of Medical Jurisprudence and Public Health and two medical societies, which, like his Royal Scottish Horticulural Society, survive into the twenty-first century (*Royal College of Physicians of Edinburgh*).

agricultural reform brought about better nutrition; disease could be effectively prevented – vaccination brought about a decline in smallpox and citrus fruits were used to abolish scurvy. Yet while some diseases declined, others increased and new ones appeared, many of these caused by the overcrowding and squalor brought about by increasing urbanisation. While the literati of medicine theorised about the causes of disease, this did not result in dramatic improvements in medical care for the ordinary Scot. Medicine did not produce an innovative intellectual giant, no Adam Smith, James Hutton or David Hume. Yet from this period emerged a large and flourishing practice in medical education, again out of all proportion to the size of the country, which resulted in generations of doctors destined to serve Britain, her armed forces and her expanding empire. There were other benefits in the form of the new dispensaries and infirmaries providing organised health care, much of it free, for the 'sick poor'; benefits came too with the origins of public health. By the end of the period, medical teaching, training and organisation had improved out of all recognition; the age of rational thinking, experiment and quest for knowledge had provided insights and set the stage for the dramatic medical and surgical innovations of the latter half of the nineteenth century.

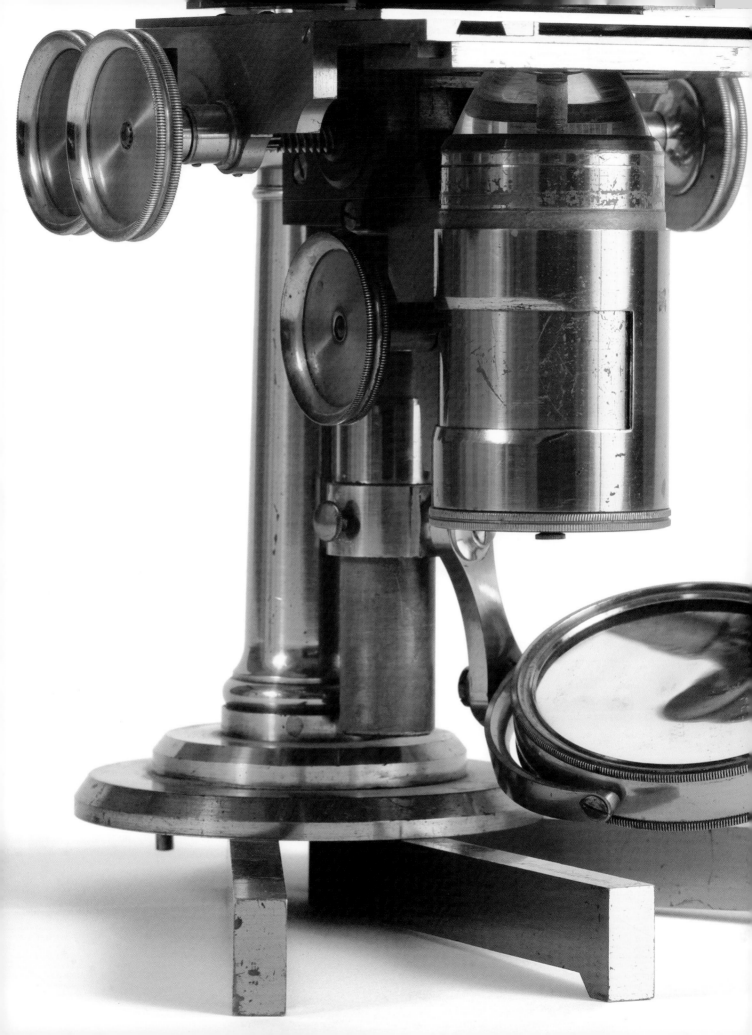

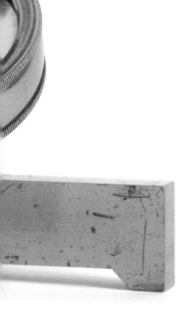

CHAPTER FOUR

INTERVENTION BY THE STATE

Morrice McCrae

———

The testimony of an eyewitness is worth more than that of all
the fathers of medicine who wrote on false information.

GARCIA D'ORTA
(1501–1568)

———

The health of the people of Britain is not properly looked after.

ANEURIN BEVAN
(1897–1960)

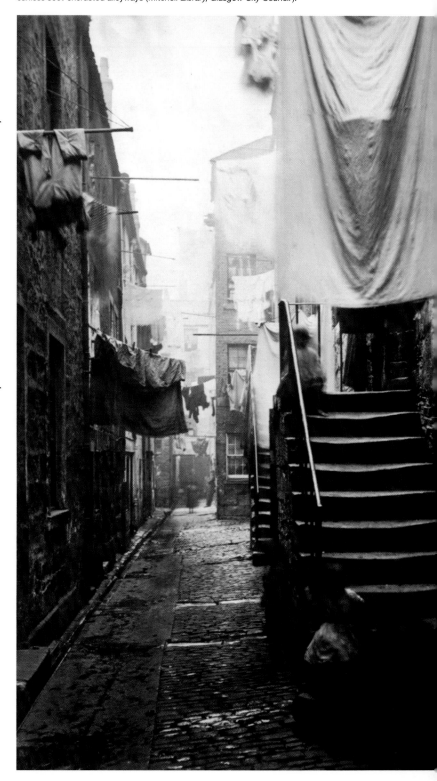

4.1 Families living in Scotland's urban slums in the nineteenth century had difficulty in keeping themselves clean. Their one or two room tenement houses had little convenient access to a supply of clean water. Soap only became easily affordable in the middle of the century. Laundry had to be hung out to dry in sunless soot-encrusted alleyways (*Mitchell Library, Glasgow City Council*).

INTRODUCTION

In 1843 Thomas Carlyle lamented that there were now in Scotland's industrial towns and cities 'scenes of woe and destitution such as the sun never saw before in the most barbarous regions where men dwelt.' For half a century Scotland's population had been growing at an unprecedented rate. Those who could no longer find employment in the modern labour-efficient commercial farms flocked from the countryside to look for work in the factories and workshops of the towns. The population of these towns first doubled and then more than trebled. But many of this new and growing urban population failed to maintain even a modestly respectable level of existence. The unemployed, the sick, the unemployable and the misanthropic crowded into slums and rookeries that came to be feared by the more well-to-do citizens as breeding grounds of violence, criminality and disease.

This degrading and divisive social problem was not unique to Scotland. It troubled the industrial towns and cities of Europe and America. It was vividly portrayed in the novels of Charles Dickens and Elizabeth Gaskell. It was debated by politicians and later studied by historians as the 'Social Question of the Nineteenth Century'. But in Scotland it was a problem that lingered long into the twentieth century, leaving behind such a legacy of poor health among the population that Scotland still remains the 'Sick Man of Western Europe'. In the history of medicine in Scotland in the hundred years that preceded the Second World War (1939–1945) there are two dominant and concurrent themes: the struggle to reduce Scotland's continuing burden of poor health and Scotland's remarkable contribution to the advance of medical science and practice.

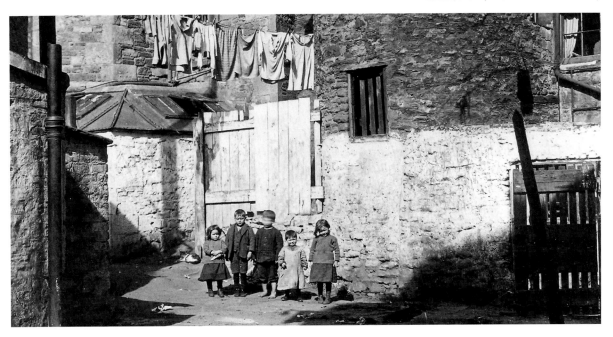

4.2 Children in Milne's Close, Overgate, Dundee, c1920 (*National Museum of Scotland*).

URBAN SICKNESS: THE RESPONSE OF THE STATE

The urbanisation of Scotland had accelerated in the first decades of the nineteenth century. By 1840, one in three of the population lived in a town and almost one in five in one of the large cities, Glasgow, Edinburgh, Dundee or Aberdeen. In less than a generation the death rate in Scotland had risen from 25 per thousand to 35 per thousand. The chief causes of death were cholera, typhus, measles, scarlet fever, diphtheria and 'consumption' (tuberculosis), all diseases fostered and made deadly by overcrowding and poor nutrition.

Life in dismal slums from which normal sunlight was excluded had led to the emergence of rickets as a major cause of sickness and deformity among children; unhygienic living conditions had inevitably resulted in a cruelly high infant mortality. And it was clear that the affliction of ill-health was at its worst in the towns.

In 1840, in his *Observations on the Management of the Poor and its Effect on the Health of the Great Towns*, W. P. Alison (1790–1859), a former president of the Royal College of Physicians of Edinburgh, insisted that the priority in improving the health of the masses in the industrial towns must be the prevention or relief of poverty. This was not a view that was shared in England.

In England the growing number of the poor was perceived as a threat to the well-being of the nation. First, the cost of maintaining the poor was thought to have become intolerable. Second, the diseases nurtured in the squalid slums of the poor were seen as a threat to the well-being of the gainfully employed majority of the public on whom the prosperity of the nation depended. To meet the first of these evils a Poor Law (Amendment) Act was passed in 1834. It was the work of a civil servant, Edwin Chadwick, a devotee of the Utilitarian principle of procuring the 'greatest benefit for the greatest number'. To reduce the cost of maintaining the nation's poor, support was only to be offered to those paupers who were willing to remain confined in a workhouse; and to keep the number seeking such help as low as possible, the workhouses were to be made as grim, forbidding and prison-like as possible.

To remove the risk of the spread of disease from the slums to the general public, Chadwick contrived the passage of a Public Health Act in 1848. Like many in England at that time, he believed that the chief source of disease was miasma, the noxious effluvium from urban

Rickets

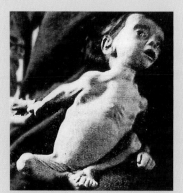

4.3 Severe rickets in infancy, often complicated by respiratory or other infections,
could result in death (*RCPEd*).

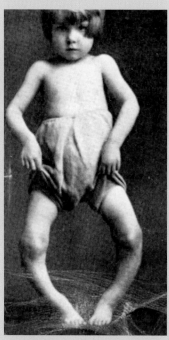

4.4 In children already old enough to stand
and walk, the weight of the body of the
upright child caused the bones of the legs
to buckle into the characteristic bowing
deformity (*from Forfar and Arneil*, Textbook
of Paediatrics, *Edinburgh, 1984*).

Rickets is usually first seen to affect children at the time when they might be expected to begin to walk. They become cross, irritable and restless. Their muscles become weak and flabby. But the chief abnormality is the distortion of their bones, most obviously the bones of the legs and the chest. The legs become bowed and the ribcage acquires a typical 'pouter pigeon' deformity. The disease is rarely fatal, but when it subsides as the child grows older or responds to active treatment, it often leaves behind deformities that persist for life.

Rickets had been known for centuries, but it became common in industrial towns in Britain, Europe and the United States in the nineteenth century. In the early twentieth century rickets had become particularly common in the industrial towns of the west of Scotland, where its incidence among children under five had risen as high as 70%.

When the Medical Research Committee was formed in 1912, one of its first projects was to study the great problem of infantile rickets, and Glasgow was chosen as the main centre for research. Leonard Finlay (1878–1947), physician at the Royal Hospital for Sick Children (and later Professor of Child Health), and Noel Paton (1859–1928), Professor of Physiology, were commissioned to carry out the research. On the basis of extensive clinical studies they concluded that, although it was well known that rickets could be cured by the oral administration of cod liver oil, it was caused by the living conditions of the children, enclosed in overcrowded tenements and without normal exposure to sunlight.

Their conclusions were effectively challenged in 1917 by Edward Mellanby in Cambridge who, in a series of laboratory studies on dogs, claimed that rickets was due to a dietary deficiency of a fat-soluble Accessory Food Factor, later identified as Vitamin D. The Medical Research Committee accepted Mellanby's results and his interpretations, and in 1920 Glasgow was dropped as its chosen centre for research on rickets. It was not until 1973 that it was shown that, even in subjects taking oral supplements of Vitamin D, over 80% of the active Vitamin D circulating in the blood was produced in the skin by the irradiation of ergosterols by sunlight.

filth. His Public Health Act made provision for a programme of sewerage and drainage which he was confident would eliminate miasma from all the towns and cities of England and Wales. Not only would slums cease to be breeding grounds of disease, the spread of disease would be entirely prevented. Chadwick had very little respect for the medical profession. He was confident that following the abolition of miasma by his programme of sanitary engineering, doctors would become redundant; doctors, he claimed, were 'necessary evils not likely to last'. In neither his Poor Law (Amendment) Act nor in his Public Health Act did Chadwick make any provision for medical services for the poor.

It had been the Government's intention that the

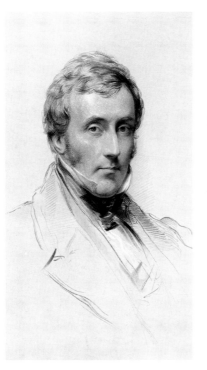

4.5 *Right.* W. P. Alison (1790–1859) was born at Boroughmuirhead on the outskirts of Edinburgh. His family members were all active supporters of social reform. He was enrolled as a student at Edinburgh University when aged only twelve and began his medical studies when aged seventeen, graduating MD in 1811. At the age of twenty-nine, he was appointed Professor of Medical Jurisprudence and Medical Police at Edinburgh University. In his most influential work, *Observations on the Management of the Poor in Scotland* (1840), he argued that the ill health suffered by the poor was not, as was commonly believed, caused by the 'miasma' rising from the rotting debris in filthy streets, but came as the result of their low pay, periods of unemployment and chronic poverty (*Wellcome Library, London*).

4.6 *Far right.* Slum landlords, who were often poor themselves, were very often reluctant to invest in costly repairs to their properties. Without the necessary financial resources, their tenements almost inevitably fell into decay (*Mitchell Library, Glasgow*).

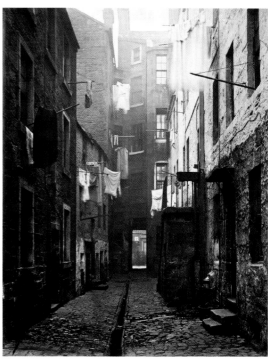

provisions of Chadwick's Poor Law (Amendment) Act and the Public Health Act of 1848 should be extended north of the Border. But this was successfully resisted by public opinion in Scotland led and inspired by W. P. Alison. Reformers in Scotland were not persuaded by Chadwick's Utilitarian ideology, and completely discounted miasma as a cause of the diseases of the poor. Since the eighteenth century medical students in Scotland had been taught that poverty – through poor diet, inadequate clothing and shelter, over-work and overcrowding – led to a state of 'debility' that was at the root of the health problems of the urban working class. Alison argued that any new Poor Law for Scotland must include support for the able-bodied poor, so that when deprived of employment for whatever reason they and their families would not be reduced through debility, depression and disease to pauperism. He stressed that appropriate support for the able-bodied poor must include medical aid when they were sick and temporarily unemployed. Equally, those who had become paupers because of ill health must have access to the medical treatment that might allow them to return to work. He proposed that new poorhouses should be built, not as the places of harsh confinement introduced in England by Chadwick but as places of refuge; and every new poorhouse was to include hospital wards to serve not only the pauper inmates but also the local poor.

However, when a Poor Law (Scotland) Amendment Act was passed in 1845, it fell far short of Alison's vision. The Act transferred responsibility for the administration of the Poor Law from the Kirk to the state. Lay Parochial Boards were set up to raise funds, by local assessment if necessary, to provide aid for the indigent poor, but not, as Alison had proposed, for the able-bodied but unemployed poor to prevent them falling into debility pauperism. However, the Act did offer those pauperised by ill health some assistance to recover their ability to work, by providing 'medicines, medical attendance, nutritious diet, cordials and clothing for such poor and in such a manner and to such an extent as seemed equitable and expedient.' In Edinburgh a Board of Supervision, chaired by Sir John McNeil, was created as an advisory body, but Parochial Boards were allowed considerable discretion in how they implemented the provisions of the Act.

In the House of Commons, Scottish members protested that the medical provisions of the Act were inadequate and in 1848 the Government agreed to make an annual grant of £10,000 to the Board of Supervision to provide a financial supplement of £20 for every parish ready to provide an equal sum to employ its own Poor Law medical officer. The Chairman of the Board of Supervision was confident that, with this inducement, parish medical officers would be established to care for the poor in every parish in Scotland. From 1848, Scotland had its first, embryo, state medical service.

THE MEDICAL PROFESSION AND MEDICAL SERVICES

In 1845 there were 1,157 medical men licensed to practice in Scotland. Of these, 557 held university medical degrees; 600 were licentiates of the Royal College of Surgeons of Edinburgh or one of the other Royal Medical Corporations. In relation to the number of its population, Scotland had more qualified medical practitioners (approximately 1 for every 2,500) than other parts of Britain and the British Empire. In addition there were many (a large but now unknowable number) men in medical practice in Scotland who had studied medicine at a university or at an extra-mural medical school but had never graduated or sought a licence from any of the many licensing bodies in Britain.

Medicine in Scotland in the nineteenth century was an overcrowded profession. Every practitioner was wholly dependent for his income on the fees he could earn from his patients; a fashionable and prestigious physician in Edinburgh might receive a fee of £300 from a single patient; a practitioner in a rural village might hope for an annual income of more than the £30 or £40 earned by the local school master but decidedly less than the stipend of £150 to £200 received by the parish minister. But there were many parts of rural Scotland where the population was widely scattered and so poor that no doctor could hope to establish a practice from which he could earn a living. The effect of the Poor Law (Scotland) Amendment Act on the provision of medical services in one such remote area became the subject of an inquiry carried out by the Royal College of Physicians of Edinburgh in 1850.

In the Highlands and Islands of Scotland the population was scattered over 14,000 square miles of rugged and difficult territory. Nevertheless, at one time it had been possible for a small number of medical men to establish modest practices at least in the market towns and larger villages. But in the economic depression that came with the end of the Napoleonic Wars in 1815 the people of the region began to suffer increasing poverty, and many of these practitioners, no longer able to make ends meet, had been forced to leave. Then, only a year after the introduction of the new Poor Law, the people of the Highlands and Islands were further 'blasted by providence'. The

Medical Graduates in Britain

From their foundation, Scotland's ancient universities had the right to grant degrees in medicine. But for some three centuries these powers were rarely exercised, and none of the Scottish universities offered students a comprehensive education in medical subjects. Scots wishing to study medicine were therefore obliged to travel to the universities of Padua and Montpellier, or later to Leiden and other universities in Northern Europe. It was not until 1726 that Edinburgh University established a faculty of medicine. The universities of Glasgow, Aberdeen and St Andrews later followed Edinburgh's lead, and by the early part of the nineteenth century all four were offering instruction in every branch of medicine. The training available at the Scottish university medical schools was not only convenient for Scottish students; its quality attracted students from every part of the English speaking world, including England itself. Oxford and Cambridge offered only theoretical library-based studies of medicine and until 1871 accepted only students who were members of the Church of England. The vast majority of England's doctors received their training at the great London teaching hospitals and were granted their licences to practice by the Royal College of Surgeons of England or the Royal College of Physicians of London. For over a hundred years, until the establishment of the English provincial university medical schools late in the nineteenth century, the majority of medical graduates practising in Britain were the products of Scottish universities.

blight that had been devastating potato crops in Ireland spread to Scotland. But the great loss of life from starvation and disease that had resulted in Ireland was not repeated in the Highlands and Islands. There the landlords had, for the most part, acted responsibly, and the Free Church of Scotland and other charitable bodies in Scotland and England had shipped in enough meal to prevent deaths from hunger and typhus. Nevertheless the famine had caused deep and widespread distress. The Royal College of Physicians in Edinburgh received reports that a major cause of that distress was the frequent inability of the people 'to procure the services of a medical man'.

An inquiry conducted by the College revealed that the 370,000 people resident in the Highlands and Islands were served by only 133 'medical men' and of these, 34 held no recognised medical qualification. The distribution of these 133 practitioners bore little relation to the parish structure of the region. No fewer than 92 parishes had no resident doctor, although several reported that, if absolutely necessary, they could call on the services of a doctor from a neighbouring parish. As many as 41 parishes were 'never visited by any regular practitioner and may therefore be regarded as destitute of medical aid'. It became clear that, in the absence of medical practitioners, the poor of the parishes looked to the parish ministers for assistance. Many of the parish ministers had attended at least some medical classes as part of their training for the ministry at Edinburgh or Glasgow and were able to provide some comfort and advice. However, in many parishes the people felt severely the want of properly skilled surgical help in such emergencies as accidents, injuries at work and abnormal obstetrical deliveries.

When the Royal College of Physicians of Edinburgh published its *Statement Regarding the Deficiency of Medical Practitioners* in 1852, it reported that in the Highlands and Islands the government scheme to recruit a medical practitioner to care for the poor in every parish had not been as successful as had been hoped. No similar investigations were carried out elsewhere in Scotland, but it may be assumed that the scheme in which the government and Sir John McNeil had such confidence was proving no more successful in other sparsely populated rural parts of Scotland.

Place of Training of Medical Graduates Practising in Britain

	Oxford/ Cambridge	Europe	Scotland
1600–1650	599	36	0
1650–1700	933	197	36
1700–1750	617	385	406
1750–1800	246	194	2,594
1800–1850	273	29	7,989

VISITS

	From	To
The first Visit in Town or advice at Practitioner's Residence,	£0 2 6	£0 10 6
Subsequent Attendance, to be according to it is length and the Social Position of the Patient,		
Night Visit	0 5 0	1 1 0
Visit to the Country, at any distance not exceeding Two Miles	0 5 0	and upwd.
For every additional Mile, from	0 1 6	0 5 0
Night Visits to Country to be Doubled.		

Every hour that the Practitioner is detained, either from urgency of the case, or desire of the Patient or Friends,   £0 2 6   0 5 0

It is understood that these Fees should be paid at them time of Visit, or when the attendance terminates.

| Ordinary Fee for Consultation | £1 0 0 | 3 3 0 |

The Fee for consultation or other Medical attendance, when the Practitioner is not the one regularly employed by the Family, is expected to be paid at the time of visit.

| Ordinary Medical Certificate, | £0 2 6 | 0 10 6 |
| Lunacy Certificate. | 1 1 0 | |

SURGICAL OPERATIONS AND MIDWIFERY

Vaccination, Extraction of Teeth, Cupping, Bleeding, and other minor Operations	£0 2 6	0 10 6
Operations of Hydrocele, Harelip, Tapping, Excision of Small Tumours, Amputation of Toes, Finger, &c	0 5 0	2 2 0
Reducing Fractures and Dislocations,	0 10 6	3 3 0
Capital Operations, viz: Amputation, Trepanning, Aneurism, Extirpation of Mamma, Lithotomy, Lithotrity,	2 2 0	21 0 0
Necessary Assistance at Operations,	1 1 0	2 2 0
Delivery in Ordinary Cases,	1 1 0	10 10 0
Do. in Difficult or Protracted Cases	1 11 6	10 10 0

In all cases of Operations and Midwifery, the Fee may be paid at the time, and to be independent of future visits.

4.7 This list of recommended doctor's fees was drawn up by the medical practitioners of the Banff, Moray and Nairn Medical Association in 1864. The list was published in the local newspapers (*reproduced from J. Jenkinson, Scottish Medical Societies, Edinburgh, 1993*).

The Regulation of the Medical Profession in Britain

In the first half of the nineteenth century, a great many of those offering medical and surgical services were unlicensed charlatans. But even among those medical practitioners who had obtained a licence to practise from a 'legitimate and proper source', there were many who were poorly educated, inadequately trained and professionally incompetent. There were no fewer than twenty different authorities in Great Britain and Ireland with the power to grant licences to practitioners. Each one set its own standards for its licentiates, and in some cases these standards were so low as to defeat the purpose of the licensing system. There were also great anomalies in the privileges and rights of the various licensing bodies. The Archbishop of Canterbury could grant a licence to practise anywhere in England, Wales or Ireland; only the Royal College of Physicians could grant a licence to practise in London; graduates of London University could practise anywhere in England except London; the Faculty of Physicians and Surgeons of Glasgow could grant a licence to practise in the counties of the see of the ancient Bishops of Glasgow; those granted (often without examination) a medical degree by St Andrews were entitled to practise anywhere in Scotland.

After many years of negotiation and controversy, a Medical Act was passed in 1858 listing the nineteen bodies with the right to grant licences to practise anywhere in Great Britain and Ireland. These were: the universities of Oxford, Cambridge, Durham and London in England; St Andrews, Glasgow, Aberdeen and Edinburgh in Scotland; the University of Dublin and Queens University of Belfast in Ireland; the Royal College of Physicians, the Royal College of Surgeons and the Society of Apothecaries in England; the Royal College of Physicians of Edinburgh, the Royal College of Surgeons of Edinburgh and the Faculty of Physicians and Surgeons of Glasgow in Scotland; The King and Queen's College of Physicians in Ireland, the Royal College of Surgeons of Ireland and the Apothecaries' Hall in Ireland. The Act also established a General Medical Council to ensure that common standards were established and maintained, and to keep a Medical Register of all those entitled to practise.

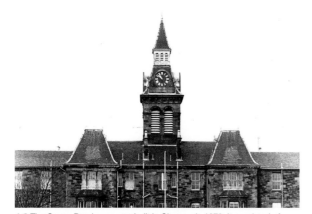

4.8 The Govan Poorhouse was built in Glasgow in 1872. It consisted of a poorhouse, a lunatic asylum and a hospital. On the creation of the National Health Service in 1948 it became the Southern General Hospital. St Cuthbert's Poorhouse, built in Edinburgh at the same time, became the Western General Hospital (*Glasgow Caledonian University*).

The measures in the Poor Law (Scotland) Amendment Act for the creation of hospital services for the poor in new large poorhouses were also falling short of expectations. Only four such poorhouses were ever built, and they were built only in Glasgow and Edinburgh. Although the Act had achieved much less than Alison and his fellow reformers had hoped, the recruitment of Poor Law medical officers in most, if not yet all, parishes in Scotland and the establishment of a permanent central Board of Supervision in Edinburgh marked the first stage in the creation of state medical services in Britain. After the creation of the National Health Service in 1948, the Govan Poor House in Glasgow became the Southern General Hospital and St Cuthbert's Poor House in Edinburgh became the Western General Hospital.

QUERIES.

1. How many Medical Men practise within the Parish of *Contin*?	*None*
2. The Names and Addresses of these.	—
3. Has the number increased or diminished of late years?	*There has never been one resident, in so far as I know*
4. Have any left the Parish since you became connected with it? If so, for what reasons?	*No*
6. Is there any complaint among the people of inadequacy in the supply of Medical aid?	*Not that I have heard. Indeed some of the people (especially those in mountainous parts) have an ignorant prejudice against medical aid.*
5. Do you know of any cases of protracted suffering, or of injury by Accident, such as might have been alleviated had proper advice been at hand?	*In a Parish from 30 to 40 miles long, without a resident medical man, such cases have no doubts occurred, and may be expected to occur again*
7. To what extent is the deficiency of qualified practitioners made up by the efforts of other parties?	*By the benevolence of certain individuals, and the services of a most skilful Physician appointed by the Parochial Board*
8. Does your experience enable you to suggest any measure—of general applicability—such as would be likely to relieve to some extent the evils (if they exist) of deficiency in the supply of Medical aid?	*No, for the Parish is chiefly Pastoral, with a scattered population. Those in the lower part of it are within 8 miles of the town of Dingwall where several medical gentlemen practise*
9. What Heritors are resident, either generally or occasionally, in your Parish?	*Sir James Mackenzie of Scatwell Bart. - Captn. Douglas of Meikle Scatwell - and Mr. Balfour of Whittingham*

C. D. Bayne Minister

4.9 *Above.* A questionnaire sent by the Royal College of Physicians of Edinburgh to ministers and to the 133 medical men known to be practising in the crofting counties of the Highlands and Islands in 1850. The aim was to assess the extent to which the people of the region had access to medical attention (*Royal College of Physicians of Edinburgh*).

4.10 *Right.* The early stethoscope was a simple wooden tube short enough to be carried under the physician's tall hat (*Wellcome Library, London*).

MEDICAL CARE IN THE EARLY NINETEENTH CENTURY

The French Revolution at the end of the eighteenth century had brought radical change in the study and practice of medicine. Hospitals were removed from the hands of the Church and the vast hospitals in Paris (totalling over 20,000 beds) came under the control of salaried clinically and academically ambitious physicians. Together they shifted the emphasis in the study of medicine from the library to the bedside, from the assimilation of the classical medical texts to the careful observation of the patient and the accumulation of personal experience of the presentation and course of their diseases. The clinical examination of patients was made more precise and informative by the introduction of new methods of examination, notably the auscultation of the chest using Laennec's stethoscope, and Auenbrugger's technique of percussion of the chest. Should the patients die, the study of their cases was completed in the post-mortem room. From the early years of the nineteenth century, students and practitioners from Europe and America flocked in their thousands to Paris to be taught this new approach to the practice of medicine. Later, from the 1840s, in university laboratories in France and Germany, animal experiments added significantly to the understanding of human physiology and disease.

The innovations in clinical examination came slowly and somewhat obliquely to Scotland. Auenbrugger (1722–1809) published his *Inventum Novum* in 1767; William Cullen (1710–1790) Professor of the Practice of Physic at

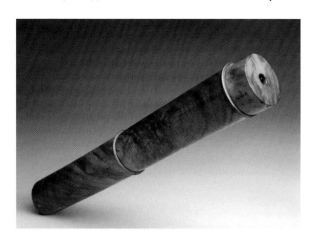

Sir James Clark (1788–1870)

Sir James Clark was born at Cullen in Aberdeenshire. After graduating MA at Aberdeen he studied medicine at Edinburgh, becoming a licentiate of the Royal College of Surgeons in 1809. He served as a surgeon in the Royal Navy until the end of the Napoleonic Wars. Thereafter he settled in Rome, where he established a practice among wealthy and fashionable British patients seeking treatment for phthisis (pulmonary tuberculosis) in the congenial climate of southern Europe. On a visit to Carlsbad he met Prince Leopold (later King of the Belgians), who appointed him as his physician. Clark returned to London in 1826, and on the recommendation of Prince Leopold, in 1834 he became physician to the Duchess of Kent and her daughter Princess Victoria; and after her succession, physician to the young Queen Victoria.

At court in 1839, Clark became involved in a major scandal. Lady Flora Hastings, a Lady-in-Waiting, was noticed to have a growing swelling of her abdomen. Although she was unmarried, it became rumoured that she was pregnant. To quash the rumours, she agreed to be examined by Sir James Clark assisted by the royal accoucheur, Sir Charles Clarke. They found that she appeared to be *virgo intacta*, but acknowledged to the Queen that this did not necessarily prove that she was not pregnant. To the great distress of the Hastings family the rumours continued. When Lady Flora Hastings died only weeks after she had been examined by Clark, it was found that she was not pregnant but had a cancer of her liver.

From the beginning the scandal had been widely reported in the press. Sir James Clark was publically disgraced, but to widespread surprise the Queen did not discharge him from her service.

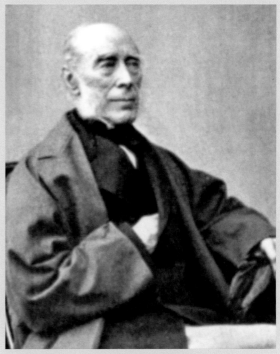

4.11 Sir James Clark (1788–1870) Physician to Queen Victoria (*Wellcome Library, London*).

Edinburgh, was not greatly impressed and the technique was not taught with any enthusiasm in Scotland until the 1820s. Rene Laennec (1781–1826) published his *Traite de l'auscultation médiate* in 1819; it was translated into English by Sir John Forbes (1787–1861), but his interest was in the pulmonary pathology described by Laennec and he had to be persuaded by his friend Sir James Clark to try Laennec's stethoscope. The use of the stethoscope added nothing to what could be heard by applying the ear to the patient's chest, but as this was disagreeable to the physician and often offensive to the patient, the stethoscope soon became popular.

However these various advances in diagnosis and in prognosis were not immediately reflected in improvements in the treatment of the common diseases of the time. Even the most successful physicians were still severely limited in what they could achieve for their patients. They could offer sound advice on the maintenance of a healthy lifestyle. When the patient was ill they could make a more accurate diagnosis than ever before. But there were no specific cures. Physicians could prescribe medicines intended to ease their patient's symptoms, but the very large number of alternative medicaments listed in the pharmacopoeias of the time indicates that only a few were effective and reliable. For many physicians it was normal practice, when one elaborate and

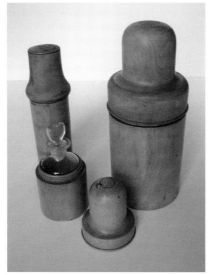

4.12 Glass medicine bottles were enclosed in wooden cases to protect them from damage when being carried in the doctor's saddlebags when he visited his patients on horseback (*Private Collection*).

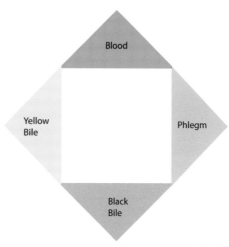

4.13 This diagram represents the supposed relationship of the four bodily humours, blood, phlegm, yellow bile and black bile, which in classical Hippocratic theory, must be kept in perfect balance to ensure good health.

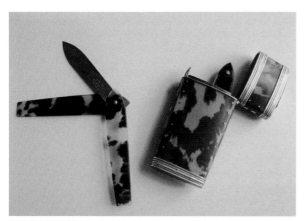

4.14 For centuries bleeding the patient by opening a vein was the recommended form of treatment for many disorders. The necessary lancets were often carried in the doctor's waistcoat pocket in an elegant case. The cases were often made of silver or, as in this case, silver-mounted tortoiseshell (*Private Collection*).

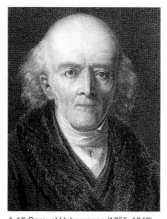

4.15 Samuel Hahnemann (1755–1843) was born in Meissen and studied medicine in Leipzig and in Vienna. In 1796, he published a principle of his own invention, based on the 'law of similarities' or 'like cures like'. In his new 'homoeopathic' system the patient was given a very highly diluted solution of a substance that was known to cause the same symptoms as those suffered in his illness. Homoeopathy is still practised to a very limited extent in Scotland (*Wellcome Library, London*).

possibly expensive medicament failed, to add another and, when that too failed, to add a third followed possibly by a fourth. Few physicians could be content with such polypharmacy; many even of the most eminent still resorted on occasion to ancient expedients based on the Hippocratic concept of disease as an imbalance of the four bodily humours – blood, phlegm, yellow bile and black bile. Patients were treated by bleeding (either by the lancet or by the application of leeches) or the administration of drugs to cause vigorous evacuation of the bowels. But some physicians, frustrated by the inadequacy of conventional therapeutics, dared to take up the unorthodox practices of homoeopathy or mesmerism.

Homoeopathy

The founder of homoeopathy, Samuel Hahnemann (1755–1843) had studied medicine at Leipzig and Vienna, but his studies had provided him with no universal principle according to which all cases of all diseases could be treated. Without such a single guiding principle he had felt unable to practise. Nevertheless he had continued to theorise and eventually formulated a principle based on two counter-intuitive ideas. First, that a disease should be treated by administering a substance that, if administered to a healthy person, would produce the same symptoms as the disease; second, that the effectiveness of such a substance would be improved, not by increasing the dose,

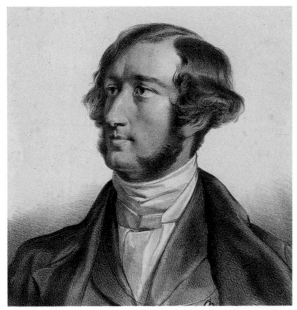

4.16 William Henderson (1810–1872) was born at Thurso in Caithness. He graduated from Edinburgh University and later studied at Paris, Berlin and Vienna. In 1842 he became Professor of Pathology at Edinburgh University and Physician at Edinburgh Royal Infirmary. Shortly after his appointment he was a convert to homoeopathy, and despite opposition, played an important part in introducing homoeopathy more widely in Britain (*Wellcome Library, London*).

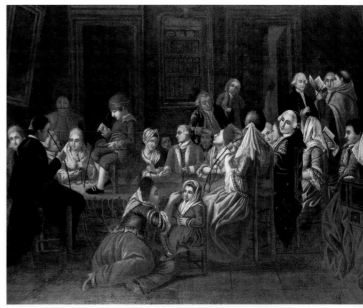

4.17 A group of mesmerised French patients. This painting shows Mesmer, background right, touching a friar with a magnetised rod. The black tubes held by other patients contain magnetised fluid. These tubes were applied to the diseased part of the body in the hope of a cure (*Wellcome Library, London*).

but by diminishing it. Armed with this principle he again took up medical practice. His ideas attracted some support among the many, both doctors and patients, who were dissatisfied with conventional forms of treatment. Most physicians of the time found Hahnemann's homoeopathy absurd, and after Hahnemann's death it came to seem even more absurd. By the late 1840s, it was accepted by even the most committed homoeopathic practitioners that the strict observance of Hahnemann's principles should not be observed in cases 'when life seems almost extinguished' or in difficult diseases such as syphilis. In such cases effective conventional treatment must be used. Nevertheless, for some homoeopathy had become not a science but a faith. In the United States, candidates for admission as members of one homoeopathic institute were required to swear 'by our Saviour Jesus Christ not to treat patients but by medicaments which are in the domain of pure homoeopathy'.

In Scotland, interest in homoeopathy centred principally in Glasgow. However, one of the first homoeopathic dispensaries was founded in Edinburgh in 1841, and it was in Edinburgh that the system was most actively resisted. Andrew Wood, secretary of the Royal College of Physi-

cians, published a pamphlet, *Homoeopathy Unmasked,* which he hoped 'would put down that miserable humbug'. However, a number of Edinburgh physicians persisted in practising as homoeopathists, and when they were joined in 1844 by William Henderson, Professor of Pathology at Edinburgh University and physician at Edinburgh Royal Infirmary, 'the consternation manifested by the Medical Faculty of the University and by the Royal College of Physicians was such as might be exhibited in ecclesiastical circles if the Professor of Divinity were to announce that he had become a Mohammedan.' James Syme, as Dean of the Faculty of Medicine, attempted to have him removed from his Chair. However, Henderson defended his position in a pamphlet, *An Inquiry into the Homoeopathic Practice of Medicine.*

After a bitter and prolonged dispute, Henderson was allowed to continue as Professor of Pathology, but he was barred from clinical teaching and patient care at Edinburgh Royal Infirmary. And in 1851, the Royal Colleges of Physicians and of Surgeons in Edinburgh and the Faculty of Physicians and Surgeons of Glasgow announced that they would decline to admit homoeopathic practitioners as Fellows, and decreed that Fellows of the Colleges and

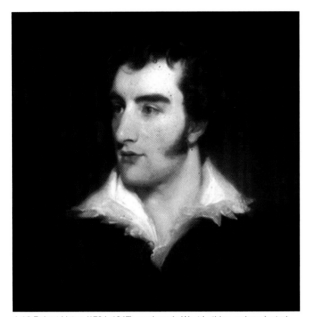

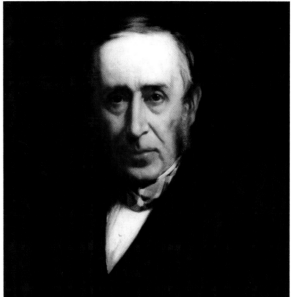

4.18 Robert Liston (1794–1847) was born in West Lothian and graduated from Edinburgh University in 1815. In 1818, after further study in London, he was appointed as a surgeon at Edinburgh Royal Infirmary. His speed and dexterity became legendary, and it was said that he could amputate a leg in 28 seconds. He was popular with his students and patients but he was quarrelsome and much disliked by his fellow surgeons. In 1834 he left Edinburgh to become Professor of Clinical Surgery at London University (*RCSEd*).

4.19 James Syme (1799–1870) was one of the leading British surgeons in the nineteenth century. He graduated MD in 1820 and quickly built up an extensive practice as a surgeon. When he failed to be appointed to the staff of Edinburgh Royal Infirmary he opened a surgical hospital of his own at Minto House. In 1833 he was appointed to the Regius Chair of Clinical Surgery at Edinburgh and to the staff of the Edinburgh Royal Infirmary (*RCSEd*).

Faculty should not meet practitioners of homoeopathy in consultation or co-operation. Nevertheless, homoeopathy continued to be practised in Scotland and homoeopathic hospitals are still supported by the National Health Service.

Mesmerism

The craze of mesmerism had its origins in the concepts of Franz Anton Mesmer, an Austrian physician practising in the 1790s. It was introduced in Britain by Professor John Elliotson of London University in 1837. At a series of meetings at University College Hospital, Elliotson 'demonstrated' that, by making certain hand movements, he was able to influence his subject's nervous system supposedly by the penetration of an invisible magnetic fluid. Elliotson's demonstrations were later exposed as fraudulent and he was forced to resign from his chair. Nevertheless, a few unorthodox surgeons found that, in some cases, mesmerism (alternatively 'animal magnetism' or 'hypnotism') seemed to be capable of inducing a degree of anaesthesia sufficient for minor operations. Two Scottish surgeons, James Braid (1795–1825), practising in Dumfries and later in Manchester, and James Esdaile (1808–1859), in India, reported considerable success in

using the technique. But in the 1840s and 1850s a number of other surgeons in Scotland who experimented in the use of mesmerism failed to repeat their experience. By then more reliable anaesthetics were being introduced.

Surgery

In the first decades of the nineteenth century, the practice of surgery was still constrained by the patients' limited capacity to endure pain. Surgeons treated patients who had suffered fractures or other accidental injuries; they opened and drained abscesses; they treated ulcers and other chronic skin disorders. They might open the bladder to remove a stone, but they would almost never dare to open any other of the body's major cavities; disorders within these closed cavities were left to the care of the practitioners in internal medicine, the physicians.

Even at the largest and most famous hospitals, only a handful of major operations (the amputation of a limb or the excision of a cancerous breast) were performed each month. Most of the most illustrious Scottish surgeons of the time are also remembered as teachers of anatomy. Those who rose to fame in the operating theatre were those who could successfully perform agonising opera-

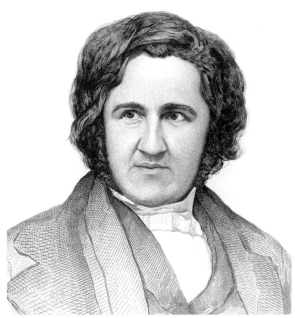

4.20 Sir James Y. Simpson Bart. (1811–1870), seen here as a young man, was born into a prosperous and socially ambitious family in West Lothian. He studied medicine at Edinburgh, graduating MD in 1832. By the age of twenty-nine he was Professor of Midwifery at Edinburgh; in 1847 he was made a Physician to Queen Victoria, in 1850 he was elected President of the Royal College of Physicians of Edinburgh and in 1866 he was made a baronet. By then he had been the most famous physician in Europe for almost forty years. He is best remembered for his pioneering of general anaesthesia, his introduction of chloroform and the use of general anaesthesia in childbirth (*RCPE*).

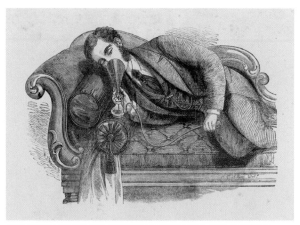

4.21 For many years, first ether, and later chloroform, were popular as recreational drugs. Illustrated is an apparatus designed and sold specifically for the recreational inhalation of chloroform (*reproduced from Linda Stratman,* Chloroform, The Quest for Oblivion. *Sutton, 2005*).

tions in the shortest possible time – Robert Liston (1794–1847), who could amputate a limb in less than a minute; James Syme (1799–1870), who could amputate at the ankle quickly and 'without a wasted word or a drop of blood' (see pp. 123–4); Sir William Fergusson Bt. (1808–77), who could extract a stone from the bladder in 30 seconds.

But whatever the speed and dexterity of the surgeon, few patients were willing to submit to surgery except in extreme necessity. Every operation offered the dreadful prospect of being forced to lie physically restrained and struggling to repress screams of agony.

General Anaesthesia

The introduction of general anaesthesia in 1847 was welcomed as a seemingly miraculous blessing. The anaesthetic properties of certain gases had first been recognised at the Pneumatic Medical Institute in Bristol where Thomas Beddoes and his assistant Humphry Davy were searching for inhalable gases that might relieve the symptoms of patients suffering from tuberculosis and other respiratory diseases. In 1800, Davy discovered that when

nitrous oxide was inhaled it had both exhilarating and analgesic effects. He suggested that it might be used to relieve the pain of very minor surgical operations; but he gave it the name 'laughing gas', and it was as 'laughing gas' that, for the next forty years and more, it was inhaled by the dashing and fashionable as an after-dinner amusement.

Meanwhile Beddoes had been investigating the medicinal properties of ether. His patients had discovered that it had soothing and mildly intoxicating effects, and it had later become a popular recreational drug in fashionable society both in Britain and America. It was not until 1846 that a dentist practising in Boston, William T. G. Morton, used it successfully to anaesthetise patients having teeth extracted. Later, at Massachusetts General Hospital, a public trial of ether as a general anaesthetic for general surgery was a complete success. The news that an inhalable gas had been found that could abolish the pain of surgery was quickly carried to Britain and Europe.

Among the first surgeons in Britain to use ether was Robert Liston, an Edinburgh graduate and formerly a successful surgeon in Edinburgh, but now Professor of

Clinical Surgery at London University (see p.*** [Chapter 3]). On 21 December 1846, Liston successfully amputated the leg of a man at the level of mid-thigh; having inhaled ether, the patient remained quiet, unresisting and oblivious of pain.

The immense significance of what had been witnessed was at once widely understood. However, many surgeons feared that to use this new and unknown drug was to add yet another risk to an already dangerous procedure. Others, particularly military surgeons, believed that the pain during operations acted as an essential stimulus to post-operative recovery; surgeons in the army of the United States were forbidden to administer ether when operating on casualties of the war with Mexico in 1846–48.

More substantial and practical objections to ether were that the gas was unpleasant and irritant to the patient's respiratory passages, and the apparatus required to administer it was clumsy, making it inconvenient for use in the patient's home. In the summer of 1847, James Y. Simpson (1811–70), Professor of Midwifery at Edinburgh, began a search for a new inhalable anaesthetic that patients would find more agreeable than ether and that their doctors would find more convenient to administer.

He explored the shelves of the university's laboratories, and took for testing samples of every volatile liquid that was to be found; friends, medical colleagues and local pharmacists suggested substances that they thought might possibly be the answer.

To test these various chemicals, Simpson chose a procedure that was foolhardy and even potentially lethal. Early in the morning or late in the evening, Simpson would meet his assistants, James Matthews Duncan (1826–1890) and George Keith (1819–1910), in the dining room of his house at 52 Queen Street, where they would pour the substances to be tested into saucers or tumblers, inhale their vapours and scribble notes on their effects.

The search had been unsuccessful until 18 October when Simpson received a visit from an old friend, David Waldie (1813–1889). They had been contemporaries as medical students at Edinburgh, but Waldie had chosen to make his career as a chemist in Liverpool. Waldie suggested to Simpson that the anaesthetic that he was searching for might be chloroform, the active component of an intoxicating cordial popular in the Eastern United States, and used in Liverpool in the treatment of asthma.

When, on 4 November 1847, a sample of chloroform supplied by Edinburgh's leading manufacturing chemists,

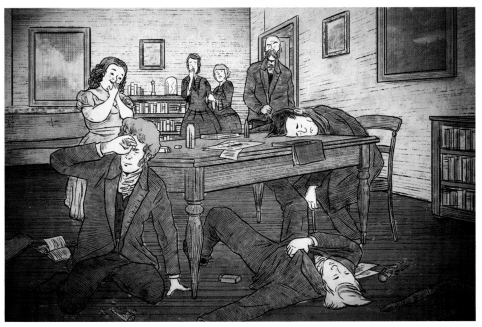

4.22 An artist's impression of the moment of discovery of the anaesthetic properties of chloroform by James Y. Simpson and his two assistants, James Matthews Duncan and George Keith. After all three have inhaled its vapour, Simpson is on his knees, Matthews Duncan is unconscious on the floor and Keith is asleep at the table. The moment was witnessed by Simpson's wife Jessie, his sister Williamina, his niece Agnes and his brother-in-law, Captain Petrie (*drawing by Dave Morrow*).

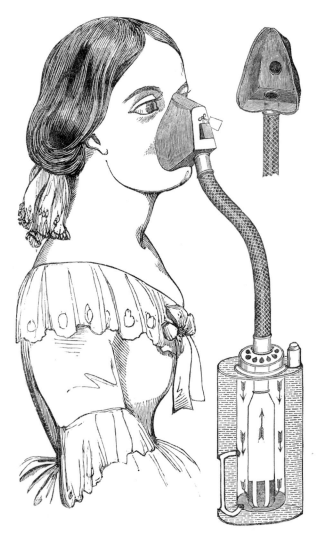

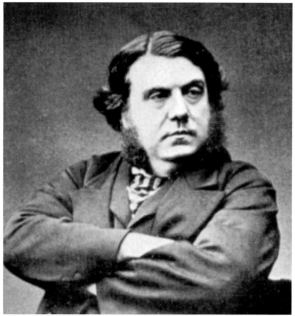

4.23 *Above.* Robert Lawson Tait (1845-1899) graduated from Edinburgh in 1866. Trained by James Y. Simpson and James Matthews Duncan, he was one of the first practising gynaecologists in Britain, introducing new operations for salpingectomy and ovariotomy. When a student he played on a similarity in appearance to claim that he was the illegitimate son of Simpson, although he was not in any way related to him. This led to a malicious rumour that Simpson had indeed fathered an illegitimate son, causing Simpson great distress (*Wellcome Library, London*).

4.24 *Left.* Simpson insisted that chloroform was best administered on a handkerchief held loosely over the patient's nose and mouth but others believed that it was necessary to use an inhaler that regulated the amount of chloroform. Illustrated is an inhaler invented in London by John Snow (*reproduced from Linda Stratman,* Chloroform, The Quest for Oblivion. *Sutton, 2005*).

Duncan, Flockhart & Co., was tested, George Keith was the first to inhale its vapour. Seeing his reaction, Simpson and Matthew Duncan immediately tried it for themselves. Simpson was the first to regain consciousness. While still on the floor he was heard to say that 'this is far stronger and better than ether.'

Six days later, on 10 November, Simpson administered chloroform for three surgical operations performed in the presence of an invited gathering of medical men at Edinburgh Royal Infirmary. This, the first public trial of his new anaesthetic, was completely successful, and that evening Simpson announced his discovery to a meeting of Edinburgh's Medico-Chirurgical Society. His success was immediately reported in the medical press, but Simpson expected that the conservative medical profession would be as over-cautious in accepting chloroform as they had been in accepting ether. Quickly, on 15 November, he published a pamphlet, *Account of a New Anaesthetic Agent as a Substitute for Sulphuric Ether in Surgery and Midwifery*, aimed chiefly at the lay public. In it he assured his readers that chloroform was 'infinitely more efficacious' than ether. It could be easily administered; it avoided the unpleasant inconveniencies of ether; it was inexpensive; and, above all, chloroform was safe: 'I tried it on myself.' Within weeks, his pamphlet had fully achieved its purpose. The general public had been alerted to his discovery of a new anaesthetic that was even better than ether, and patients were already demanding that their doctors should always have it available and should be ready to make full use of it. By the end of the year, established manufacturers were finding it difficult to satisfy the demand for chloroform, and new firms were being set up to produce it. Chloroform was already on its way to becoming the most widely used general anaesthetic in the British Empire, in Europe and in many parts of the United States.

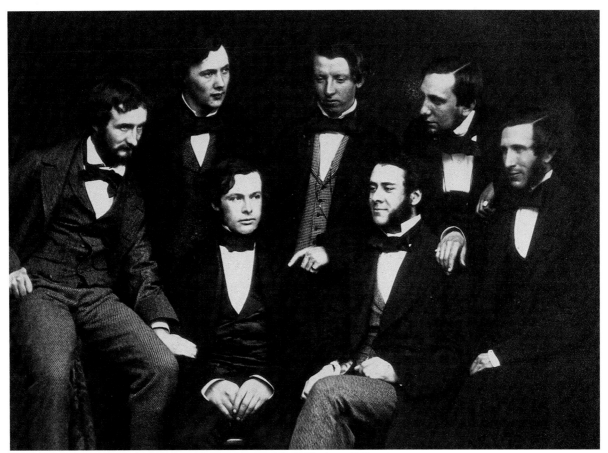

4.25 Resident House Surgeons at Edinburgh Royal Infirmary in 1854. John Beddoe (seated left), John Kirk (back row), Joseph Lister (seated in front row), George Pringle (back row), David Christison (seated), Patrick Heron Watson (back row), Alexander Struthers (seated right). Of those present only Lister, a Quaker, did not go as a volunteer surgeon to attend the sick and wounded in the 'Russian War' in the Crimea (*Wellcome Library, London*).

Anaesthesia in Surgery

The introduction of first ether and then chloroform as general anaesthetics transformed the practice of surgery. Under anaesthesia, operations were less hurried and much less stressful for the patients; survival rates after surgery improved sharply. Since operations could now be performed without pain, patients became more ready to accept the surgical treatment their disorders required. And surgeons could now devise new, more invasive, more complex and therefore more prolonged operations that would previously have been unthinkable. Scottish surgeons were quick to take advantage of the possibilities offered by general anaesthesia. Robert Lawson Tait (1845–99) was the first surgeon in Britain to remove an acutely inflamed appendix and the first to be successful in operating on the gall bladder to remove gall stones; John Lizars (1787–1860) was the first surgeon in Britain to open the abdomen to remove a tumour of the ovary.

Anaesthesia in Obstetrics

Within a week of his discovery of chloroform, Simpson had used it successfully in a number of difficult and life-threatening cases of childbirth. It soon became clear that other obstetricians needed little persuasion to use chloroform in prolonged and painful deliveries, especially when instruments were to be used. However, Simpson went on to advocate the use of chloroform to alleviate the pains of normal childbirth. Some obstetricians protested that to do so was to interfere quite improperly with what was a perfectly natural function. It was a view that Simpson briskly dismissed; however he expected that he would be confronted by another and a much more powerful objection. In 1847 he had used ether in a few cases of normal delivery, and a number of his professional colleagues had protested that to banish the pain suffered during parturition was contrary to religion and the express commands of Scripture. He had expected that after the publication of his *Account* of the uses of chloroform in 1848, this objection would be repeated and would be put forward more forcefully. He therefore prepared to meet the torrent of protest that he thought must surely come. In December 1848 he published a carefully argued pamphlet, his *Answer to the Religious Objections Advanced Against the Employment of Anaesthetic Agents in Midwifery and Surgery*, again aimed principally at the lay public; the pamphlet was published in Edinburgh and London and thousands of copies were sold. But to his surprise, the torrent of objections to his use of chloroform in normal childbirth did not arrive. Theologians and leaders of the Church of Scotland, the Free Church of Scotland and the Episcopal Church in Scotland all wrote to congratulate him. The Archbishop of Canterbury and the Moderator of the Church of Scotland also expressed approval of his arguments presented in his *Answer*. Simpson was soon able to write to a friend in London that 'the religious opposition to chloroform has ceased among us.' In 1853 Queen Victoria inhaled chloroform during the birth of Prince Leopold and again in 1857 at the birth of Princess Beatrice.

Anaesthesia and Gynaecology

In Scotland, as elsewhere, the great majority of cases of childbirth were conducted at home with the assistance of a midwife who had no skills in repairing the damage of traumatic deliveries. In the nineteenth century, even the most fashionable and successful of specialist obstetricians in Britain were still physician-accoucheurs with no training in surgery. Their principal objective was to make the whole business of childbirth as painless as possible. Tears of the perineum caused during difficult deliveries were therefore often left unrepaired by surgery, and nothing was done except to approximate the sides of the tear by tying the patient's legs together and 'to hope for the best'. Similarly few attempts had ever been made to close tears that created open wounds allowing the bladder to open into the vagina (vesico-vaginal fistulas) leaving many women suffering urinary incontinence and distressing discomfort for the rest of their lives. And prolapse of the uterus, one of the disabilities that afflicted women after repeated pregnancies, was routinely relieved only by pads and pessaries and the result was rarely satisfactory.

Obstetricians did treat the 'diseases of women', but these were restricted only to the disorders of menstruation, displacements of the uterus and the pains usually attributed to inflammation of the uterus. The treatments used were pessaries, clysters, blisters, setons and cauterisation of the cervix. Even in Scotland, where most obstetricians had some formal training in surgery, major procedures, including caesarean section, were carried out very rarely and only by practising surgeons.

'Chloroform Syncope'

As chloroform came into widespread use in general surgery, reports began to appear in the medical press of isolated cases of sudden, unexpected and inexplicable deaths during induction of chloroform anaesthesia; these events became labelled 'chloroform syncope'. Simpson claimed that these deaths were the result of improper and inexpert technique in administering the anaesthetic; he claimed that they never occurred in Edinburgh where the university medical school gave formal courses of instruction on the practice of chloroform anaesthesia. But several clinicians attributed the deaths to an unfortunate and unpredictable idiosyncrasy suffered by a small number of patients. The incidence of these deaths was very low, but obstetricians, especially in the United States, declared that even if the incidence was as low as one in a thousand they would never use chloroform to relieve the pain of such a natural process as normal childbirth. 'Chloroform syncope' was later discovered to be caused by ventricular fibrillation, but the controversy over the use of chloroform during normal deliveries continued well into the twentieth century.

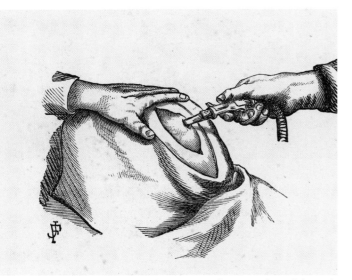

4.26 Ovarian cyst being drained by means of a trocar and cannula inserted through the abdominal wall (*reproduced from T. Spenser Wells,* Diseases of the Ovaries, *London, 1872*).

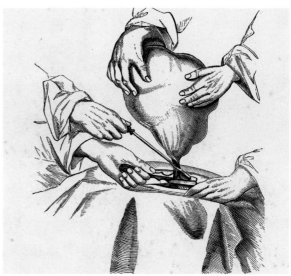

4.27 Ovarian cyst being removed through an open wound into the cavity of the abdomen (*reproduced from T. Spenser Wells,* Diseases of the Ovaries, *London, 1872*).

In Britain it had been the practice to treat cases of ovarian cysts by the insertion of a needle and cannula through the wall of the vagina or the abdomen to tap the cyst, and withdraw as much as possible of its content; iodine, port wine and water, rose leaves in wine or even pure alcohol was then injected into the cyst in an attempt to prevent the further accumulation of fluid. But in three cases between 1809 and 1817, Ephraim McDowell, an American surgeon who had studied in Edinburgh under John Bell (see p. 121), excised ovarian cysts completely through abdominal incisions; however two of his patients died. The first ovariotomy in Britain was performed in 1842 when Charles Clay (1802–93), an Edinburgh-trained surgeon practising in Manchester, removed an ovarian cyst weighing 36 lbs. He continued to perform the operation during the next two years, but without the benefit of general anaesthesia his mortality rate was over 50%, and the *Lancet* concluded that such a risk could not be justified. From 1857, Spencer Wells in London succeeded in performing a series of ovariotomies under general anaesthesia with a much lower post-operative mortality. From 1862 even better results were achieved by the Edinburgh surgeon, Thomas Keith. Keith had been trained by James Syme, and had learned from him the value of maintaining a high standard of cleanliness in the operating room but especially in the immediate area of the surgical wound; his post-operative mortality remained low. By 1863 the *Lancet* had been won over, and gave the new gynaecological operation of ovariotomy its blessing.

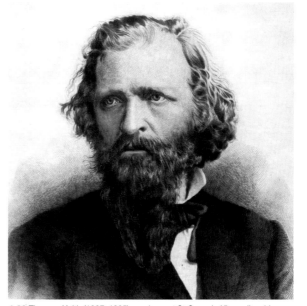

4.28 Thomas Keith (1827–1895) was born at St Cyrus in Kincardineshire. He trained as an apprentice to J. Y. Simpson, as the last doctor to be trained by apprenticeship in Edinburgh. He later became one of the leading gynaecological surgeons of his time (*RCSEd*).

Significantly, the word gynaecology had been first used in 1847, the year in which general anaesthesia came into general use. It was from that time that in Edinburgh, James Y. Simpson, as Professor of Midwifery, had encouraged Thomas Keith and all his students to think beyond the traditional limits of obstetrical practice and to take up the new invasive gynaecological operations that the intro-

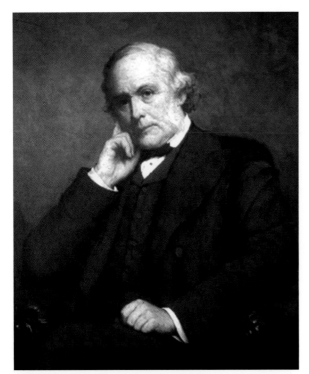

4.29 Joseph Lister (1927–1912) was born into a Quaker family in Essex. His father was a wine merchant and amateur scientist. Lister was educated in England and graduated from London University which, unlike Oxford and Cambridge at that time, was open to Quakers. He was advised to go for further training in surgery under Professor James Syme in Edinburgh, became Syme's assistant at Edinburgh Royal Infirmary and later married his daughter. In 1860 he was appointed Regius Professor of Surgery at Glasgow. Later he became Professor of Clinical Surgery at Edinburgh and, later still, Professor of Clinical Surgery at King's College, London (*Wellcome Library, London*).

duction of general anaesthesia had made possible. Under anaesthesia the tears of the perineum caused by traumatic delivery could be painlessly repaired at once. And it was he who persuaded them that to open the peritoneal cavity was not as dangerous as had been thought and, under anaesthesia, tumours of the ovaries or uterus could be excised. In the middle years of the nineteenth century, gynaecology had at least reached its infancy.

Antiseptic Surgery

In the middle years of the nineteenth century, surgical and gynaecological operations were best carried out in the patient's home. Amputations performed even in the largest and most prestigious of hospitals carried a mortality rate of over 40%; when performed in a suitable room in the patient's home, the same operation had a mortality rate of less than 10%. Similarly, mothers delivered of their children in a maternity hospital were ten times more like to die than mothers delivered at home. The majority of

deaths following surgery or childbirth were due to 'fever', surgical fever or puerperal fever.

Although Gordon's ideas had not been widely accepted, a few obstetricians and surgeons had taken notice. In 1842 in London, Thomas Watson (1792–1882) recommended hand-washing in a solution of chlorine to prevent the practitioner from becoming 'the vehicle of contagion and death between one patient and another.' In Edinburgh James Syme (1799–1870), to prevent the spread of infection, insisted on cleanliness by the generous use of cold water. In Boston in 1843, Oliver Wendell Holmes (1809–1894) published his essay on *The Contagiousness of Puerperal Fever*. Then in 1847, Ignaz Semmelweis (1818–1865), an obstetrician at the Lying-In Hospital in Vienna, demonstrated that the maternal mortality from puerperal fever in his wards could be reduced from 30% to 3% by ensuring that medical students washed their hands in a solution of chloride of lime before examining their patients. It had occurred to him that his students went each morning from the post-mortem room, where they had examined the bodies of patients who had died of puerperal fever, directly to the labour room, where they made vaginal examinations of women in labour. This had suggested to him that it was the 'cadaverous particles' still adhering to the hands of his students that had transferred the disease to patients in his ward. However, further experience showed that puerperal fever could afflict women in his ward who could not possibly have been inoculated with material carried from the post-mortem room; he therefore conceded that puerperal fever could be carried to new patients not only by cadaveric particles but also by other 'morbid matter'.

Lister's Research

Meanwhile Joseph Lister (1827–1912) was taking his own rather different approach to the problem of hospital fever. As a medical student at London University, the young Lister became interested in the inflammation that so often led to the decomposition of the tissue of wounds. Later, as a house surgeon at King's College Hospital in London, he had further practical experience of gangrene, the mortification of tissue that rotted away the wounds and led to the deaths of so many patients after surgery. In 1852,

William Sharpey

William Sharpey (1802–1880) was born in Arbroath. He studied medicine at Edinburgh University, graduating in 1823. After practising for a time in Arbroath, in 1831 he became a successful lecturer in anatomy at Edinburgh. In 1836 he was invited to accept the Chair of Anatomy and Physiology at the University of London. In 1840 vigorous attempts by his friends and admirers were made to secure his election as Professor of the Practice of Medicine at Edinburgh. The efforts failed, but for forty years thereafter, as Professor of Physiology in London, he continued to exercise great power and influence in the medical and scientific world. He became a Fellow of the Royal Society in 1839 and its secretary from 1853 until 1872. He is now remembered as the Father of Modern Physiology.

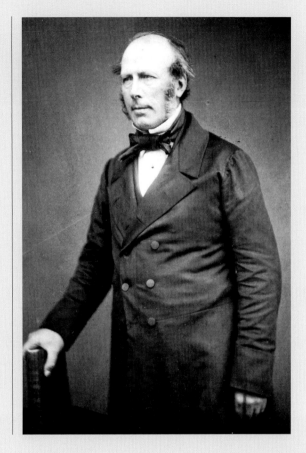

4.30 Sir William Sharpey, FRS (*Wellcome Library, London*).

on the advice of his Professor of Physiology, William Sharpey (1802–1880), he became a pupil of James Syme, Professor of Surgery at Edinburgh. Later he became Syme's house surgeon and later still his assistant. In 1855, he was appointed Lecturer in Surgery at Edinburgh and was in a position to resume his work on the inflammation and mortification of wounds. His animal experiments, carried out at his home or in abattoirs in Edinburgh, led to his election as a Fellow of the Royal Society in 1860.

In 1861 Lister was appointed Professor of Surgery at Glasgow. The chair of Surgery at Glasgow did not carry an automatic appointment as surgeon to Glasgow Royal Infirmary, and for over a year Lister was able to devote much of his time to his animal experiments; later, in 1862, when he was at last appointed as a surgeon at the Infirmary, he was able to conduct clinical trials in his wards. At Glasgow Royal Infirmary at that time, little attention was paid to cleanliness. Fever, pyaemia and gangrene were never absent from the wards and at times they became

epidemic. In his wards, Lister introduced a regime of 'rigorous cleanliness' that demanded clean towels, clean dressings and the liberal use of soap and water. The effect was negligible; surgical fever and gangrene continued as before. Lister now looked to his laboratory to find some other means to reduce that mortality. His researches had made little progress until, in 1865, he read a paper 'Rescherches sur la Putrefaction', written two years earlier in Lille by Louis Pasteur (1822–1895). Pasteur had first proved that the primary agents in the fermentation of wine, in milk and in butter were minute living micro-organisms (alternatively 'germs' or 'microbes'); he had then demonstrated that microbes of many kinds were present everywhere in the air; later still he showed that microbes were not only the agents of fermentation but also the agents of the putrefaction of dead animal material. It seemed to Lister that microbes might also be responsible for the putrefaction of devitalised human flesh; his work now was to find a chemical to destroy microbes before

Sir Alexander Ogston

Alexander Ogston (1844–1929) Professor of Surgery at Aberdeen University (1882–1909) was an early convert to Lister's antiseptic surgery, introducing the use of the carbolic spray in Aberdeen. Before being appointed to his chair he had made his own studies of wound infection. In 1880–82 he examined the bacteria in specimens of pus taken from a series of 100 wound abscesses and was able to describe a previously unidentified bacterium which he named staphylococcus aureus.

Ogston also had a distinguished career as a general surgeon, becoming Surgeon in Ordinary to Queen Victoria, King Edward VII and King George V. He was knighted in 1912.

For many years he had contributed to military surgery, serving in General Gordon's campaign in Sudan in 1884 and the Boer War in 1899–1902. His military experiences led him to become a leading and successful advocate for the creation of the Royal Army Medical Corps.

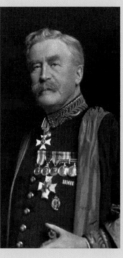
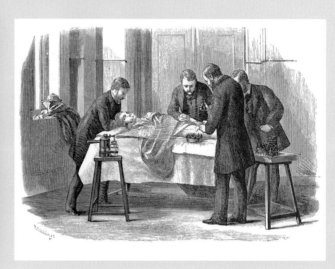

4.31 *Right.* Sir Alexander Ogston (*Wellcome Library, London*). He was one of the first surgeons in Scotland to adopt Lister's principles. *Far right.* Ogston (third from the left) is seen operating under a spray of carbolic at Aberdeen Royal Infirmary (*Aberdeen City Library*).

they were able to reach the partially devitalised human flesh at the sites of surgical operations. He discovered that in Carlisle, the local authority had been successful in suppressing the smell of decaying sewage by treating it with carbolic acid.

From March 1865, Lister began to apply a dressing soaked in a solution of carbolic acid in twenty parts of water on the wounds of his patients to prevent germs from gaining access to the temporarily damaged tissues. The effect was just as he had hoped; in every case the patient's wound had healed without evidence of suppuration. In September 1867, he published his early results in a series of articles on the *Antiseptic Principle of the Practice of Surgery* in the *British Medical Journal.* Over the next three years, his wards were said to enjoy 'immunity from the ordinary evils of surgical hospitals'. In 1869, Lister was appointed Professor of Surgery at Edinburgh. There he continued his work on antisepsis. Two medical students

suggested that even better results would be achieved by using a spray of carbolic acid to remove the microbes from the air surrounding the patient on the operating table. This idea was quickly adopted and for a time the use of the carbolic spray was actively promoted. But experience showed that the little that was gained did not compensate for the inconvenience and discomfort it caused the staff in the operating theatre, and it fell out of use. Lister continued to make further cautious improvements to his antiseptic procedures, but although his results seemed to offer an effective answer to hospital fever, several very influential surgeons continued to be sceptical.

Aseptic Surgery

Lister's methods were only slowly adopted over a period of twenty years and by the end of that time his methods were already being challenged by one his former students. From 1877, William Macewen (1848–1924), then a lecturer

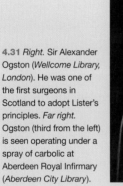

174

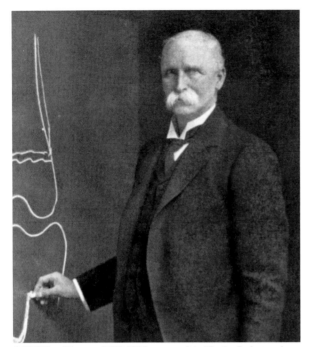

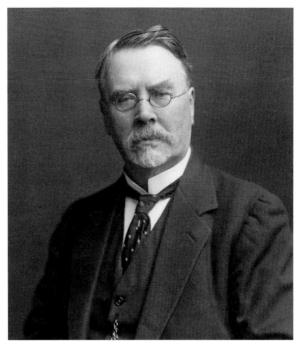

4.32 William Macewen (1848–1924) was appointed Regius Professor of Clinical Surgery at Glasgow University in 1892 and knighted in 1902. He became widely celebrated as a pioneer of brain surgery, bone graft surgery (especially the correction of bone deformities resulting from childhood rickets) and thoracic surgery (*Wellcome Library, London*).

4.33 Murdoch Cameron (1847–1930) was Regius Professor of Midwifery at Glasgow University from 1894 until 1926. He was a pioneer of antiseptic surgery and became internationally famous in 1888 when he performed the first successful Caesarean section under antiseptic conditions at Glasgow Royal Maternity Hospital (*Wellcome Library, London*).

on surgery at Glasgow University, abandoned the use of chemical (and often irritating) antiseptics such as carbolic acid, and used heat to sterilise the instruments, towels and dressings used during operations, and insisted on deep scrubbing of the hands and arms by all those taking part; within a few years his system of aseptic surgery had replaced antiseptic surgery.

Macewen, (later Sir William Macewen, Regius Professor of Surgery at Glasgow) took full advantage of the development of general anaesthesia and of his aseptic system to widen the scope of surgery. He ventured into neurosurgery; he was the first to operate on a series of brain abscesses in 1876 and he successfully removed a brain tumour in 1878. He developed new orthopaedic techniques for the correction of bone deformities caused by rickets; his studies of bone growth led to the discovery that bones grow at the line of the epiphyseal line and not at the bone end; in 1879 he performed the first bone graft, a technique that allowed him to insert small portions of bone into the limb bones. He performed the first pneumonectomy, the removal of a tuberculous lung. In 1888, at Glasgow Royal Maternity Hospital, Murdoch Cameron (later Professor of Midwifery at Glasgow) followed Macewen's adventurous lead,

performing the first caesarean section to be carried out under aseptic conditions.

By the end of the nineteenth century, surgery in Scotland had been transformed. Since the introduction of chloroform anaesthesia, the number of operations performed in the country's hospitals had multiplied by a factor of almost twenty. In the first twenty years the overall mortality from hospital surgery had increased slightly as more operations were performed, some much more radical and hazardous than had formerly been thought possible. It was not until later in the century, when antiseptic and then aseptic surgery were introduced (see below) that mortality fell dramatically to a small fraction of the rate in the 1850s.

Unfortunately there was no such improvement in maternal mortality, which had many causes other than puerperal fever. The overall maternal mortality in some maternity hospitals continued to be as high as 10%. However, very few normal deliveries were conducted in hospital, and domiciliary deliveries continued to be relatively safe. In Scotland the overall maternal mortality rate at the end of the nineteenth century was still a little over 5 per 1000, just as it had been in 1850.

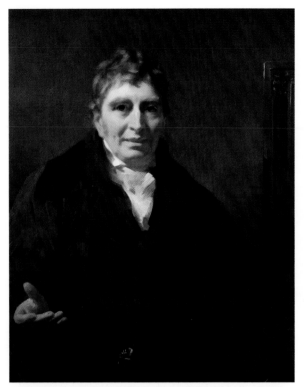

4.34 Andrew Duncan (1744–1828) was born at Crail in Fife, where his father was a merchant. At the age of fourteen he became a student at St Andrews University, taking his MA degree in 1762. He then studied medicine at Edinburgh, where he was taught by Alexander Monro *secundus*, Joseph Black, John Gregory and William Cullen. At Edinburgh he also became strongly influenced by the philosophy and sociology of David Hume, Adam Smith and Adam Ferguson, then at the height of their powers. He became Professor of the Institute of Medicine at Edinburgh in 1790, Professor of Materia Medica and Physician to the King in 1821 (*RCPE*).

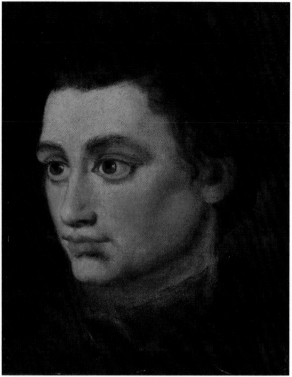

4.35 The poet Robert Fergusson (1750–1774) was educated at St Andrews University then lived a somewhat Bohemian life in Edinburgh. He published a collection of his work in 1773. After suffering a head injury in 1774, he was incarcerated with the pauper lunatics in Edinburgh's primitive Bedlam, and died soon after. It was his death in such appalling circumstances that led eventually to the foundation of Edinburgh Lunatic Asylum in 1813. Oil on paper by Alexander Runciman, *c*1772 (*Scottish National Portrait Gallery*).

PSYCHIATRY

At the beginning of the nineteenth century, the laws governing the care and the custody of the insane in Scotland had not changed since the fourteenth century. By a statute of Robert I (1274–1329) the care of those of 'fatuous mind' was the responsibility of the family; the care and management of the 'furious' (potentially violent) insane was likewise the responsibility of the family but, when the family failed, responsibility devolved on the sheriff of the county, the 'Crown having the sole power of coercing by fetters.' In the first years of the nineteenth century, families who could afford the high fees might devolve the care of their fatuous, deviant or simply inconvenient relatives to a private asylum operating for profit; the great majority of families, however, chose either to care for their fatuous relatives at home or left them free to fend for themselves. Only a few families had the resources to confine their 'furious' relations at home or could find a private asylum willing to accept them; the great majority of the difficult, disorderly or dangerous insane in Scotland were incarcerated in some public institution. In Edinburgh, the furious were committed to 'Bedlam' (Darien House, a charity institution); in Glasgow they were confined in cells set aside for the purpose in the Town's Hospital; but where there were no public asylums, the 'furious' were incarcerated along with the criminals in the country's jails and tolbooths. In Perth, the tolbooth was a dark and wretched building in the middle of the town; at Inverness the mad were confined in a vault between the second and third arches of the old bridge over the Tay.

Asylums and Legislation

In October 1774, the Edinburgh physician, Andrew Duncan was distressed to find his mentally disturbed and dying friend, the poet Robert Fergusson, confined in

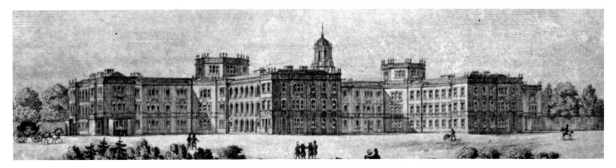

4.36 *Above*. The Crichton Institute was founded at Dumfries in 1839 by the widow of James Crichton who had made his fortune as a trader in India and China. The Crichton Royal Hospital, as it later became known, became a leader in practising a new 'moral treatment' of insanity. Patients were to be managed with 'kindness and occupation', rather than simply incarcerated as before (*Wellcome Library, London*).

4.37 *Right*. Alexander Morison (1779–1866) was a pioneer of psychiatric medicine. This portrait was painted against the background of his estate at Newhaven, near Edinburgh, by Richard Dadd, one of his patients at Bethlem Asylum in Surrey. Dadd had murdered his father, believing him to be the devil. He had never visited Scotland but based the background of the portrait on a sketch by Morison's daughter. The two female figures in the painting may be based on photographs of Newhaven fishwives taken by Hill and Adamson (*National Gallery of Scotland*).

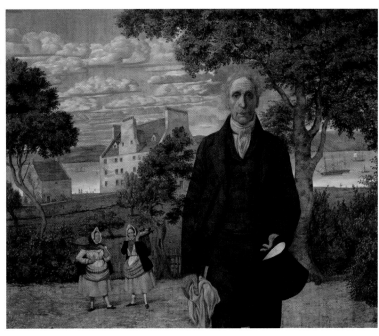

squalor in Darien House. When he became President of the Royal College of Physicians in 1790, Duncan launched a public campaign for the establishment of a Lunatic Asylum in Edinburgh on the model of the asylum already founded by Mrs Carnegie of Charlton in Montrose for the treatment of both private patients and the insane poor. By 1845 there were seven such asylums in Scotland: Montrose Royal Asylum (founded in 1781), Aberdeen Royal Asylum (1800), Royal Edinburgh Asylum (1813), Glasgow Royal Asylum (1814), Dundee Royal Asylum (1820), Perth Royal Asylum (1820) and Crichton Royal Asylum (1839) at Dumfries. They represented a significant step in the progress of the care of the insane in Scotland. Nevertheless the treatment was still inhumane. A Justice of the Peace who had visited many asylums in both Scotland and England in the early years of the nineteenth century wrote that in both countries, 'lunatics were kept constantly chained to the wall in dark cells and had nothing to lie on

but straw. The keepers visited them, whip in hand, and lashed them into obedience.'

In June 1815, the Lord Advocate secured new legislation for Scotland: *An Act to Regulate Madhouses in Scotland*, that made provision for the medical inspection of all establishments for the insane in Scotland. However, there were then very few members of the medical profession ready to devote their careers, or indeed any great part of their time, to the care of the insane. Among the earliest and most prominent of the physicians to do so was Alexander Morison. After graduating at Edinburgh in 1799, he had spent two years in London with his friend at the Westminster Hospital, the Scottish physician Sir Alexander Crichton (1763–1856). Crichton, who had long experience in the care of the insane, had recently published a book on *The Nature and Origins of Mental Derangement*. Morison did not pursue his interest in the subject further at that time. But when a Bill presented to Parliament in

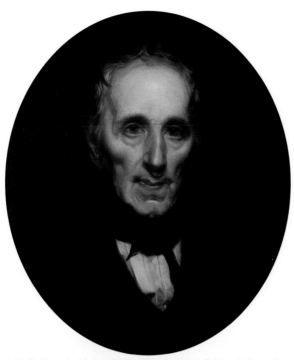

4.38 Sir Alexander Morison (1779–1866) was born in Edinburgh. He studied medicine at Edinburgh University, graduating in 1799. He practised as a general physician in London until 1810, when he was appointed inspecting physician to the madhouses in Surrey, and thereafter became one of the first physicians in Britain to devote his career entirely to the care of the insane. He became consulting physician to the Hanwell Asylum and the Bethlem Royal Hospital in London in 1832, and wrote many books on mental disease (*RCPEd*).

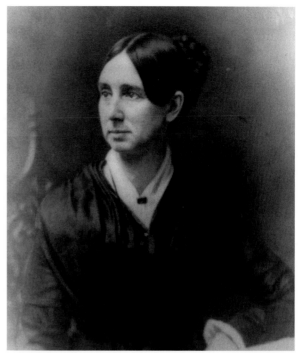

4.39 Dorothea Lynde Dix (1802–1887) was born in Hampden, Maine. At the age of twelve she escaped from her alcoholic and abusive father to live with a wealthy aunt in Boston. She opened schools for young ladies in Boston but had to give them up after periods of ill-health. She travelled to England, where she became interested in new forms of treatment for the insane. For almost four years, she toured and inspected madhouses and asylums in Britain, writing reports that were submitted to the House of Commons.

1816 proposed the appointment of salaried Commissioners in Lunacy to oversee asylums and the welfare of the mentally ill in England, he became determined to become one of the Commissioners. Although the Bill failed, he nevertheless travelled to Paris to spend time attending the clinics of Jean Esquirol at the Salpêtrière.

When Morison visited Paris in 1818, Esquirol was already attracting large numbers of students to study his new, more humane, 'moral treatment' of insanity. Essential to moral treatment was the abandonment of physical restraint; the asylums were to be made as comfortable and as unlike a prison as possible, and staffed by attendants in whom 'mildness and command of temper were as indispensable as strength and firmness'. Under constant supervision, the patients were to be encouraged to occupy themselves in as normal a way as possible.

Morison returned to London, where he continued to practise as a physician with modest success until, in 1823, one of his patients, the widow of the banker Thomas Coutts, offered to fund the creation of a chair in mental disorders at Edinburgh University. The offer was rejected by the University. Morison was undeterred. He hired a classroom at the University and in November 1823 he became the first man in Britain to devote a complete course of lectures to the management of the insane. In the years that followed, the attendance at his lectures grew, and the number of lectures in each series increased from eleven to eighteen. He also published three editions of his *Outlines of Mental Diseases for the Use of Students* in which he recommended that the patient should be restrained by wrist and ankle manacles until the active stages of the illness had been subdued. Only then were the shackles to be removed and moral treatment begun.

'Moral' management

Alexander Morison's views on the management of the insane were influential for a time, but from 1834 they were overtaken by those of W.A.F. Browne, the new superintendent of the Royal Mental Hospital at Montrose. At Montrose, Browne had created what be believed to be the ideal environment for the 'moral' and physical management of the insane. Chains, manacles and straight-jackets and all other means of physical restraint were banned completely. The patients were housed as comfortably as possible; modern gas lighting was installed everywhere in the asylum; the exercise areas were liberally planted with flowers and shrubs; there was divine service every Sunday. The patients were treated as much in the manner of a rational being as their state of mind would allow. And they were encouraged to collaborate in managing their own recovery in an early form of group therapy. In 1838, Browne was invited to become superintendent of the new Crichton Royal Asylum at Dumfries, then the most generously endowed asylum in Britain and one of the best endowed in Europe. His methods began to be adopted in other forward-looking asylums in Scotland.

However, in 1838 there were still few asylums in Scotland, although elsewhere in Britain social reformers had long been intent on confining the insane in institutions. The primary purpose of these early reformers was to rescue the insane from the neglect, hardship and abuse that they suffered when at liberty in the community. At the same time they had in mind the need to remove the threat that their presence in the community posed to morality and social order: 'It is not calculated to improve morals, that half naked maniacs should haunt our paths with tendencies as well as aspects of satyrs. Unchecked, uncontrolled they obey the injunction to multiply their own kind. Reason or religion cannot reach them and they are abandoned to the dominion of sin.'

It was not until 1841 that an Act of Parliament gave sheriffs in Scotland powers to commit to an institution any furious or fatuous person thought to be 'in a state threatening to the lieges'. By 1851, the number of lunatics confined in public institutions in Scotland had increased to 3,486, approximately 600 more than the number left at large in the community. Unfortunately, however, the reforms that Browne had introduced to Scotland had not yet been adopted by all those entrusted with the management of the insane. In some of Scotland's asylums treatment was deplorable. And outside the asylums the state of the insane continued to be as bad as it had ever been.

In 1855, Britain was visited by Dorothea Lynde Dix, a formidable American philanthropist who had devoted herself to the improvement of the care of the insane. In Scotland, her suspicions were first aroused by the great difficulty she had in gaining access to several of the lunatic asylums. When she was eventually allowed entry, she found the inmates in a most miserable state. She immediately travelled to London and confronted the Home Secretary. He found her account so startling that, in April 1855, a Royal Commission was appointed 'to inquire into the condition of lunatic asylums in Scotland and the existing state of the Law in that country in reference to lunatics and lunatic asylum.' Following its report an *Act for the Regulation of Care and Treatment of Lunatics and for the Provision Maintenance and Regulation of Lunatic Asylums in Scotland* was passed in August 1857.

The Act made provision for the appointment of a Board of Commissioners in Lunacy for Scotland with powers to grant (or withdraw) licences to the proprietors of *private* asylums; with powers to have private asylums visited and inspected regularly by the sheriff of the county or his deputy; and to have the right to visit private asylums as they saw fit. The Act divided Scotland into districts; each district was to have a District Board, and each District Board was to provide a District Asylum. These *public* asylums were to be visited and inspected regularly by the sheriff of the county or his deputy; and the Board was to have the right to visit private asylums as it saw fit.

Patients were to be admitted to public and private asylums by order of a sheriff on medical certificates specifying the facts on which the opinion of insanity was founded. And a medical practitioner was to be resident in every asylum licensed for a hundred patients or more; a physician was to visit daily those for more than fifty patients; those for fifty or less were to be visited twice every week.

The increase in the number of public asylums, both north and south of the Border, created many new and more reputable posts for doctors. That all asylums in Britain were now open to the scrutiny and discipline of Boards of Commissioners relieved much of the medical profession's longstanding suspicion and disapproval of the methods employed by asylum doctors; and as salaried officials of the state, mad-doctors (or alienists as many now preferred to be called) no longer had to endure the low status associated with employment in trade.

Craiglockhart War Hospital for Officers

On the outbreak of war in 1914, the poet Siegfried Sassoon volunteered for service in the army. In France, as an officer in the Royal Welch Fusiliers, he showed conspicuous gallantry and was awarded the Military Cross. However, by 1917 he had become disillusioned by the conduct of the war, and at the end of a short period of leave in England he threw away his Military Cross, and encouraged by George Bernard Shaw and Lady Ottoline Morrell, he refused to return to his regiment. In a letter to his commanding officer he protested that what had begun as a war of defence had become a 'war of aggression and conquest'. The Secretary of State for War decided that he should not be court-martialed but should be sent to the Craiglockhart War Hospital for Officers in Edinburgh. There, with his fellow poet, Wilfred Owen, he was treated by W.H.R. Rivers for 'shell shock', the name recently given by Rivers for the severe mental trauma suffered by many soldiers in battle, a condition that had not previously been regarded as an illness.

Craiglockhart is now one of the buildings on the campus of Edinburgh Napier University.

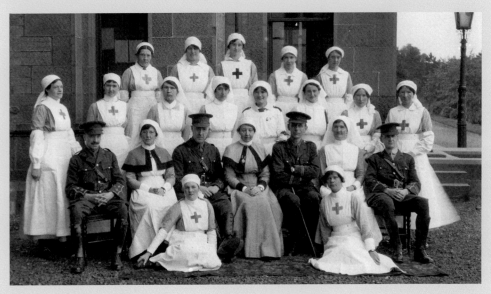

4.40 Staff of the Craiglockhart War Hospital for Officers (*Edinburgh Napier University*).

PUBLIC HEALTH

By the second half of the nineteenth century the industrialisation and urbanisation of Scotland was entering a second phase. The manufacture of textiles was taking second place to heavy industries based on coal, iron and steel. Towns and villages across central Scotland were being changed beyond recognition. Towns that had been little more than hamlets in 1800, and had become textile towns of several thousand inhabitants by the 1840s, now grew even more rapidly into coal and iron towns with 'the ramshackle and dangerous character of frontier towns'. Villages that had been quite unaffected by industrialisation in the first half of the century now suddenly grew into major centres for the production of iron and steel. Glasgow, already the overcrowded industrial megalopolis of Scotland, suffered a massive increase in the numbers of its starving poor in the aftermath of the great Potato Famine in Ireland. In this famine, visited on Ireland from 1845, over a million died. A further million emigrated to escape the miseries at home; those who could afford the fare took passage across the Atlantic; those for whom that small sum was too great went to Liverpool; but the utterly destitute crowded into Glasgow.

Living conditions in Scotland's towns and cities were now worse than in comparable towns in England or elsewhere in Europe. Much of the housing was of very poor quality, and as the population continued to increase and

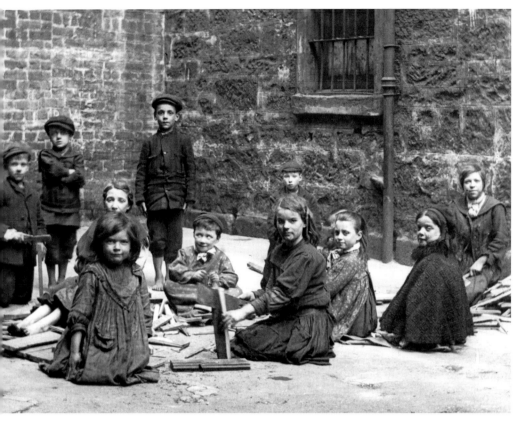

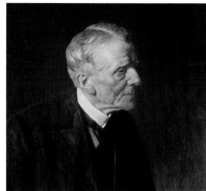

4.41 *Above*. Sir Henry Littlejohn (1826–1914) was a graduate of Edinburgh University. He trained as a surgeon, becoming lecturer at the Royal College of Surgeons of Edinburgh. In 1897 he was appointed Professor of Medical Jurisprudence at Edinburgh University. For many years he served as Police Surgeon for Edinburgh and Medical Advisor to the Crown in Scotland, and was called as an expert witness in several notable criminal trials. However, he is best remembered as a reformer in the field of Public Health, becoming President of the Institute of Public Health in 1893 (*Scottish National Portrait Gallery*).

4.42 *Left*. Children in a city street in 1910 chopping sticks to be sold, for a few pennies, as kindling in the surrounding tenements (*Mitchell Library, Glasgow*).

the numbers seeking employment in the industrial towns continued to grow, overcrowding became an ever more severe problem well into the twentieth century. Between the two World Wars, 32% of Scottish households (50% in Glasgow) lived in dwellings of one or two rooms. Working conditions were often deplorable. For those employed in the new heavy industries, working conditions were particularly hazardous; the mortality rate among iron and steel workers was more than 50% higher than among fishermen.

As the industrialisation of Scotland continued into the second half of the century and Britain became more prosperous, wages for those in regular employment improved; a gradual and slow fall in the death rate in Scotland (21 per thousand in 1855 to 18 per thousand in 1900) has been attributed to an improvement in the general diet. But the cost of living was high (relative to wages in Scotland's low wage economy) and recurring periods of economic depression caused widespread unemployment. Poverty, inadequate housing and overcrowding continued. The consequences were most severe where living conditions were worst; the infant mortality rate was almost three times higher in Glasgow than in rural Scotland and the maternal mortality rate in the rapidly growing steel towns

was twice the national average. As the century progressed, the health and fitness of the great mass of the population in Scotland continued to deteriorate.

Public Health Legislation

After the creation of the Board of Supervision in 1845, successive governments proved reluctant to intervene further in the promotion of public health. In 1856 the Board of Supervision was formally recognised as the central public health authority in Scotland, but its functions continued to be only advisory. From 1856, a series of Nuisance Removal Acts made temporary provisions to meet crises such as epidemics; but the Acts made it clear that, except during these sporadic interventions by central government, responsibility for the promotion of public health remained with the local authorities. Of these Glasgow was particularly active; it created the Loch Katrine scheme which supplied the city with clean water through 50 miles of pipes, and it installed 100 miles of sewers. Among the important innovations made by the most progressive local authorities was the appointment of Medical Officers of Health to advise them on the measures required for the promotion of public health. The first Medical Officer of Health was Henry Littlejohn (1826–

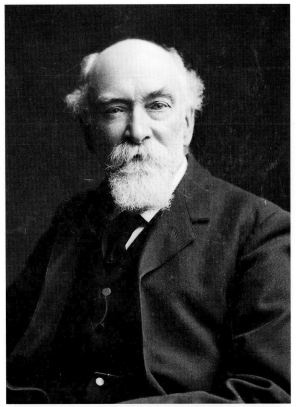

4.43 James Burn Russell (1837–1904) was born and educated in Glasgow, graduating MD from Glasgow University in 1858. After an appointment as assistant surgeon on HMS *Agamemnon*, he became physician to Glasgow's City Poorhouse and Physician Superintendent of Glasgow's fever hospitals, an experience that convinced him of the need for great improvement in the living conditions of the city's poor. He became Glasgow's first Medical Officer of Health in 1872 and campaigned successfully for efficient sanitation, pollution control and slum clearance. He made his international reputation by introducing compulsory notification of infectious disease (*Wellcome Library, London*).

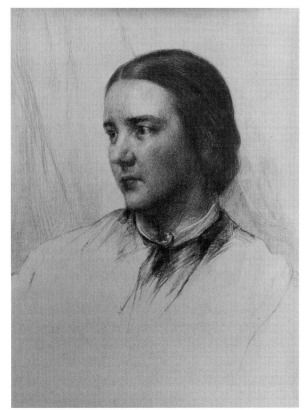

4.44 Sophia Jex Blake (1840–1912), was born in Hastings, the daughter of a successful barrister. Her struggle to enable women to study and qualify as doctors was eventually successful, despite vigorous opposition from the all-male student body and many of the teaching staff of Edinburgh University, where she and her friends were studying. At her instigation, a Bill was introduced in Parliament that would empower all medical training bodies to admit women, and an Act was passed in 1876. Sophia Jex Blake qualified as a doctor in Dublin in 1877 (*Edinburgh University Library*).

1914) appointed for Edinburgh in 1862. The appointment of other distinguished and highly effective Medical Officers of Health followed – James Burn Russell (1837–1904) for Glasgow, Matthew Hay (1855–1932) for Aberdeen and W. Leslie Mackenzie for Leith (1862–1935). These and other Medical Officers of Health, and the Health Committees of the local authorities that had appointed them, were responsible for such innovations as the notification of disease, the establishment of fever hospitals, the control and prevention of gross overcrowding, installation of drainage systems in burghs and in populous rural areas beyond burgh administration, child welfare schemes, provision of free and safe milk for the infants of the poor and the gathering of reliable health statistics. Eventually a Local Government Act in 1889 and a Public Health Act in 1897 brought together the piecemeal legislation that had gone before, making it general and obligatory rather than

local and only enabling and, in place of the Board of Supervision, established the Local Government Board as the central health authority for Scotland.

During the second half of the nineteenth century much was achieved, but it served to contain the threats to the health of the great mass of the public rather than to eliminate them. Infant mortality actually increased from 121 per 1000 live births to 134. Maternal mortality continued at 5 or more per 1000 births. Life expectancy at birth continued to be approximately 41 years for males and 43.3 for females until 1870, when it began to improve as deaths from typhus, smallpox, scarlet fever and diphtheria all declined. Over 7,000 deaths each year from pulmonary tuberculosis made it the commonest cause of death in young adults. In the years between 1850 and 1890 the overall annual death rate in Scotland had changed only from 20.8 to 19.2.

Medical Education for Women

The first woman medical graduate to be licensed to practise in Britain was Elizabeth Blackwell (1821–1910). After graduating from Geneva College, New York, in 1849, she had travelled to Europe for two years of further study. Her reception in Paris was hostile. In London, she was treated mostly as an interesting anomaly, but she did succeed in working for a short time with James Paget at St Bartholomew's Hospital. In 1851, she returned to America; but when she later came briefly to London to lecture, she became, on 1 January 1859, the first woman to have her name entered in the Medical Register in Britain. While in London she had met and inspired Elizabeth Garret (1812–1893), the daughter of a wealthy businessman, to follow her example and study medicine. However, no medical school in Britain would accept Garret as a student. After years of private study, in 1865 she persuaded a very reluctant Society of Apothecaries to allow her to take its examinations for a licence to practice as an apothecary. On the strength of that licence, in 1866 she opened a dispensary for women and children in London. Then in 1870, having learned French for the purpose, she was granted a medical degree by the Sorbonne in Paris. In 1874 she founded the London School of Medicine for Women.

By then another woman had joined the battle. Sophia Jex-Blake (1840–1912) was the daughter of a successful barrister. Her parents held very traditional views on education, and it was only with reluctance that in 1858 they allowed her to attend classes at Queen's College, London. Sophia proved to be an outstanding pupil, and was later asked to join the staff of the College as a tutor of mathematics. Her parents considered it inappropriate for a middle-class woman to work, and only gave their approval on condition that she did not receive a salary.

In 1862 Jex-Blake travelled to the United States, where she became an assistant administrator at the New England Hospital for Women. She had hoped to study at a medical school in the United States, but in 1868 her father died. She returned to England to be with her mother, but she was still determined to qualify as a doctor. This proved to be difficult. Oxford, Cambridge and London Universities all proved unhelpful. She later wrote: 'My thoughts turned to Scotland, to which so much credit is always given for its enlightened views respecting education and where the universities boast of their freedom from ecclesiastical and other trammels. I therefore made my first application to the University of Edinburgh.'

The 'Edinburgh Seven'

At Edinburgh, her application to attend classes on medicine at the University was accepted by the Medical Faculty and by the Senate, but their decision was overturned by the University Court. The Court did not rule on the question whether women should or should not be taught in the medical classes of the University, but it refused to make some temporary arrangement for the benefit of only one woman. Jex-Blake now recruited six other women, and together they applied, this time not for permission to attend lectures, but for the right to matriculate and attend all the classes and examinations required for a degree in medicine. In July 1869, the Medical Faculty, the Senate and the University Court all agreed to their application. However, by the terms of the agreement, university lecturers were permitted to admit women to their classes but not obliged to admit them. And the majority of the student body were strongly opposed to the admission of women. Less than half of the students who began to study medicine at Edinburgh University ever succeeded in graduating; those who did entered an overcrowded profession, and most faced years of struggle and hardship. They were not at all eager to welcome competition from women, and they had purchasing power. Lecturers received their fees, not from the university but directly from the students. Lecturers who made themselves unpopular with the student body were therefore likely to suffer a loss in income; many found it politic to refuse to teach women.

While Jex-Blake and her colleagues found it difficult to find university lecturers willing to teach them in the classroom, they were able to enrol in the equivalent classes at the extra-mural school of Edinburgh's Royal Colleges of Physicians and Surgeons. However, they were unable to overcome a campaign to exclude them from clinical teaching at the Royal Infirmary, and from taking the examination necessary for graduation. On a number of issues their battles were fought out in the law courts. The publicity brought them the support of the public in Edinburgh, and

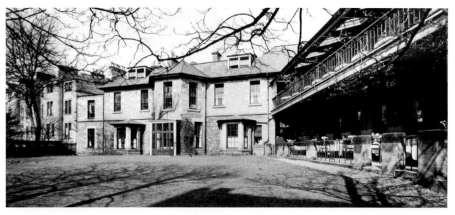

4.45 Bruntsfield Hospital continued as a hospital for women and children after the creation of the NHS but was eventually closed in 1989.

the lay press was generally sympathetic to their ambitions. Within the University their cause was loyally promoted by David Masson (1822–1907), the Professor of Rhetoric and Sir J. Y. Simpson, Professor of Midwifery, but their advocacy was overwhelmed by the implacable hostility of Sir Robert Christison (1797–1882), Professor of Materia Medica, Physician to the Queen in Scotland and President of the Royal Society of Edinburgh. Christison was a member of every committee and every administrative body of importance in Edinburgh medicine, and he had the backing of some of Edinburgh's most eminent medical men, including the new Professor of Surgery, Joseph Lister. Unable to overcome the opposition orchestrated by Christison, in March 1874 Jex-Blake and her colleagues abandoned their attempt to qualify for entry to the medical profession as graduates of Edinburgh University.

Jex-Blake returned to London. There she joined with (the now married) Elizabeth Garrett Anderson in founding the London School of Medicine for Women, and became one of its first students. In January 1877, she graduated MD at Berne, and in May she qualified for entry on the Medical Register by passing the examination for the licence of the Kings and Queen's College of Physicians in Dublin. In June 1878 she returned to Edinburgh and set up practice at 4 Manor Place as Scotland's first woman doctor. In 1881, she suffered a period of depression that lasted for two years. She then returned to Edinburgh and medical practice, now at her home, Bruntsfield Lodge. She established a small dispensary in Manor Place; then in 1885 she set up a larger dispensary at Bruntsfield that included a five-bed hospital ward.

The Edinburgh School of Medicine for Women

By 1885 the medical scene was quite changed. Christison had died in 1882 and Lister had left Edinburgh for London. Together the Edinburgh Colleges and the

Glasgow Faculty had introduced a Triple Qualification that was open to women. In 1887, Sophia Jex-Blake was able to reassemble several of those who had supported her in her struggles a decade before. They now formed a Committee to help her establish a medical school for women in Scotland. Leith Hospital, which in the 1860s and 1870s had been too small to provide proper clinical experience for students, had been enlarged and had been accredited by the Edinburgh Colleges; in the 1880s the staff of the hospital were very ready to welcome women students. It was now possible to establish a medical school for women that offered a complete medical training. The Edinburgh School of Medicine for Women opened at 1 Surgeons Square in October 1887. In its first years the new school had to overcome some administrative difficulties, but it soon seemed successfully established. However, Jex-Blake's autocratic style of management soon came to be resented by a number of her students. When, in the summer of 1889, two students, the sisters Grace and Martha Cadell, were expelled for 'insubordination', resentment became open rebellion. With the support of several of their fellow students, the Cadell sisters took legal action against Jex-Blake's medical school. In November the court found in favour of the Cadells and the sisters were each awarded £50 in damages. The Edinburgh School of Medicine for Women did not recover, and in 1898 it was closed. However, an alternative school was already in place. One of the students who had rebelled in support of the Cadell sisters was Elsie Inglis. With the help of her father, she had founded the Scottish Association for the Medical Education of Women; by the autumn of 1889 the Association had founded the Medical College for Women. Even in its first years there was no shortage of students; in 1900, the number of students who registered to qualify for entry on the Medical Register was 28, more than the total number registering at St Andrews and half as many as at Aberdeen.

BRITAIN'S FIRST MEDICAL RESEARCH LABORATORY

Scientific laboratories had not played any great part in the progress of medicine in nineteenth-century Britain. Important advances had been made in medical understanding and practice, but these had come chiefly from observations and experience at the bedside and from the verdicts of the post-mortem room. As late as 1876, the bacteriological studies that were so important for Lister's work on antiseptic surgery were still being carried on in a small passage behind the operating theatre in Edinburgh Royal Infirmary, where there was only the simplest of laboratory equipment. Edinburgh University was better provided with laboratory facilities than any other medical school in Britain, but these were used almost exclusively for the instruction of medical students. In medical science Edinburgh could not pretend to compete with Germany.

From the 1840s Germany had become the major centre for scientific research and education, attracting students from all over the world. In the restructuring of the German states during the years that followed the Napoleonic Wars and the collapse of the Napoleonic empire, the leading universities were transformed from independent corporate bodies to state institutions. The governments in each of the German states gained control over academic appointments and were able to shift the emphasis in academic activities away from the traditional pre-eminence of pedagogy towards the establishment of research institutes and commissioned research programmes that would yield practical returns. New scientific methods in chemistry and physics were developed in well-equipped laboratories and were later soon applied to physiology. In Germany, experimental physiology soon replaced clinical trial and pathological anatomy to form the basis of a new scientific and experimental medicine.

In 1886 in Edinburgh, a group of eighteen Fellows of the Royal College of Physicians, determined to be part of this new experimental medicine, proposed that their College should 'establish and maintain a laboratory to prosecute original research'. All but five had studied as postgraduates at medical science laboratories in Vienna, Berlin, Heidelberg, Frankfurt, Prague or Paris, and had already published work in prestigious scientific journals.

For a time the Council of the College was reluctant to invest such a substantial proportion of College funds on the project, but at a meeting in December, the proposal received the unanimous support of all the Fellows.

The College Laboratory, commissioned in August 1887, was the first medical research laboratory to be established in Britain. It was housed conveniently close to Edinburgh Royal Infirmary at 7 Lauriston Lane, a building of sixteen rooms on three floors, with a large detached hall in the courtyard behind. The hall was equipped for work on experimental physiology; other rooms were for

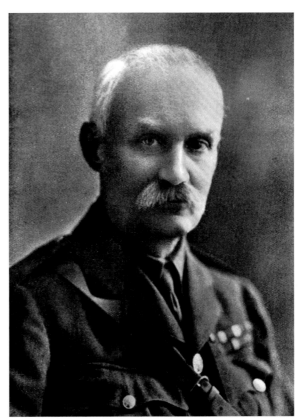

4.46 Sir German Sims Woodhead (1855–1921) was the first Superintendent of the Research Laboratory of the Royal College of Physicians of Edinburgh. He was educated at Huddersfield College and Edinburgh University, going on to study bacteriology under Robert Koch in Berlin and Louis Pasteur in Paris. Returning to Edinburgh, he became first assistant to the Professor of Pathology at Edinburgh, publishing his *Practical Pathology* in 1883 and *Practical Mycology*, the first textbook of bacteriology in English, in 1885 (*Wellcome Library, London*).

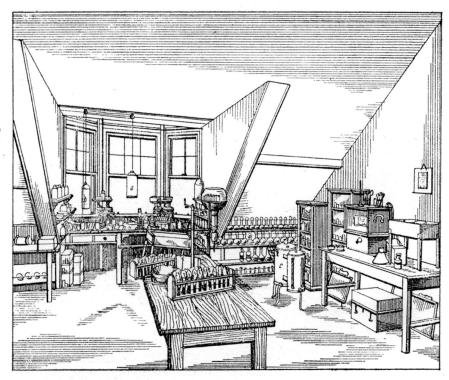

4.47 The Research Laboratory of the Royal College Physicians of Edinburgh occupied sixteen rooms. Illustrated here is the room equipped for bacteriological experiments (*RCPEd*).

histology, chemistry and bacteriology. There were offices, a workshop, a photographic room and a common room; one large room was furnished for the reception and examination of patients.

It soon became clear that larger premises were needed, and in November 1895 the College bought Darien House in Forrest Road, again conveniently near the Royal Infirmary. In its new and larger premises, new skills were developed and made available, and demands on the services of the Laboratory continued to increase. Within a very few years further expansion was being inhibited by lack of funds. From 1899, the Royal College of Surgeons, a few of whose Fellows made regular use of the Laboratory's facilities, made an annual contribution toward its running costs.

Nevertheless, research and development remained the chief preoccupations of the Laboratory. Between its foundation and 1950, the results of the researches carried out in the Laboratory were reported in 624 articles published in British and European medical and scientific journals. Over a third of these articles appeared in journals of particular interest to medical scientists – *Journal of Physiology, Journal of Anatomy and Physiology, Journal of Pathology and Bacteriology, Journal of the Chemical Society, Biochemical Journal, Nature* and others. In these publications the career scientists working in the Laboratory made impor-

tant contributions to comparative anatomy, the physiology of the nervous system, the endocrine glands, metabolism and nutrition.

The career scientists who directed these studies made up only a small minority of those working in the Laboratory. The physicians, surgeons and obstetricians who made up the majority of the Laboratory's researchers directed their attention to the pressing medical concerns of the times. In the spring of 1894, a trial at the Pasteur Institute in Paris had shown that the administration of the appropriate antitoxin serum was a very effective treatment for diphtheria. The College decided that, although it would inevitably interfere with its research work, the Laboratory should as quickly as possible produce a supply of the antitoxin for general use. The Laboratory continued to be the chief source of antitoxin in Scotland until a commercial antitoxin serum became available in 1898.

In the first years of the twentieth century, the Laboratory published important work on milk-borne bovine tuberculosis in children and on the tuberculosis of bones and joints. There were several investigations into the diseases associated with poverty – malnutrition, anaemia, and vitamin deficiencies. There were very relevant studies of the physiology and pathology of pregnancy and childbirth. In all, some 400 articles on these contemporary and pressing medical problems were published in the leading medical journals of the time. Within its first thirty years the College Laboratory's medical scientists, working in collaboration with clinicians devoting part of their time to laboratory research, contributed more to the advance of medical science than all four of Scotland's universities, and had gained for the Laboratory a reputation as one of the foremost centres of medical research in Britain.

Because of its reputation, the Laboratory was commissioned to carry out investigations for the government and other public bodies. These commissions led to the publication of: *Report on the Air of Coal Mines* (1888) for the Mining Institute of Scotland; *An Investigation into the Life History of the Salmon in Fresh Water* (1898) for the Fisheries Board; *Report on Prison Dietaries* (1899) for the Prison Commission; *A Study of the Diet of the Labouring Classes in Edinburgh* (1900) for Edinburgh Town Council; *Observations on the Movement of Pollution in the Tyne* (1901) for local authorities in Northumberland; *Famine Foods: The Nutritive Value of Some Uncultivated Foods Used during Recent Famines* (1903) for the India Office; *Report on an Outbreak of Scarlet Fever Associated with Milk Supply* (1910) for the Local Government Board of Scotland; and *Observations on the Pathology of Trench Foot* (1915) for the War Office.

In 1912 the Royal College of Surgeons of Edinburgh had proposed the creation of a research institute as a memorial to Lord Lister. In March 1913, representatives of the Royal College of Surgeons, the Royal College of Physicians and Edinburgh University prepared a draft scheme for what was to be called the 'Edinburgh Lister Institute of Pathology'. The building was to become part of the University and would house the university departments of pathology and bacteriology; it was to absorb the work of the Colleges' Research Laboratory and the Fellows of the Colleges were to retain their right to work there. In July 1914 a site was acquired for £50,000, but the plan had to be set aside until the end of World War I. In 1919 the scheme was revived, and efforts began to find the necessary finance, estimated at £250,000.

In 1920 the Rockefeller Foundation of New York had begun to make its great philanthropic contribution to the reconstruction of Europe. Among its schemes was one for reinvigorating medical education and improving patient care by establishing 'a community of interest between the biological basic sciences, organised professional medicine, and university education'. The Foundation Division of Medical Education was created to bring the leading centres of medical education in Europe into line with the best in the United States. In 1921, one of the European centres visited by representatives of the Foundation was Edinburgh. The University drew up a document, its 'Scheme of Extension and Development', in which the proposed Lister Institute was presented as part of its plan for future growth. However the Foundation's representatives found this continuation of the historic interdependence of four avowedly independent institutions – Edinburgh University, the Royal College of Physicians, the Edinburgh Royal Infirmary and the Royal College of Surgeons – bizarre and undesirable. They therefore gave their support directly to the development of the University's departments of pathology and bacteriology, but offered no support to the proposed Lister Institute or to the Colleges' Research Laboratory. The Colleges' Laboratory was later rescued from its increasing financial difficulties in 1933, when the Carnegie Trustees for the Universities of Scotland bought the Laboratory from the College and assumed responsibility for the whole cost of its maintenance. This financial support made it possible for the Laboratory to continue its free diagnostic service reporting on bacteriological, histological and biochemical specimens submitted by medical practitioners in Edinburgh or elsewhere. This arrangement with the Carnegie Trust continued until 1950.

Throughout the Laboratory's sixty years of achievement, clinicians and laboratory scientists worked in close and active partnership. In Britain, this merging of the world of the laboratory with the world of the consulting room was unique. In England, there was not only geographical separation of the medical laboratories of Oxford and Cambridge from the leading teaching hospitals of London, there was also a conscious distancing of the clinician from the medical scientist that persisted well into the twentieth century. In an address to the Royal Medical Society in Edinburgh in 1936, Lord Horder, Physician to the King and to St Bartholomew's Hospital, insisted that the practice of medicine did not require the

Tropical Medicine: Sir Patrick Manson and Malaria

In the last years of the nineteenth century, 20% of British medical graduates were practising overseas in tropical or subtropical climates, and of these the majority were graduates of Scottish universities. One of the most distinguished was Patrick Manson (1844–1922). Manson was born at Old Meldrum in Aberdeenshire, the son of John Manson of Fingask, a bonnet laird and manager of the local bank. Manson graduated in medicine from Aberdeen University in 1865, and after a short spell as a medical assistant at an asylum, he joined the Chinese Imperial Maritime Customs Service as Medical Officer, first in Formosa, later at Amoy and, later still, in Hong Kong. In China he soon acquired extensive experience of elephantiasis (Lymphatic Filariasis) in which parasitic

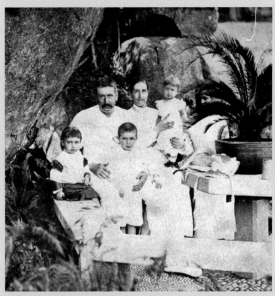

4.48 Sir Patrick Manson (1844–1922) (*Wellcome Library, London*).

worms produce an inflammation and obstruction of the lymphatic vessels that leads to extreme enlargement of the affected area, most commonly the limbs. After years of research, he proved that the disease was transmitted by the bites of a mosquito, *Culex fatigans*. Manson went on to speculate that malaria might be transmitted in the same way. However, the idea that elephantiasis, malaria or any other disease could be transmitted by an animal vector was new, and for a time it was vigorously resisted by the medical establishment. Nevertheless, Manson persisted. In 1890 he returned to Britain to continue his work at the Seamen's Hospital in London, and four years later he published a full account of his ideas on the relationship between the mosquito and malaria.

Later that year he was visited by Ronald Ross, a Staff Surgeon in the Indian Medical Service on leave from Bangalore. Ross had been conducting his own research on malaria, but had been sceptical of the idea that it was transmitted by mosquitoes. But after meeting Manson, he wrote 'My doubts are now removed.' With some initial guidance from Manson, Ross began his work to prove that the mosquito was the vector of malaria. His investigations were unsuccessful until in 1898 he discovered that the vector was not the common brown mosquito (*Culex fatigans*) but the anopheline mosquito (*Anopheles gambia*), a discovery for which he was awarded the Nobel Prize. Manson did not share in the award, but he went on to found the London School of Tropical Medicine and is still regarded as the Father of Tropical Medicine.

sanction of science but must be 'inductive and empirical'. However he stressed to his Scottish audience that his was the English tradition, 'not the tradition of your country'. It was a difference that was reflected in the academic careers of many Scottish trained clinicians and medical scientists. The empirical physicians and surgeons who dominated the leading teaching hospitals in England were intent on creating their students, and therefore their potential successors, in their own image. Careers in laboratory science or in academic medicine and surgery were

not presented as carrying the same prestige as success in fashionable clinical practice. The opposite was the case in the university medical schools in Scotland. There the most ambitious students very often chose to make their careers in the academic world. Trained in Edinburgh at the College Laboratory, or later in research orientated university departments established at Glasgow and Edinburgh, many were appointed to university chairs in laboratory medicine or in clinical medicine or surgery.

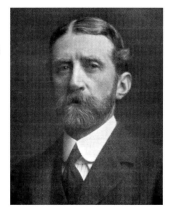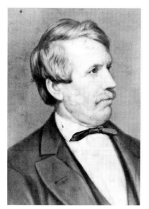

4.49 *Right.* Diarmid Noel Paton (1859–1928) succeeded German Sims Woodhead as Superintendent of the Research Laboratory of the Royal College of Physicians in 1890. The son of the painter Sir Joseph Noel Paton, he was educated at Edinburgh Academy and Edinburgh University, graduating BSc in 1881 and MB CM in 1882. After studying in Europe, he was awarded a fellowship in the physiology department of Edinburgh University. He then set up in private practice as a physician, but retired from practice when he became Superintendent of the Research Laboratory in 1890. He later became Regius Professor of Physiology at Glasgow University (*RCPSG*).

4.50 *Far right.* David Livingstone (1813–73). Explorer and medical missionary (*Library of Congress, USA*).

Later prestigious appointments of members of the Research Laboratory

Medical Science

R. Barry, Professor of Anatomy, Melbourne

E. P. Cathcart, Professor of Physiology, Glasgow

J. N. Davidson, Professor of Biochemistry, Glasgow

W. S. Greenfield, Professor of Pathology, Cambridge

W. O. Cormack, Professor of Biochemistry, Aberdeen

S. McDonald, Professor of Pathology, Durham

J. Miller, Professor of Pathology, Queen's, Ontario

D. Noel Paton, Professor of Physiology, Glasgow

J. Ritchie, Professor of Bacteriology, Oxford

T. Shennan, Professor of Pathology, Aberdeen

Sir G. M. Woodhead, Professor of Pathology, Cambridge

C.Y. Yang, Professor of Pathology, Hong Kong

Clinical Medicine and Surgery

F. D. Boyd, Professor of Clinical Medicine, Edinburgh

Sir John Fraser, Professor of Clinical Surgery, Edinburgh

G. L. Gulland, Professor of Medicine, Edinburgh

R. T. Ritchie, Professor of Medicine, Edinburgh

R. Stockman, Professor of Materia Medica, Glasgow

H. A. Thomson, Professor of Surgery, Edinburgh

Sir John Batty Tuke, President Royal College of Physicians, Edinburgh

Sir Byrom Branwell, President Royal College of Physicians, Edinburgh

A. H. Freeland Barbour, President Royal College of Physicians, Edinburgh

G. Lovell Gulland, President Royal College of Physicians, Edinburgh

Alexander Goodall, President Royal College of Physicians, Edinburgh

MEDICAL MISSIONARIES

Having acquired a vast empire, Victorian Britain dreamed not only of ruling the world but of redeeming it. From 1860 until 1960, Scottish medical missionaries served in Africa, China, India, the Middle East, the Pacific Islands and the Caribbean. During the greater part of that time they, together with other Christian missions, provided the peoples of Africa with a prototype health service, while the various colonial governments did little or nothing. The most remarkable medical missionaries to Africa in those years were David Livingstone and Neil Macvicar.

David Livingstone

David Livingstone (1813–1873) was born in Blantyre, Lanarkshire, on 19 March 1813 into a family that had left the poverty of the Hebridean island of Ulva to find employment in the new cotton mills of central Scotland. Livingstone attended a local school until the age of 10; from then until he was 26 he was employed in a cotton mill, first as a 'piecer' (re-tying broken threads) and later as a spinner. During these years he took full advantage of the evening classes that his employer offered to all his workers and by the age of 21 he was preparing for a life as a medical missionary. He continued to save what he could from his wages, until in 1836 he could afford to enrol as a medical student at Anderson's University in Glasgow. There he studied anatomy, physiology, chemistry, materia medica, the principles of surgery and the theory of medicine. At the same time he attended Greek and theology classes at Glasgow University. In the summer months between academic years he returned to work in the Blantyre cotton mill.

In 1838, Livingstone was accepted for training by the London Missionary Society, and financed by the Society

Anderson's University was founded by the will of John Anderson, MA FRS (1726–1796) Professor of Natural Philosophy at Glasgow University from 1760 until his death. Anderson believed that a knowledge of the principles of natural philosophy would be invaluable to many of the craftsmen, engineers and mechanics who were then vital to the development of Glasgow's new industries, but for whom a university education was not possible. During his thirty-six year tenure of his chair at Glasgow University, he held open and free evening classes on natural philosophy every Tuesday and Thursday during the academic year. When he died in January 1796, he left everything he owned 'to the public, for the good of mankind, and the improvement of science, in an institution to be denominated "Anderson's University".' His foundation was at first known as Anderson's Institution. In 1828 the name was changed to Anderson's University, and in 1877, by Act of Parliament, it became Anderson's College.

It had been John Anderson's intention that his university should have all four of the faculties offered by the other universities in Scotland at that time – Arts, Medicine, Law and Theology. However funds were never adequate for the establishment of faculties of Law or Theology. Chairs of Midwifery, Materia Medica and the Practice of Medicine were instituted in 1828, followed by Medical Jurisprudence in 1831, Institutes of Medicine (Physiology) in 1849 and Ophthalmic Medicine and Surgery in 1869. The Medical School did not offer any clinical teaching. Students were therefore obliged to seek clinical experience in hospitals in Glasgow or elsewhere before presenting themselves for examination for a licence to practice from one or other of the Royal Colleges (or Faculties) of Medicine and Surgery. Nevertheless, Anderson's University (or College) was for many years a highly regarded extra-mural school providing a medical education for those who could not afford a place at one of the ancient universities.

However, in the 1920s, the number enrolling to study medicine at Anderson's College was in sharp decline, until a quota system introduced in the United States reduced the numbers of Jewish students being admitted to American medical schools. By 1929 many of these excluded Jewish students had begun to make their way to medical schools in Scotland. The number studying at Anderson's College reached 253 in 1938.

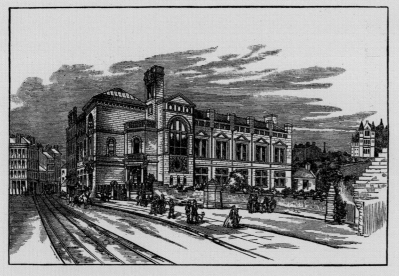

4.51 Anderson's University in Glasgow.

Year	1930	1931	1932	1933	1934	1935	1936	1937	1938
Number	24	40	66	71	89	123	168	196	253

American Jewish Medical Students at Anderson's College, Glasgow

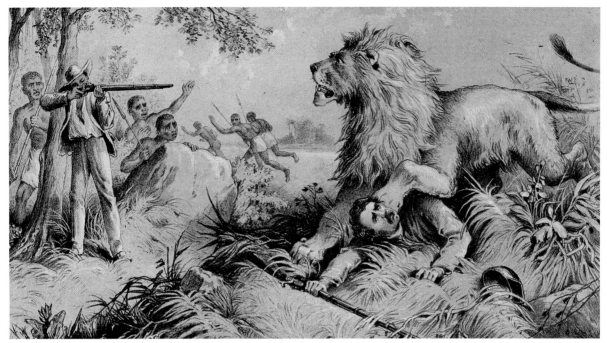

4.52 On one of his long and hazardous treks, David Livingstone was attacked by a lion. He suffered a fracture of his humerus which failed to heal normally, leaving him with an unstable and much weakened left arm (*reproduced from David Livingstone, Missionary Travels and Researches in South Africa*).

he moved to London to complete his medical training at Charing Cross Hospital, St Bartholomew's Hospital and Moorfields Hospital. In November 1840 he obtained his licence to practise from the Royal Faculty of Physicians and Surgeons of Glasgow. He was sent as an assistant to the mission station established ten years earlier at Kuruman, to the north of the Orange River, 500 miles from Cape Town. For three years he played his part in the work of the mission, but he became dissatisfied by his life caring for the medical needs of a small, unambitious and settled Christian community. In 1844, he was given permission to move 250 miles to the north-east to establish a small mission in the remote district of Mobotswa. From there he began his 'itinerating' (his word for travelling) even further to the north, to find new African communities and bring them into the orbit of the Christian missions.

His 'itinerating' led him into the heart of a vast area of Africa still thought of in Britain as *terra incognita*. There he found a large native population, its traditional way of life troubled and degraded by the activities of Portuguese slave traders. Livingstone decided that these and all the peoples of central Africa could best be saved by the twin forces of Christianity and commerce. The presence of missionaries and honest traders would lead to the estab-

lishment of an ethical and profitable form of commerce that would undercut and end the slave trade, allowing the development of a peaceful, prosperous and free African society. Livingstone believed that, as his mission, he had been called to open up a route that would provide prospective ethical traders with ready access into the heart of Africa.

In October 1852 he marched north across the Kalahari Desert to Linyanti in central Africa, twelve hundred miles north of Cape Town. From Linyanti he searched for possible routes to the coast. First he explored the difficult and treacherous thousand miles to the west coast at Loanda. When that search proved unsuccessful, he explored the equally difficult eight hundred miles to the east coast at Quilemane. When he reached there in May 1856, he had once again failed to find the route he was seeking. But reports of his explorations had made him a celebrity. HMS *Frolic* was at hand to carry him to Mauritius, and from there he was taken by steamer and by rail to London. In Britain he was welcomed as a hero and showered with honours.

Livingstone was exhausted and unwell, but he was determined to return to Africa. Since the London Missionary Society would not countenance any further 'adventures', he looked to the British government for

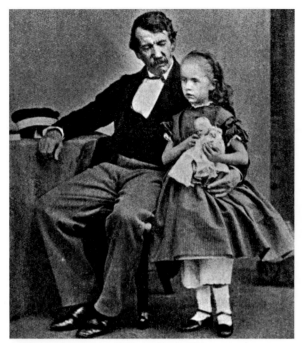

4.53 Livingstone at home with his daughter (*corbisimages.com*).

support. The government proposed that he should lead a large expedition of over two hundred officers and ratings of the Royal Navy into the valley of the Zambesi. Livingstone refused to be associated with what appeared to be a British attempt to take possession of central Africa. In March 1858 he set out with a much smaller party to navigate and explore the Zambesi as another possible commercial route into the interior. But the expedition was a disaster, and in 1864 Livingstone was recalled by the British Government.

Livingstone was still determined to return to Africa. In 1866 he was granted £500 by the Royal Geographical Society and £500 from the Foreign Office to explore the upper reaches of the Nile. As his search blundered on, his few European companions gradually left him; he lost all contact with the outside world until he was 'discovered' by Henry Morton Stanley in October 1871. Thereafter he remained in Africa until his death in 1873.

During his years in Africa, Livingstone had 'discovered' Victoria Falls, Lake Ngami, Lake Malawi, and Lake Bangweulu; he had defined the extent of Lake Tanganyika and Lake Mweru. He had explored the course of several rivers and mapped parts of central Africa for the first time. But his mission to save the people of central Africa by bringing them Christianity and commerce had failed.

Neil Macvicar (1871–1949)

Neil Macvicar's mission took a quite different course. He was born in 1871 at Manor, near Peebles in Scotland, where his father was parish minister. On leaving school he was apprenticed to a firm of lawyers in Peebles, but he soon became determined to become a medical missionary. On completing his legal apprenticeship he studied medicine at Edinburgh University. He was the outstanding student of his year, graduating M.B., C.M. with first-class honours in 1893. After serving as house physician and house surgeon at Edinburgh Royal Infirmary, in 1895 he was appointed medical officer to the Blantyre Mission of the Church of Scotland in Nyasaland (Malawi). There he immediately began to build a comprehensive health service, based on a central hospital in Blantyre linked to a series of peripheral rural dispensaries run by African 'medical assistants' trained at the central hospital. This scheme was adopted by other medical missions and much later by the colonial government.

In 1900, Macvicar returned to Scotland, and after a further period of study (taking his Diploma in Public Health), in 1902 he was appointed medical officer to the Victoria Hospital at Lovedale in Cape Colony. The hospital had been established in 1898 but had been closed during the Boer War. Macvicar gradually built up the hospital to a total complement of 170 beds. However he found it impossible in the 'white'-dominated medical world of Cape Colony to employ locally trained medical assistants to establish and run peripheral dispensaries.

In 1903, in face of strong opposition from both European and Bantu sections of the population, he began the training of Bantu girls as nurses, hundreds of whom were later employed throughout the Union of South Africa. In 1909 he began to lecture on public health, founding the South African Health Society and editing its journal *The Health Magazine* until his death in 1949. As a missionary Neil Macvicar had focused on the provision of essential health services for the native population of a colonial Africa. This was in sharp contrast with the intention of his illustrious predecessor, David Livingstone, whose aim was to help establish a prosperous non-colonial Christian Africa.

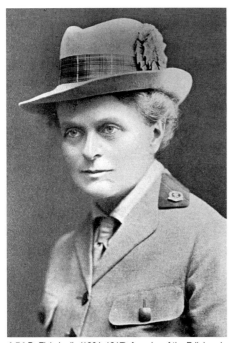

4.54 Dr Elsie Inglis (1864–1917), founder of the Edinburgh Maternity Hospice in 1899, the forerunner of the Elsie Inglis Memorial Maternity Hospital.

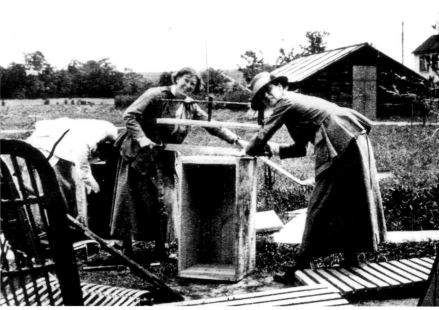

4.55 Doctors making furniture at a Scottish Women's Hospitals camp at Villers Cotterets, France (*Mitchell Library, Glasgow*).

WOMEN'S HOSPITALS

By 1914, there were fifteen hospitals in Britain founded and staffed entirely by women. They were promoted in the belief that the medical care provided by women-run hospitals was more appropriate to female patients' needs than that provided in male-staffed hospitals. Women's hospitals also provided a means of opening career possibilities for women graduates, as in the early years of the twentieth century women were still effectively excluded from the staff of the country's prestigious voluntary hospitals; they also offered training opportunities for young medical graduates. The Glasgow Private Hospital for Women (15 beds) was founded in 1903 by two women general practitioners, but had male specialists as consultants. The Dundee Private Hospital for Women (6 beds) was founded by two female general practitioners, but received the female patients of practitioners of either sex. The two hospitals in Edinburgh, the Edinburgh Hospital for Women and Children (5 beds, later 60 beds) founded by Jex-Blake in 1885, and the Edinburgh Maternity Hospice (13 beds) founded by Elsie Inglis in 1899, were both staffed entirely by women. By 1914 women doctors in Scotland had been providing hospital services for almost twenty years, but they had treated only women and children. That limitation was breached in 1914.

Within weeks of the outbreak of the Great War, Dr Elsie Inglis (1864–1917) offered her services to the army as a military surgeon.

Elsie Inglis was born into a family with long and distinguished associations with India. Her great-grandfather had been secretary to Warren Hastings, the first Governor General of India. Her father had been a director of the East India Company before being appointed Chief Commissioner of Oudh. Elsie Inglis, the sixth of eight children, was born at Niani Tal in the foothills of the Himalayas.

When her father retired in 1875, the family returned to Edinburgh. Elsie was educated privately, and even as a very young woman she became actively involved in the Women's Suffrage movement. At the age of 21 she enrolled as a student at Sophia Jex-Blake's Edinburgh School of Medicine for Women. Following a disagreement with Sophia Jex-Blake, she and her father launched the Scottish Association for the Medical Education of Women, which created a new Medical College for Women in Chambers Street in Edinburgh. Elsie Inglis continued her studies there and later completed her surgical training under Sir William Macewen at Glasgow Royal Infirmary. In 1892 she qualified to practise as a licentiate of the Royal College of Physicians of Edinburgh, the Royal College of Surgeons of Edinburgh and the Royal Faculty of Physicians and

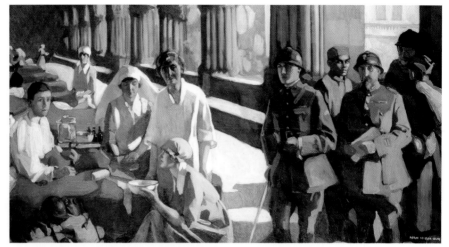

4.56 A painting by Norah Neilson Gray of the Scottish Women's Hospital at Royaumont, north of Paris. The woman doctor in the foreground is Frances Ivens, Chief Medical Officer at Royaumont throughout the war. She was awarded Legion d'Honneur and Croix de Guerre for her services. After the war she became a consultant in obstetrics and gynaecology in Liverpool.

Surgeons of Glasgow. After spending some time at Elizabeth Garret Anderson's New Hospital for Women in London and at the Rotunda Hospital in Dublin, she set up in general practice in Edinburgh with Dr Jessie MacGregor and opened a maternity hospital for poor women (later the Elsie Inglis Maternity Hospital). In 1905 she was appointed consultant at the Edinburgh Hospital for Women and Children at Bruntsfield.

The Scottish Women's Hospitals

When she offered her services to the army at Edinburgh Castle in 1914, Elsie was 50 years old and already unwell. Her offer was refused; she was advised to 'go home and sit still'. This she was unwilling to do. She was Honorary Secretary of the Scottish Federation of Women's Suffrage Societies, and at the next meeting of its committee she proposed that the Federation should raise a fully-equipped military hospital staffed entirely by women; since the British army had been so unwelcoming it was agreed that the hospital should be offered to one of the allies, Belgium, France or Serbia. The scheme was adopted and later expanded by the National Union of Women's Suffrage Societies in London, and thereafter much of its funding came from England. Nevertheless, since the proposal had come from Scotland, the title 'Scottish Women's Hospitals' was agreed and the headquarters were established in St Andrew Square in Edinburgh.

Before a Scottish Women's Hospital (SWH) could be sent there, Belgium had already been overrun by the German armies. When the first SWH arrived in Calais in November 1914, Belgian casualties were flowing in and within days they had been further afflicted by an outbreak of typhoid. In December the SWH moved to Royaumont, 25 miles north of Paris, where it continued to receive floods of casualties up to and beyond the Great Push of July 1916. A SWH sent to Serbia in December 1914 at first found few wounded, but was confronted by an extensive outbreak of typhus. Special fever hospitals were set up, but when, in 1915, Serbia began to collapse before the forces of Austria, Germany and Bulgaria, the number of casualties vastly increased. An additional SWH dispatched to help in December 1915 was diverted to Malta to take care of casualties evacuated from the disastrous Gallipoli campaign.

By the end of the Great War, SWHs had served with distinction in France, Serbia, Siberia, Russia, Bulgaria, Malta, Corsica and Greece. Elsie Inglis had remained in Edinburgh to direct the operation of her scheme. But in April 1915 the Chief Medical Officer of the principal SWH in Serbia became ill. Elsie Inglis immediately took her place, and thereafter took personal charge of the treatment of the sick and the wounded in the war zones of Eastern Europe until February 1916. Many believed that her achievements ranked with those of Florence Nightingale. However Florence Nightingale survived for long enough to press home the lessons that had been learnt in the Crimea. In contrast, when the Great War came to an end in 1918, Elsie Inglis had already been dead for a year.

In England, the great teaching hospitals that had opened their doors to women during the war were quick to close them again when the war ended. In Scotland, the university medical schools continued to admit women as they had done since the 1890s; but the career opportunities open to women graduating in Scotland were now no greater than they had been before Elsie Inglis had demonstrated the potential of women doctors in providing excellent hospital services even in the most difficult of circumstances.

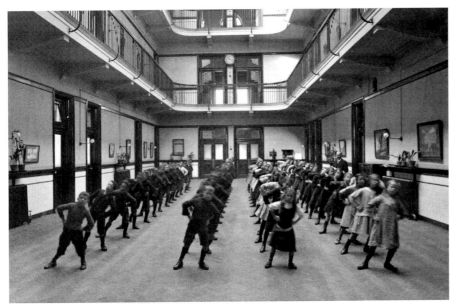

4.57 Alarmed at the extremely poor level of physical fitness among recruits for service in the Boer War, the government set up an Inter-departmental Committee on Physical Deterioration in 1902. One of its recommendations was that physical education should be part of the curriculum in British schools. Shown here is a physical education class ('drill') at London Road Public School in Glasgow (*Glasgow City Council Archives*).

STATE PROMOTION OF EFFICIENCY AND HEALTH

At the end of the nineteenth century, Britain was the most powerful nation in the world with an empire that reached round the globe. It owed its position to the wealth created by its resources of iron and coal, the productivity of its heavy industries and its dominance of world trade. In 1890 Britain still produced and exported more coal, more steel and more ships than any other nation. But in 1900, while Britain's annual output of coal had risen to 219 million tons, America produced 268 tons; Britain now produced 5 million tons of steel but Germany produced 6 million tons, already owned two million tons of merchant shipping and had a 20% share of world trade. Britain was in danger of falling behind, and many blamed this on deficiencies in the strength and energy of the workforce. Britain had recently become engaged in a 'small' war with the Boer population of South Africa; after two and a half years Britain, although claiming victory, had been frequently defeated, humiliated and discredited in the eyes of the major nations of Europe. The generals blamed the qualities of their men. Yet the men had been the fittest available. Of the many thousands who had volunteered to fight, as many as 73% had to be rejected as unfit.

At the beginning of the twentieth century, the political classes became suddenly afraid that Britain was losing its place in the world because of a loss of fitness, vigour and efficiency in its people. In his Rectorial Address at Glasgow University in 1900, Lord Rosebery launched a drive for National Efficiency. For a time National Efficiency became an attractive and adaptable, even if very uncertain, ideology which grouped together all manner of projects intended to rescue the nation from decline.

In most fields of activity the drive for 'Efficiency' soon died out, but the promotion of National Efficiency by improving the physical fitness of the people attracted more lasting attention. In 1902 the Secretary for Scotland set up a Royal Commission on Physical Training to discover whether the promotion of physical education in Scotland's schools would improve 'national strength'. The investigation was conducted by Leslie Mackenzie, Medical Officer of Health for Leith, and Professor Matthew Hay, Medical Officer of Health for Aberdeen. They found that there could be a place for physical education in schools, but that such a programme would be pointless while so many of the children were undernourished and hungry. The government took no action on their report in 1903, but three years later a Glasgow-born Member of Parliament, Arthur Henderson, raised the matter in the House of Commons. An Education (Provision of Meals) Act followed in 1906, and in 1908 legislation 'for attending to the health and physical condition of children in Public Elementary Schools' established the School Health Service in Scotland.

In the years that followed, other methods of achieving improvement in the strength, fitness and quality of the nation were promoted by the state.

EUGENICS

Francis Galton (1822–1911) first introduced the concept of eugenics in 1883 in his *Inheritance of Human Faculties*. His idea was that the quality of the race could be improved by selective breeding to get rid of the undesirables (negative breeding) and multiply the desirables (positive breeding). Some 200 people came together, forming the Eugenics Society to promote the idea. It soon became apparent that positive breeding was impracticable, since there was no agreement on which were the desirable qualities to be encouraged. Negative breeding was more feasible, but it met with strong ethical objections. Laws had already been passed in California, Canada, Sweden and Switzerland to provide for the sterilisation of defective subjects. In Britain no such laws were ever passed, but in 1913 a Mental Deficiency Act was passed to make it compulsory for the feeble-minded, idiots, imbeciles, and moral imbeciles (including habitual drunkards) to be institutionalised and segregated by sex to prevent them from breeding. The law could not be implemented during the First World War, and later became impossible to put into practice, as Britain's doctors refused to certify children as 'defective' against the wishes of their parents.

IMPROVED MATERNITY SERVICES

In 1880, maternal mortality was still high in all social classes, and particularly high in lying-in hospitals where the death rate could be ten times that for deliveries at home. The introduction of first antiseptic and later aseptic techniques brought a general reduction in deaths from puerperal sepsis and a spectacular reduction in maternal deaths in hospital. By 1900 the risk of death from puerperal fever was for the first time lower in hospitals than in home deliveries. It was assumed that the maternity mortality rate (MMR) in home deliveries could be further improved by more general and more rigorous application of hospital practices. In 1902 a Maternity Act was intended to ensure that hospital-trained midwives would be more generally available for home deliveries. Contrary to expectation, the MMR increased, and by 1918 in Scotland it had reached 7 per thousand births. Moves were made to increase the participation of general practitioners in home deliveries. Again this brought no improvement. In 1935 a *Report on Maternal Morbidity and Mortality in Scotland* concluded that 'the general level of antenatal care is unsatisfactory' and 'there is no doubt that one of the most disquieting features of present day obstetrics is hurried and unnecessarily meddlesome midwifery.' In 1935, while in England it was 4.2, the MMR in Scotland was 6.2 (in Renfrewshire it was 8.5 and in Coatbridge, at the centre of the iron and steel industry, it was 12). That year an experiment in Wales showed that the number of maternal deaths could be dramatically reduced by the distribution of food to women attending antenatal clinics. The distribution of free food to pregnant women did not, however, become an accepted practice.

IMPROVED INFANT WELFARE

The high infant mortality that accompanied the industri-alisation of Britain reached its peak in the 1870s. In Scot-land the Infant Mortality Rate (IMR), even at its worst in Glasgow and Dundee, was never as high as in England. But in the last decades of the century the IMR declined more rapidly in England than in Scotland. By 1910 the rate was equal in the two countries. But the rate was still appalling, at 110 per thousand live births.

The greatest immediate cause of death was the summer plague of infective infant diarrhoea. In 1901, William Robertson, the Medical Officer of Health for Leith, persuaded his local authority to introduce a scheme that had proved successful in France. A 'Milk Depot' was set up in Leith at which mothers were supplied with 'clean' milk, and where the growth and health of their infants was carefully monitored. The scheme was judged to be a success, and it was copied in Glasgow and Dundee. However, the effect of the schemes on the IMR was never measured.

At that time the gathering of statistics on infant deaths was unsatisfactory. It was generally understood that deaths were particularly common among illegitimate infants and among infants who had fallen victim to 'baby farming' (the boarding out of unwanted new-born infants) although no reliable statistics were available. A.C. Chalmers, Medical Officer of Health in Glasgow, led a campaign that led to the passing of the Notification of Births Act in 1907. The information gathered prompted Edinburgh to appoint the first health visitor, and by 1910 this single official was assisted by 300 volunteers. Gradu-ally other local authorities in Scotland followed this lead.

In the early months of the First World War, the IMR rose to 125.5 per thousand births, reversing the earlier trend. In 1915 the government made the Notification of Births compulsory, and offered a 50% grant to support Milk Depots and empowered local authorities 'to make such arrangements as they think fit and be sanctioned by us for the attending to the health of expectant mothers and nursing mothers and of children under the age of five years.' Local authorities varied in their response to this opportunity, but overall the move proved successful. By the end of the war the IMR had fallen to 77.

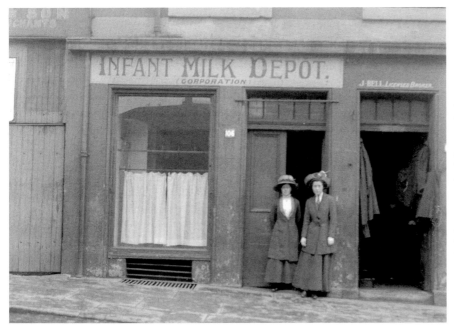

4.58 By the end of the nineteenth century, the appallingly high Infant Mortality Rate in Britain had given rise to fears that there would be a dangerous weakening of the nation. The major cause of infant deaths at that time was infective 'summer diarrhoea'. In 1901 William Robertson, Medical Officer of Health for Leith, established a Milk Depot to provide free 'clean' uncontaminated milk for the children of the poor, the chief victims of 'summer diarrhoea'. Milk Depots were later established elsewhere in Scotland. Illustrated here is the depot established in Cowcaddens Street in Glasgow (*Glasgow City Council Archives*).

MEDICAL CARE FOR THE INDUSTRIAL WORKFORCE:
THE NATIONAL HEALTH INSURANCE SCHEME

The recommendations of a Royal Commission on the Poor Laws and Relief of Distress, after two years of vigorous debate, led in 1911 to the introduction to Parliament of Lloyd George's National Insurance Bill. At its first reading, it was found to include a scheme for National Health Insurance. The proposal came as a 'bolt from the blue'. From January 1912, the Act brought in an insurance scheme, compulsory for persons employed under a contract of service in manual labour but open on a voluntary basis to non-manual workers whose annual income did not exceed £160. Together the insured person and his employer were to pay 7d (7 pence) per week (6d for a woman) and the state added a contribution of 2d. In addition to a cash benefit during periods of incapacity for work

and a maternity benefit of £2, to be paid on the confinement of an insured woman or the wife of an insured man, every insured person (but not his wife or children) was entitled to medical treatment by a doctor included on a 'panel' of accredited general practitioners. Every qualified medical practitioner had the right to be included in this panel of insurance medical practitioners and to enrol up to 2,500 insured persons on his list, and for each one he would receive a capitation fee of nine shillings. The scheme was generally popular in Scotland, but its contribution to the health of the working population was negligible. It displaced local schemes that had been in place for many years, schemes that had provided medical attendance not only for the worker but also his wife and children.

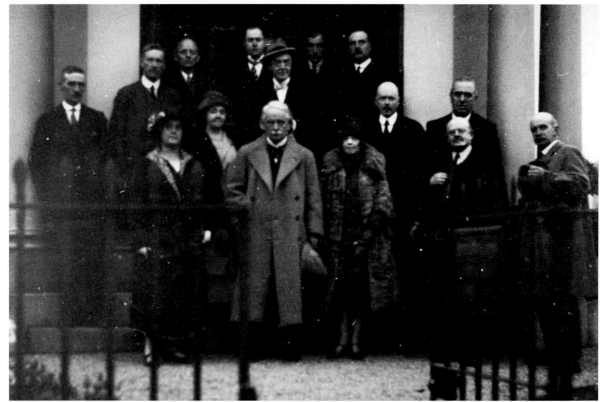

4.59 David Lloyd George at Burns' Mausoleum, Dumfries, in 1925. David Lloyd George was no longer Prime Minister but remained a popular figure when he visited Dumfries in 1925. He gave a speech in the town's drill hall to a capacity audience before visiting the grave of Robert Burns at the mausoleum in St Michael's Churchyard, Dumfries (*Dumfries and Galloway Museums Service*).

HIGHLANDS AND ISLANDS MEDICAL SERVICE

There was a large part of Scotland where the National Health Insurance Scheme was unworkable. In the Crofting Counties of the Highlands and Islands, the great majority of the workers were independent crofters, with no contracts of labour and no employers to share the cost of the contribution to the Scheme; crofters were almost by definition poor and even the few pennies of a weekly contribution could not be afforded.

On 11 July 1912 the Chancellor of the Exchequer set a committee, the Dewar Committee, to report on the provision of medical attention in the Highlands and Islands and to advise on the best method of securing an adequate medical service in the region. The Dewar Committee found that medical services there were very near to collapse and that government intervention was now essential. In an appendix to the report Leslie Mackenzie (Medical Officer of Health for Leith and a member of the Committee) set out a *Scheme for the Administrative Consolidation of Medical Services in the Highlands and Islands*.

Later in December 1913 the Secretary for Scotland announced a grant of £42,000 to finance a Highlands and Islands Medical Service and the establishment of a Highland and Islands Medical Board to administer it. All eight members of the Board were familiar with the way of life in the Highlands and Islands, and six were doctors with experience in the administration of medical services. The Board was made responsible for the provision of medical

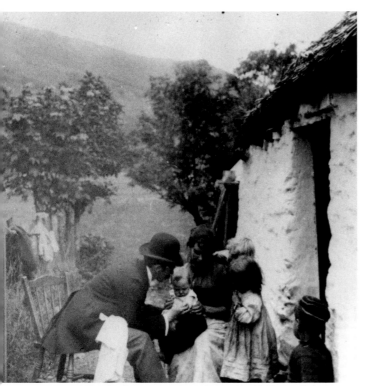

4.60 Lachlan Grant, a general practitioner of the Highland and Islands Medical Service, is seen here examining a sick child. Since the examination would have been difficult in the dark interior of the 'black house', the child has been has been taken outdoors (*Scottish Life Archive, National Museums of Scotland*).

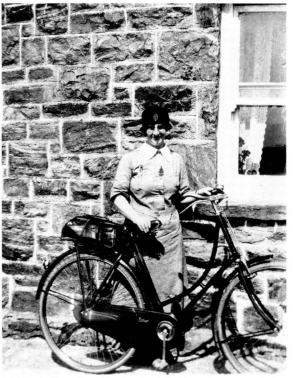

4.61 District Nurse, Ness, Isle of Lewis, 1930s. The nurses were recruited through the Queen's Jubilee Institute for Nurses. Most were issued with bicycles, although some had motorcycles which they found particularly suitable for the terrain they had to cover (*Scottish Life Archive, National Museum of Scotland*).

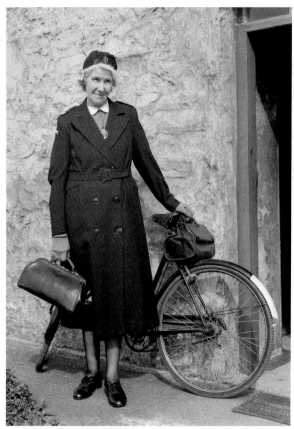

4.62 Margaret Cairns, District Nurse, Fair Isle, Shetland, 1956. The introduction of the National Health Service (Scotland) Act 1947 made it compulsory for every County and City Council to provide the services of District Nurses, although as a result of the Highlands and Islands Medical scheme, many were already in place (*Scottish Life Archive, National Museum of Scotland*).

care to a population of 285,000 people scattered over 14,000 square miles of difficult country. It found an imaginative way in which to make best use of a very small budget. Payment of general practitioners by capitation fee, as in the new National Health Insurance Scheme, was seen as inappropriate. It would have operated much to the advantage of practitioners in the more populous areas who had easy access to comparatively large numbers of patients without heavy expenditure on travel. Payment by salary would have been difficult to adjust to reflect the unequal demands of very different practices and would have acted as a disincentive to the doctors' effort and initiative, especially in caring for their most remote patients. In the

scheme adopted by the Board, Treasury funds were used to subsidise practice expenses rather than to contribute directly to the doctor's income. Each practice received a grant calculated to reflect its particular operating expenses, such as the distribution of free medicines and the cost of travel. Where necessary, the doctor was assisted in buying his own motor boat, motor car or whatever means of travel was appropriate. Provision was made either for the improvement of the houses already occupied by doctors or for the building of new ones. In calculating the grant for each practice, care was taken to ensure that the doctor's income would not fall below a reasonable minimum. In return the doctors were required to 'visit systematically those requiring medical attention, including Poor Law and insured persons and also to undertake such Public Health duties as were required.' For patients not insured or entitled to treatment under the Poor Law, doctors were allowed to charge fees of 5s (five shillings) for a first visit and 2/6 (two shillings and sixpence) for subsequent visits; the fee for midwifery was set at one pound. It was understood, however, that, based on previous experience in the region, it was unlikely that these fees would ever be paid. Grants were planned to meet the cost of patients' travel for necessary specialist services in Aberdeen, Glasgow or Edinburgh.

Full implementation of the scheme was interrupted by the First World War. Then, in August 1919, the administration of the Highlands and Islands Medical Service was taken over by the newly created Scottish Health Board in Edinburgh. Thereafter the service developed steadily. There was no difficulty in recruiting medical staff. District Nurses were employed to manage and supervise the treatment of patients in their homes. From 1924, six cottage hospitals were upgraded and specialist services were introduced; consultant surgeons were appointed at five of these hospitals and consultant physicians from Aberdeen held regular outpatients clinics at each one. When necessary, from 1933 an Air Ambulance Service flew patients to teaching hospitals in Glasgow. The Highlands and Islands Medical Service proved to be successful and greatly valued by the people of the region it served. It became the model for medical services introduced in remote parts of Australia and the United States.

MEDICINE FOR THE TWENTIETH CENTURY

General Practice

In the first half of the twentieth century, four out of five members of the medical profession in Scotland were general practitioners. General practice was still a business, and fees charged by practitioners remained much as they had been in the 1890s. Each practitioner was, of course, at liberty to set his own rates but broadly, fees tended to be set in relation to house rentals, which were taken as a reflection of the income of the patients. It was assumed that the medical needs of patients paying less than £10 in rent, approximately a quarter of the population, would be supplied by the Poor Law, by one of Scotland's 1,300 Friendly Societies or by one of the many less formal 'clubs' which collected a modest weekly contribution (usually a penny for an adult and a halfpenny for a child); alternatively, such poor patients might consult a sixpenny doctor. ('Four pence for the medicine, six pence if I examine you.') For patients who seemed sufficiently well-housed, the usual fee was 2/6 (two shillings and sixpence) for each home visit, rising in the most affluent suburbs to 7/6 (seven shillings and sixpence) or even 10/6 (ten shillings and sixpence). A midwifery fee in a working class community was usually one pound or 15 shillings; in more affluent areas, three to five guineas was generally thought to be more appropriate. After 1919, most practitioners' incomes were enhanced by participation in the National Health Insurance Scheme, and many were further supplemented by appointments to insurance companies, industrial firms, private schools, police forces, Friendly Societies or one of the new state medical services. However, general practitioners continued to depend for at least two-thirds of their income on the fees paid by their patients; and since medicine was a crowded profession, there was intense competition in an open medical market. As a result fees, and therefore general practitioners' incomes, did not tend to rise with time. Few general practitioners were able to achieve an income of much more than £1,000 a year.

Very few general practices were based in purpose-built premises. General practitioners worked at and from home, usually without paid ancillary help. Once a practitioner was well established, he might advertise for an assistant 'with a view to partnership', although early in the century that full partnership might only be achieved after ten years. As practices expanded after the introduction of the National Health Insurance Scheme, partnerships became more common, but even in the 1930s only one in four general practitioners were partners. General practitioners were expected to provide a twenty-four hours a day, seven days a week service. The scope of that service varied. Since the Medical Act of 1858, every practitioner listed in the Medical Register maintained by the General Medical Council had been trained in medicine, surgery and midwifery and was entitled to practise in any of these fields according to his own assessment of his abilities. The distinction between general practitioner and hospital consultant was not absolute. Consultants had often made a living in general practice while struggling to establish themselves in their chosen specialist field, and had continued thereafter to act as general practitioners to a few well-chosen families. In the 1920s and 1930s, most general practitioners were able to deal with the vast majority of cases that came their way, but in difficult or unusual cases it was open to them to call in a consultant (for an additional fee) to see the patient in his or her home or to refer the patient to an appropriate hospital.

Hospital Practice

At the beginning of the twentieth century there were 21 general infirmaries, the largest in Edinburgh, Glasgow and Aberdeen. In the cities these were supplemented by 20 specialist hospitals – for women, for children, for midwifery, for cancer and for eye or ear, nose and throat surgery. Across the country in rural areas there were more than 40 cottage hospitals. Together these various hospitals provided accommodation for some 5,500 patients. The infirmaries and specialist hospitals were voluntary hospitals, staffed by leading physicians and surgeons who gave their services free, and supported in part by donations and bequests. The hospitals' regular funding, however, came from the collection of subscriptions, which entitled the subscribers to recommend patients for admission. Many of these 'subscribers' were not individuals but groups of

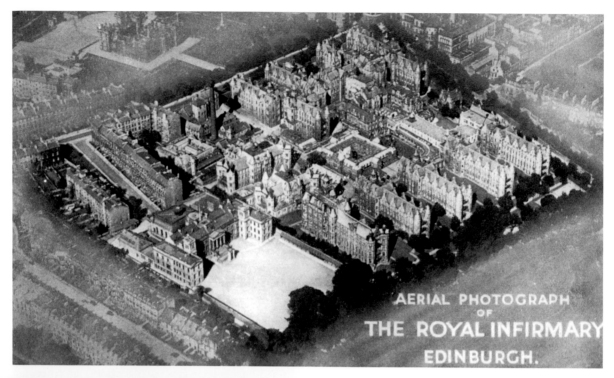

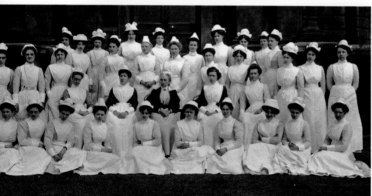

4.63 *Top.* Edinburgh Royal Infirmary, built in 1879. It was designed, not as a single very large block, but as a series of pavilions connected by corridors at street level. This was a layout proposed by Professor J.Y. Simpson to prevent, or at least limit, the transmission of infection from one ward to another.

4.64 *Above.* The nursing staff of Glasgow Royal Infirmary. The Matron, Rebecca Strong (centre), was born in London in 1843. In 1867 she became a pupil at Florence Nightingales' school for nurses at St Thomas's Hospital in London. She was appointed Nursing Superintendent (Matron) at Glasgow Royal Infirmary in 1879. In the following years she improved the accommodation of the patients and the working conditions of the nursing staff. She persuaded the Board to provide the nurses with suitable uniforms for the first time. However when in 1885 she failed to persuade the Board to build a nurses home she resigned. In 1891 she was only persuaded to return after a nursing home had at last been provided. With the encouragement of Sir William Macewen, the Professor of Clinical Surgery at the Royal Infirmary Medical School, she established a very successful nursing school which became the model for nursing schools elsewhere in Britain and overseas.

workers in mills, factories or other industrial firms, who clubbed together to make themselves eligible for treatment at a voluntary hospital of their choice. A number of business firms became subscribers in order to find proper hospital care for their employees and a few Poor Law authorities also became subscribers in order to find proper hospital care for their dependants.

The Public Health (Scotland) Act of 1897 had made it mandatory for local authorities, singly or in partnership with others, to establish hospitals for infectious fevers. And after the Poor Law responsibilities of Parochial Boards were transferred to elected local authority councils, some councils used their powers to establish new general and specialist hospitals of their own; the new authority in Glasgow was particularly active, building Stobhill Hospital (1,800 beds with a further 200 for tuberculosis), the Western District Hospital (320 beds) and the Eastern District Hospital (312 beds).

Although the early decades of the twentieth century saw a remarkable increase in the number of hospitals and hospital beds in Scotland, not every hospital was well-staffed or generously equipped. Hospital services in Scotland were still led and inspired by the large voluntary infirmaries that served as teaching hospitals for the medical schools of Aberdeen, Edinburgh, Glasgow and St Andrews. In these hospitals, the greatest advances were being achieved in surgery. The sudden adoption of general

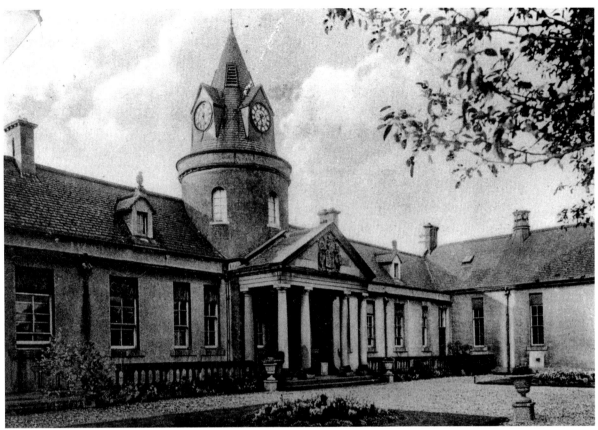

4.65 Randolph Wemyss Memorial Hospital, Buckhaven

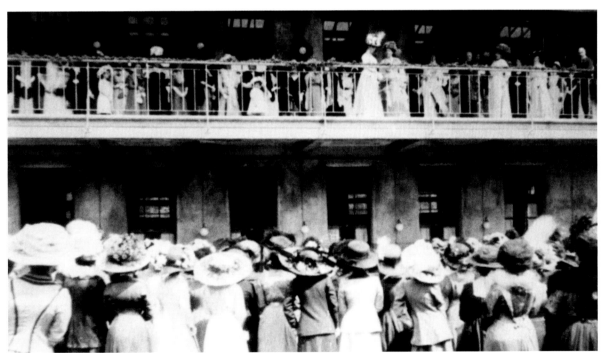

4.66 Sophia Jex Blake bought Bruntsfield Lodge in Whitehouse Loan, Edinburgh, in 1883. In 1885 it became the Edinburgh Hospital and Dispensary for Women and Children, later known as Bruntsfield Hospital. Until it became part of the National Health Service in 1948, Bruntsfield Hospital was staffed entirely by women doctors. This picture shows Queen Mary opening an extension to Bruntsfield Hospital in 1911. The hospital finally closed in 1989.

anaesthesia in the middle years of the nineteenth century and later the more gradual introduction of, first, antiseptic and then aseptic techniques had led to a vast expansion of the field of surgery. By 1865 the number of operations carried out each year at Glasgow's teaching hospitals had already increased to 310; in 1900 that number had become 4,531. In the nineteenth century appendicitis, then treated by frequent enemas and the generous use of opium, had carried a mortality of up to 70 %; in the first years of the twentieth century, appendicitis could be treated surgically with very little risk of death. Children crippled by rickets could have their distorted bones broken and reshaped; abdominal hernias that had once been a distressing inconvenience to be tolerated for a lifetime could now be easily corrected; and new operations could be devised and performed within the abdomen, within the chest and even within the cranium.

Advances in medicine were not so immediately and so obviously of advantage to the patient. But research in medical science led to some remarkable discoveries in the fields of radiology, cardiology and endocrinology. Scottish scientists and clinicians played some part.

Radiology

The world's first X-ray department was established by John Macintyre (1859–1928) at Glasgow Royal Infirmary in 1896. Macintyre was born in Glasgow and trained initially as an electrical engineer. He later studied medicine, graduating from Glasgow University in 1882. Thereafter he spent some time visiting hospitals in Vienna and elsewhere in Europe. On his return to Glasgow he held junior appointments at Glasgow Royal Infirmary and lectured on anatomy at St Mungo's College of Medicine before being appointed an ear, nose and throat surgeon at the Royal Infirmary. At the same time he was also appointed as the Infirmary's Consulting Medical Electrician.

When William Röntgen announced his discovery of X-rays in December 1895, he sent a copy of his paper to Lord Kelvin, who passed it to Macintyre. In March 1896 the managers of the Infirmary gave Macintyre permission to set up an X-ray branch of his electrical department. One of his many innovations, made with the co-operation

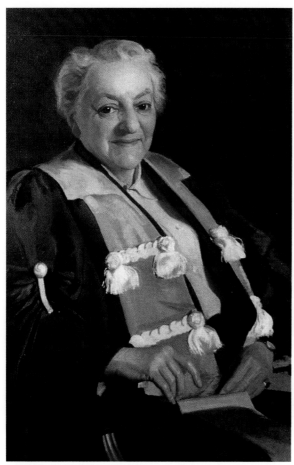

4.67 Gertrude Herzfeld (1890–1981) was, in 1920, the first woman to take her seat as a Fellow of the Royal College of Surgeons of Edinburgh. She was born in London, her parents having recently emigrated from Austria, and studied medicine at Edinburgh University, graduating in 1814. She became the first woman House Surgeon at Edinburgh Royal Infirmary. During World War I, she served in the Royal Army Medical Corps at Aldershot. Aferwards she became Assistant Surgeon at the Royal Hospital for Sick Children and Bruntsfield Hospital in Edinburgh. In 1925 she was appointed consultant to both these hospitals. She was later elected President of the Women's Medical Federation (*RCSEd*).

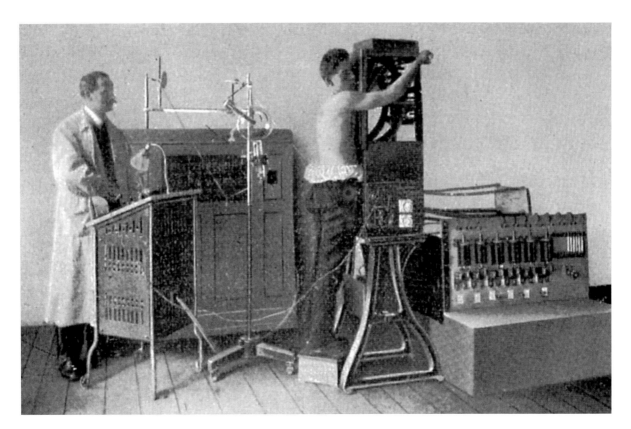

of Lord Kelvin, was a remarkable X-ray cine film of a moving frog's leg. At the inaugural meeting of the Röntgen Society (later the Royal Institute of Radiology), he was acknowledged as one of 'the earliest and most successful practitioners of the new art'.

Cardiology

Between 1882 and 1925 the orientation and practice of cardiology was transformed by Sir James Mackenzie (1853–1925). Mackenzie was born in Perthshire. After graduating MD from Edinburgh, he set up in practice as a general practitioner in Burnley in Lancashire, and for the next twenty years he combined practice with research work in cardiology. At that time cardiac ischemia and cardiac infarction had not yet been recognised as major health problems. Cardiology still centred on the abnormalities of the valves and structure of the heart; auscultation and the interpretation of heart murmurs were still the essential components of the examination of the patient. Mackenzie changed the focus of cardiological study to the function rather than the structure of the heart. He gave great attention to evidence of heart failure and he invented a polygraph which he used to study the rhythm of the heart by recording the arterial and venous pulses at various parts of the body. He was able to distinguish innocent arrhyth-

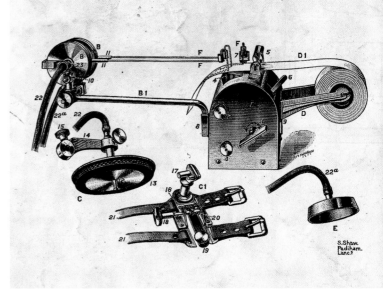

4.68 *Top.* Only surviving image of Britain's first hospital X-ray Department, established at Glasgow Royal Infirmary in 1896 by John Macintyre with the support and encouragement of Lord Kelvin (*Greater Glasgow and Clyde Archives*).

4.69 *Above.* The polygraph invented by Sir James Mackenzie (1853–1925) and used in his original studies of cardiac arrhythmias (*reproduced from* Sir James Mackenzie, The Future of Medicine, *London, 1919*).

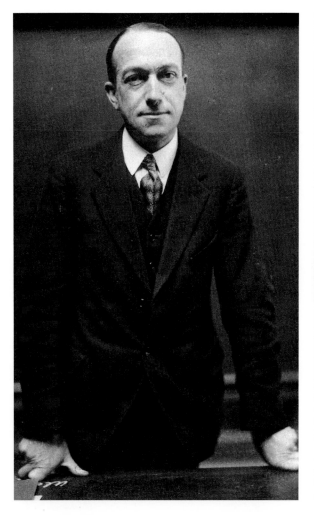

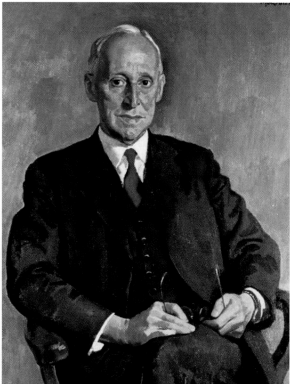

4.70 *Left.* Sir David Wilkie (1882–1938) who established in Scotland a new scientific tradition of discipline and criticism in surgical research and clinical practice.

4.71 *Above.* Sir Charles Illingworth (1899–1991), Regius Professor of Surgery at Glasgow University, who created at the University and the Western Infirmary, Glasgow, a department that became recognised as a world leader in surgical research and training (*RCPEd*).

mias from arrhythmias of pathological significance. He went on to establish the part that digitalis could play in treating those irregularities which impaired the function of the heart. In 1907 he moved to London to create a cardiology department at the London Hospital and to practise at 133 Harley Street. In 1915 he was knighted and made a Fellow of the Royal Society. In 1915 he returned to Scotland to establish a Clinical Research Institute at St Andrews. By then Mackenzie had already inspired a new generation of cardiologists in Britain, Europe and America.

Research-Based Systematic Surgery

In the years immediately following the First World War, the Rockefeller Foundation was intent, as they saw it, on dragging medical schools in Britain into the modern world. At Edinburgh in 1919, the Foundation supported the appointment of Jonathan Meakins (1882–1959) as the first Christison Professor of Therapeutics. He created a Biochemical Department which provided a diagnostic

testing service for the Royal Infirmary, but which was primarily a centre for research, now regarded as the true symbol of modernity. When Alexis Thomson, the Professor of Systematic Surgery, resigned in 1923, the Foundation offered to support the appointment of a successor who would also create a research laboratory and make research his chief commitment. In 1924 David Wilkie, then an assistant surgeon at Edinburgh Royal Infirmary, was the chosen candidate.

David Wilkie (1882–1938) was born in Kirriemuir, the son of a wealthy jute merchant. He was educated at Edinburgh Academy and Edinburgh University. He graduated first in 1904, adding the degrees of MD and ChM in 1909. His first appointment was to Leith Hospital, and during his years there his contributions to the surgical literature earned him election to the elite Moynihan Chirurgical Club.

During the First World War he served as a surgeon in the Royal Navy. On his return to Edinburgh he became

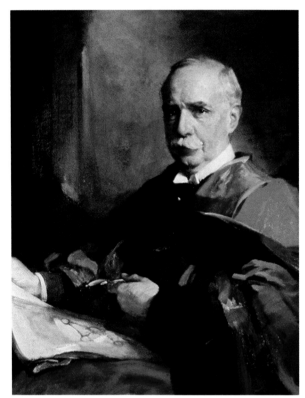

4.72 Sir Robert Philip (1857–1939) was born in Govan in Glasgow and graduated from Edinburgh University in 1882. He studied in Germany just after Robert Koch, in Berlin, had identified the bacteria responsible for pulmonary tuberculosis ('consumption'). In Edinburgh in 1887, he founded the first Dispensary for Consumption, and later established the Victoria Hospital for Consumption at Craigleith in Edinburgh (*RCPEd*).

assistant surgeon at the Royal Infirmary and a highly successful lecturer at the extramural school. Following his election to the Chair of Systematic Surgery he established a research department in a building formerly used for teaching anatomy to female students. It was equipped with an operating theatre, an X-ray unit and a photographic department. Another floor was added, and it became the best equipped surgical research department outside the USA. When he died at the early age of 52, he passed on his methods and his principles to his pupils, notably Charles Illingworth (1899–1991), William Wilson (1897–74) and Ian Aird (1905–62), who in turn passed them on to a new generation of surgeons in Britain and Australia.

Infectious Disease

Deaths from the acute infectious diseases declined steadily during the first half of the twentieth century. The decline was already well under way before immunisation against

diphtheria, tetanus and whooping cough had become widely available in the 1920s, and also many years before the discovery of antibiotics. By 1945 the number of deaths from measles, whooping cough, scarlet fever, and diphtheria was less than a fifth of the number in 1900. The decline was probably due principally to some general improvement in living standards and in the quality of care provided in the new local authority fever hospitals; but probably it was also due in part to a decline in the virulence of the diseases themselves.

Tuberculosis

Tuberculosis, however, remained the commonest single cause of the death of young adults. In Edinburgh in 1887 Robert Philip (1857–1939), later Sir Robert, had introduced a scheme for the treatment of pulmonary tuberculosis, not designed for the wealthy who could afford treatment in health resorts in the mountains of Switzerland, but for the general public. Anyone thought to be suffering from the disease could be referred to a public dispensary for diagnosis and assessment; if they were found to have active disease their families, and as far as possible their close contacts, were also assessed. All those found to be at an early stage of the disease were isolated as in-patients in a sanatorium to prevent the spread of the disease; those who improved as a result of rest and a sound diet were later transferred to a 'colony' for gradual return towards normal activities under supervision at home; those who were judged unlikely to recover were admitted to a 'tuberculosis hospital' for terminal care.

However, many of those diagnosed at the dispensary refused admission. Although aware of the potential health benefits, men were reluctant to give up work and the responsibility of providing for their families; mothers were equally reluctant to abandon the day-to-day care of their children. As many as 50% refused admission and, of those who agreed, many later found that they could not tolerate the hospital regime and discharged themselves.

For some years Philip's system was regarded as no more than a visionary concept. Then in 1911, the new National Health Insurance Scheme included a sanatorium benefit; later, a Department of Health Committee, reviewing that benefit, recommended that Philip's scheme should be adopted throughout Britain. In 1929, when the Scottish Board of Health was replaced by the Department of Health for Scotland, there were 39 dispensaries and 119 hospitals and sanatoriums with a total of over 5,000 beds in Scotland.

By 1933 the death rate from pulmonary tuberculosis in Scotland had fallen to 78 per thousand from 170 per thousand at the beginning of the century, but in the distress and widespread unemployment of the Depression the incidence had begun to rise again. And now, because of an even greater reluctance to admit even to the possibility of having contracted tuberculosis, the diagnosis was often delayed until the disease had reached 'a stage when the response to treatment is slow or negligible'. The true incidence of pulmonary tuberculosis was therefore unknown, but there could be no doubt that it was a major and uncontrolled problem.

Endocrinology

Claude Bernard, a Professor of Physiology in Paris between 1855 and 1878, launched the modern experimental study of the role of internal secretions (hormones) in the regulation of metabolism and the 'internal environment' of the body. His most famous earliest studies were on the regulation of carbohydrate metabolism, studies that proved important in the search for the cause of diabetes mellitus. The role of insulin was finally established in 1921 in a laboratory directed by John Macleod.

John Macleod (1876–1935) was born at Clunie in Perthshire and graduated in medicine at Aberdeen University in 1899. He returned to Aberdeen as Professor of Physiology in 1928. In the years between he had studied at Leipzig, taught at London University, and been Professor of Physiology at what later became Case Western Reserve University in Ohio. In 1921 he was Professor of Physiology at the University of Toronto, where he was investigating carbohydrate metabolism and the part played in its regulation by internal secretions.

Schafer (later Sir Edward Sharpey-Schafer) had already put forward his theory that diabetes mellitus was caused by the lack of a protein hormone (which he called 'insulin') secreted by the islets of Langerhans in the pancreas. Experimental attempts to treat diabetes by

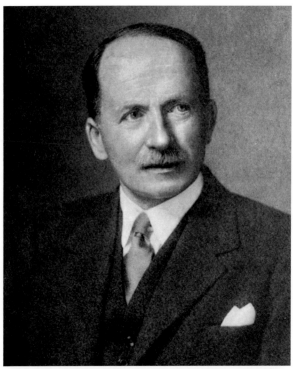

4.73 John Macleod (1876–1935) was born at Cluny, near Dunkeld. He graduated from Aberdeen University in 1899. He held a variety of posts in Canada and the USA, and at the University of Toronto in 1921, working with Frederick Banting and Charles Best, he discovered insulin, for which he was awarded the Nobel Prize in 1923 (*Aberdeen Medico-Chirurgical Society*).

feeding patients fresh pancreas had failed, it was assumed because the 'insulin' was destroyed by the proteolytic enzyme, trypsin, produced in the main body of the pancreas. In the summer of 1921, Macleod encouraged his research student, Fredrick Banting, to conduct a series of animal experiments that Banting thought might overcome this problem. Banting and his laboratory assistant, Charles Best, used ligatures to close off the pancreatic duct of a number of dogs; the trypsin-producing tissues in the pancreas quickly degenerated, leaving the insulin-producing tissue intact. It then became possible to extract the insulin from the islets of Langerhans free from the action of trypsin.

This observation quickly led to the extraction of clinically useful quantities of insulin from fresh bovine carcasses. Insulin became the first hormone to be used in pure isolated form in the treatment of diabetes, and in 1923 Macleod and Banting were jointly awarded the Nobel Prize for Medicine. Before their success the only useful treatment for diabetes mellitus had been the liberal administration of opium; now regular injections of insulin provided, not a cure, but an effective long-term treatment for diabetes mellitus.

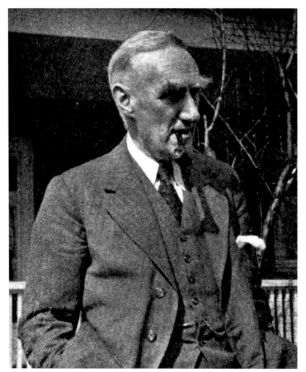

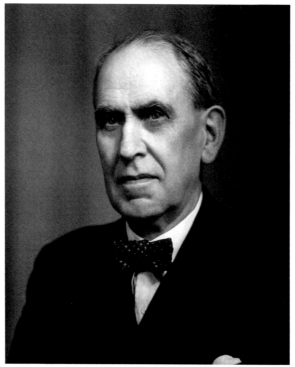

4.74 Sir John Boyd Orr (later Baron Boyd-Orr), CH, DSO, MC, FRS (1880–1971) was born in Kilmaurs in Ayrshire. He graduated BSc from Glasgow University in 1910 and MB ChB in 1912. After service in World War I, he returned to Aberdeen where he established the Rowett Research Institute. His research showed that much of the British working class was badly fed and that this was due, not to fecklessness, as was widely assumed, but to poverty. After World War II he became the first Director General of the United Nations Food and Agriculture Organisation and, in 1949, he was awarded a Nobel Prize.

4.75 Professor Edward Cathcart (1877–1954) graduated from Glasgow University in 1900. Originally intending to specialise in clinical medicine, he then decided to make his career as a medical scientist. After World War One he was appointed Professor of Physiology at Glasgow University. In 1935 he became Chairman of the Committee on Scottish Health Services. The Committee published a report (the Cathcart Report) in 1936, which proved invaluable in providing information for planning the National Health Service (*Wellcome Library, London*).

THE CATHCART REPORT

In 1933 Britain had not yet begun to recover from the Great Depression, and its industrial communities were still suffering massive unemployment and poverty. An investigation by John Boyd Orr, Director of the Rowett Research Institute in Aberdeen, found that 47% of the people of Scotland could not afford a diet that provided an adequate level of nutrition. However, for the government an even more pressing problem was the continuing financial crisis. A third of government spending was still taken up in repaying the charges on debts accumulated during the First World War, a problem now made worse by the spiralling cost of supporting the vast and increasing number of the unemployed. The Chancellor of the Exchequer, looking urgently for a reduction in public expenditure, appointed separate committees for England and Wales and for Scotland to look for possible economies in local government spending. The English committee

made no firm recommendations. The committee for Scotland (the Lovat Committee) found opportunities for economies in a number of services, but not in local authority health services. In its investigation of the health services, the Lovat Committee found evidence of poor organisation and waste of resources. In June 1933, Godfrey Collins, the Secretary of State for Scotland, appointed a committee 'to review the existing state health services in Scotland in the light of modern conditions and knowledge and to make recommendations on any changes in policy and organisation that may be considered necessary for the promotion of efficiency and economy.' The Committee was chaired by E.P. Cathcart, Professor of Physiology at Glasgow University, and every one of its ten members had already made a significant contribution to the improvement of public service. From the beginning the Committee made it clear that their ultimate aim was 'to secure the health of the people'. The Cathcart Committee therefore decided not to confine its attentions to the state health services since any review would be impossible without taking account of general practitioners in private practice, the voluntary hospitals and the many other private and voluntary agencies that were concerned with health.

In Parliament the Prime Minister, Stanley Baldwin, had claimed that during the years of the Depression the health of the nation was 'wonderfully well maintained'. This was at odds with public perception in Scotland. In attempting to assess the true state of the health of the population the Cathcart Committee found itself hampered by the inadequacy of the available statistics. Death rates were published annually by the Registrar General for Scotland, but the cause of death was frequently omitted and in many instances the diagnosis was grossly inaccurate; and in any case death rates did not reflect the incidence of serious but non-fatal illness in the population. A Morbidity Statistics Scheme had been launched in Scotland in 1930, but it recorded only incapacitating illness in the working population. It had been intended that the School Medical Service should report on the health of the nation's children, but its examinations had been reduced to mere inspections that gathered information about the appearance of the children rather than their health. In the absence of reliable statistics, the Committee collected anecdotal evidence from a large number of experienced and highly respected medical witnesses. These witnesses were in no doubt that in the 1930s there was a great and increasing mass of sickness and defects among the people of Scotland.

The Minister of Health had also claimed that during the Depression the state medical services were 'fully effective'. This was not confirmed by the investigations of the Cathcart Committee. In 1936, its reports on the state health services were damning.

The Poor Law medical service was found to be generally unsatisfactory, and suffered the difficulties inherent in maintaining a service only for people when they were destitute. A separate hospital service for the sick poor was undesirable, and a separate domiciliary medical service for the sick poor was equally undesirable. Both should be abolished.

The local authority infectious disease services, although passively accepted by the public, had not reached an acceptable standard. The infectious diseases hospitals should not be maintained merely as places for isolation but should serve as centres for expert treatment. Many of the existing hospitals were clearly unsuitable and should be replaced.

The tuberculosis service should be reformed to give greater emphasis to support for patients and their families at home. The out-patient services should continue on Philip's model but the tuberculosis dispensaries should be sited in local authority medical centres. The quality of services in the various institutions was frequently inadequate; they should be overhauled. And specialist staff and specialist equipment should be provided in new regional centres.

The School Medical Service had not fulfilled its intended purpose. Its medical services should be transferred to local authority clinics alongside maternity and child welfare clinics. Its welfare services were also found to be unsatisfactory; the infant mortality rate of 110 per thousand live births was unacceptably high. It was recommended that out-patient clinics for children under five should be combined with those for school children in a single local authority service for children of every age.

The loss of young mothers from the disorders of childbirth was described as a scandal; the Maternal Mortality Rate was increasing and in places was now as high as 12 per thousand births. A new comprehensive maternity service should be created in which general practitioners provided continuous supervision throughout pregnancy and delivery, supported by the services of fully trained midwives and the advice of consultant obstetricians at local authority clinics.

The National Health Insurance Scheme provided a service to a very large section of Scottish society but that service was strictly limited, and for many families its introduction had resulted in a reduction of care. Before 1913 a great many workmen had contributed by weekly deductions from their wages to a scheme that provided medical care for both themselves and their families. These schemes had been displaced by the National Health Insurance Scheme, and families now went without medical provision unless the workman made an additional subscription to

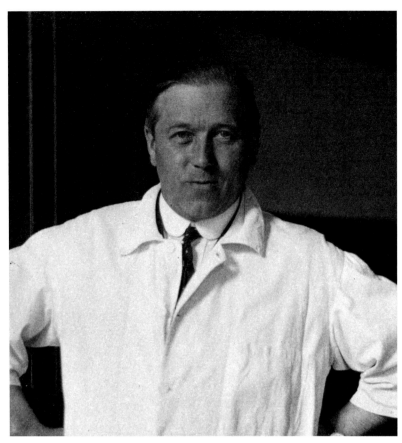

4.76 Sir John Fraser, Bt. (1885–1947) was born at Tain and educated at Tain Academy and Edinburgh University. After graduating with honours in 1907, he held resident posts at Edinburgh Royal Infirmary and the Royal Hospital for Sick Children. He then became assistant to Professor Harold Styles, and it was with his encouragement that he embarked on his historic studies of bone and joint tuberculosis in children, studies that showed for the first time that the cause of the disease, in the great majority of cases, was the bovine strain of the tubercle carried and spread in milk. His work led to the passing of legislation to eliminate the tubercle bacillus from the nation's milk supply. In 1924, he became Professor of Clinical Surgery at Edinburgh and, in 1944, Principal of the University of Edinburgh (*RCSEd*).

one of the schemes organised by general practitioners, by trade unions or by other bodies. The Cathcart Committee recommended that the services of the National Health Insurance scheme should be extended, not only to families, but to 'all classes in need', and administered by the state through the local authorities.

The reorganisation and improvement of local hospitals promised in 1929 had been slow and disappointing. The Cathcart Committee recommended that the local authority hospitals should be brought up to a standard that would fit them to play an equal part in a new integrated hospital service for Scotland. 'All hospitals whether managed by a statutory body or by a voluntary board of management should be regarded as one service.' The voluntary hospitals, although in no danger of collapse, were under increasing financial pressure. In ten years the annual number of in-patients had increased by almost 25% and the number of out-patients by 50%. The Cathcart Committee proposed that they should be granted immunity from legal and succession duties and remission from local rates, and should receive a grant in support of their teaching facilities.

In July 1936 the *Report of the Committee on Scottish*

Health Services (The Cathcart Report) was well received. In welcoming it, the *Scotsman* was clear that what was being proposed was 'a State Medical Service'. The *British Medical Journal* was equally positive: 'this publication should mark the setting up, at no distant date, of a comprehensive national health service.' But in 1936 the attention of the public was taken up by Mussolini's invasion of Abyssinia and the failure of the League of Nations. An arms race had begun, and Europe was already moving towards war. No action was taken on the Cathcart Report in 1936, but when the Report of the Committee on Social Insurance and Allied Services (Beveridge Report), with its plans for what was to become known as the 'Welfare State', was published in 1942, it was found to assume the creation of a free and comprehensive health service. The government promptly accepted the proposals of the Beveridge Report in full, and in doing so it accepted that a comprehensive free health service must be created. In London, the Ministry of Health had made no plans for such a service. However, the recommendations of the Cathcart Report were at hand, and they immediately became the basis for the urgent planning of the National Health Service.

YOUR HEALTH *Service*

HOW IT WILL
WORK IN
SCOTLAND

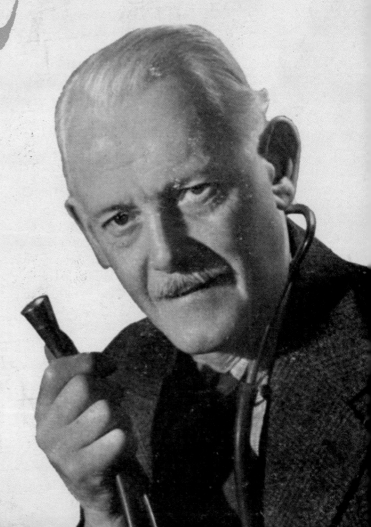

CHAPTER FIVE

HEALTH AND HEALTH CARE FROM THE MID-TWENTIETH CENTURY

David Hamilton

'The collective principle asserts that . . . no society can
legitimately call itself civilised if a sick person is denied
medical aid because of lack of means.'

ANEURIN BEVAN
In Place of Fear
1952

INTRODUCTION

In mid-century, the war in Europe changed everything, and in post-war Britain a new order resulted. Before World War Two there had been stirrings in Scotland for changes in health care provision, and the Highlands and Islands Medical Service (HIMS) had been a successful early experiment. Following this, the Cathcart Report of 1936 had planned a health service for Scotland with a distinctively Scottish flavour, but in the late 1930s continuing economic difficulties prevented the implementation of any plans for change. After the war, though Britain was no wealthier, the will for action existed.

From 1945, health care was a national priority, and the new National Health Service, brought in by the Labour government elected after the war, was to last well beyond the life span of other nationally-run industries and services created at that time. To outsiders, the NHS became associated closely with the British way of life, and it was judged to be a particular success in Scotland. The 1946 NHS legislation had some Scottish nuances which allowed a distinctive 'Scottish-ness' to be detectible in the health care systems which followed. These differences were seen at the time simply as fading vestiges of earlier pre-war arrangements, but when devolution of political power to Scotland came in 1997, the earlier separate thinking re-emerged. National events influenced health matters. In the immediate post-war period, defence budget needs were high and soon led to limits in the NHS budget. The discovery of major oil fields in the North Sea in 1969 eased the demands on the public purse, but the OPEC Oil Crisis of 1973 and the recession in the 2010s had important consequences for health spending and policy. Joining the European Economic Community (later called the EC and then renamed as the EU) meant that Britain 'shared sovereignty' on many matters, controversially including working conditions, notably after the Treaty of Maastricht in 1992. Within Britain, in 1999 Scotland gained a parliament with some devolved powers, including control over the health care budget and policy.

In the post-war period, there was a remarkable reduction in infectious disease brought about by a complex synergy of the effects of new antibiotics, new immunisation measures and better social conditions. Health in Scotland showed steady improvement as judged by the traditional indices such as life expectancy, which increased by ten years in the period 1950 to 2000, and infant mortality fell in the same period from 39 per 1,000 deaths in the first year of life to 6 per 1,000. Methods of health care changed significantly, and many new potent drugs emerged from research findings then developed by the pharmaceutical companies. New surgical procedures had important effects and there was a growing emphasis on safety in surgery. Patients became better informed and more assertive, and took an increasing interest in the quality of the health care offered. By the end of the century, the challenges of new patterns of disease emerged, with heart and lung disease rising in importance, and the special needs of the oldest age group in the population became an issue. The long standing concern in Scotland for under-nutrition diminished and was replaced imperceptibly by a focus on obesity and faulty diet. These new problems were often worse in Scotland than the rest of the UK, and compared unfavourably with other European countries. But in research and development, Scotland had a major role in the post-war rapid advances internationally in medical science. Added to this, Scottish medical education and medical practice retained their traditional strengths.

In all of these aspects of Scottish health care, seen against the international background and with some emphasis on the users' experience, it is convenient to look first at events from mid-century until the mid-1970s. The era which followed was subtly different for both providers and recipients of health care.

Wartime

Preparations for Britain's defence started early. The German use of poison gas in the First World War was not forgotten and the entire British population was issued with gas masks from September 1938. When air raids on industrial Scotland were judged to be likely, mass evacuation of children out of industrial areas, notably Glasgow, was arranged; and starting as early as September 1939, they were moved to distant villages and towns and taken in to

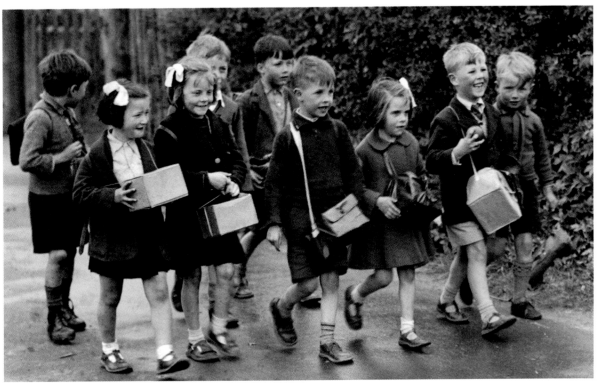

5.1 *Above*. Gas masks. Young evacuees heading off in 1939 to new temporary homes, carrying their masks in boxes (*Fergusson Gallery, Perth*).

5.2 *Below*. Rationing. The wartime ration books had coloured coupons to be handed over at the time of purchase – red for meat, blue for fat and yellow for clothing (*Orkney Archives*).

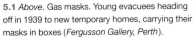

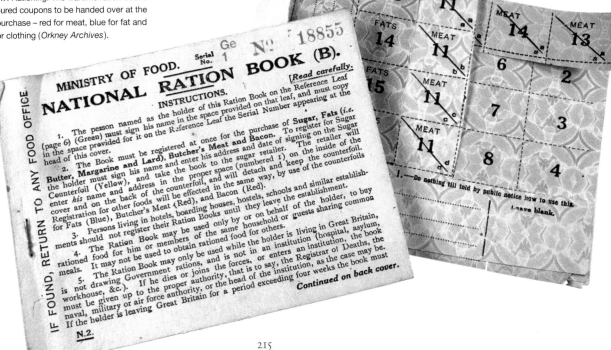

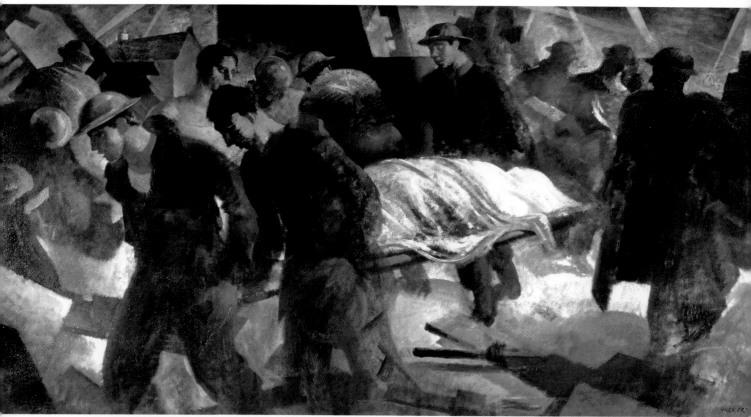

5.3 Bombing of Scotland. This painting, 'The Stretcher Bearers', is held by the Royal College of Physicians and Surgeons of Glasgow. The emergency services are shown dealing with the destruction of lives and housing in the Clydebank Blitz of March 1941 (*RCPSG*).

any houses with spare rooms. 175,000 children were moved quickly at the start of the War, but all had returned by 1943 after the air raids ceased.

The poor health of these evacuated children, often from the slums, was noted, and emphasised some of the needs of the times. Many of the children were poorly clothed and undernourished, and 30% had infestations. The skin disease impetigo was also common. Their problems on arrival strained the 'Dunkirk spirit' in the well-off host towns, and a Medical Officer of Health noted wryly that this sudden mixing of the classes 'jolted social complacency'. This gave a wider understanding of the importance of public health and support grew for a comprehensive health service.

Since the nation was hugely dependent on imports of essential supplies, food rationing was required from January 1940. Basic human nutritional needs were easily calculated from Boyd Orr's earlier studies, and rational allocations made. Some items were excluded, notably fish and potatoes, and haggis and black pudding were also exempt. Clothing was rationed, as was petrol, though doctors had a special allowance.

By September 1940, after Germany's failed attempt to destroy the RAF and its southern airfields during the Battle of Britain, German tactics switched to bombing cities and industrial areas in Britain. London was attacked for 57 consecutive nights starting in September 1940. Six months later, night bombing of industrial and military targets in Scotland commenced, and Clydebank, Glasgow and Greenock were targeted, as was Aberdeen later. The attacks on Clydebank shipyards and munitions factories on the nights of 13 and 14 March caused the greatest density of damage of all the raids on Britain. Though wartime secrecy concealed details of the effects of these raids at the time, few houses were unaffected, with 358 killed, many injured and over 35,000 made homeless. The emergency services were overwhelmed by the scale of the casualties. Five days later, at Clydebank, a mass grave was used for burial of the bodies not initially identified.

POST-WAR PLANS

In 1942, when the war with Germany began to run in favour of the Allies, thoughts turned to plans for post-war reconstruction. The needs of war meant that central planning was accepted. In this collectivist mood, bold social change was possible, and this included plans for a national health service. National morale was boosted by the crucial El Alamein victory, and shortly after, in late 1942, William Beveridge, who had been asked to chair an Interdepartmental Committee on the needs and scope of 'social insurance', produced his famous Report. Beveridge did not disappoint: expectations had been raised by the common effort and sacrifices during the war. His unusually vivid discourse famously promised new freedom from the five

'Giant Evils' of 'want, ignorance, disease, squalor and idleness'. The language of the Report was influenced by Edinburgh's Jessy Mair, later his wife, who urged him to imbue his proposals with a 'Cromwellian and Messianic spirit'. During the writing of the Report, they spent time at Boat of Garten in the Highlands in the summer of 1942.

The Report was not well received by ministers, since its radical thinking was seen as 'ambitious but impractical'; however Beveridge's supporters skilfully publicised his plans, even printing a summary for wider readership. Soon after, Churchill was prepared to accept that something had to be done, and he gave undertakings that there would be new post-war health and welfare schemes. Churchill used,

Archibald J. Cronin

Archibald J. Cronin (1896–1981), the author, was born at Cardross near Glasgow. His medical studies in Glasgow were interrupted by war service as an assistant naval surgeon, but he graduated in 1919 and then had hospital posts in Glasgow and elsewhere. In 1921 he moved to the Welsh coalmining town of Tredegar. He returned to Scotland in 1930 as a result of health problems, and there, with the aid of Dumbarton's Public Library, he wrote his first novel. Following this success, his second novel *The Citadel* portrayed a doctor struggling against the cynicism and greed of a polluting factory. It also described shady London private medical practice, and advocated a free public health service. The novel was Gollancz the publisher's bestselling title ever.

In 1939 Cronin moved to America, and films of his novels used star casts including Robert Donat, Margaret Lockwood and Gregory Peck. When *The Citadel* was filmed, the American Medical Association attempted to curb its support for 'socialised medicine'. Cronin's books were published in Germany as propaganda against decadent Britain, and the novels had official support in the Soviet

Union. In 1946 he moved to Montreux in Switzerland. His autobiography, *Adventures in Two Worlds* (1952) had less social comment, and its homely tales of Scottish general practice were adapted for television as 'Dr Finlay's Casebook' which ran from 1962 to 1971, being revived twice later.

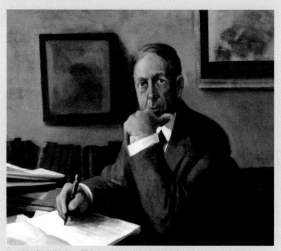

5.4 Medical fiction. This portrait of Archibald Cronin was acquired by the West Dunbartonshire Council, recalling Cronin's use of their library during the writing of *Hatter's Castle*, his first novel (*West Dunbartonshire Libraries and Museums*).

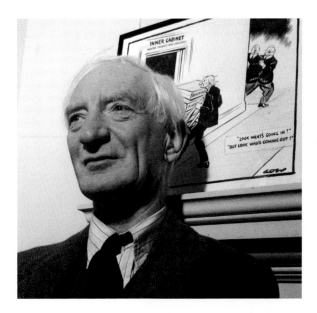

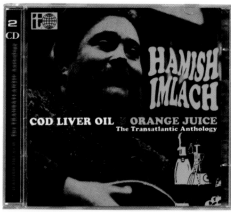

5.5 *Left*. The Welfare State. William Beveridge (1879–1963) is seen with one of the many newspaper cartoons praising his Report and its plans for a new social order post-war (*Imperial War Museum*).

5.6 *Above*. Cod Liver Oil. World War Two nutritional support was fondly remembered later in popular culture (*Castle Music*).

for the first time, the 'cradle to grave' description of the venture.

Popular opinion in Britain regarding health care was influenced by the highly successful pre-war novel *The Citadel* (1937), written by the Glasgow-trained doctor Archibald J. Cronin. Cronin had moved to Tredegar in Wales in 1921, and for two years his career overlapped that of Aneurin Bevan, who later brought in the NHS. Though not known to be close at that time, both were left-leaning, both had deep social consciences, and Cronin was medical officer to the local working man's Medical Aid Society, the successful 'socialised' medical aid scheme in Tredegar.

Health in Wartime
Scotland's health during the war showed marked changes. Perhaps surprisingly, the infant mortality rate (IMR) fell, and by 1945 had shown one of the sharpest declines ever. A possible explanation was that adequate essential nutrition was attainable for all through the new rationing system, and that family income was assisted by wartime full employment, which included plenty of work for women. Milk sales in particular rose, to the pleasure of the nutritionists, and cod liver oil and orange juice were distributed free to children to provide vitamins. These supplements are recalled with nostalgia as part of the wartime experience, but are a reminder that the health of all could be the responsibility of the State. These nutritional supplements were also given to expectant women, and the phrase 'cod liver oil and orange juice' entered Scottish popular culture and ballads as an indirect reference to pregnancy.

But the Scottish IMR, even with its wartime fall, was now worse than in England, and was higher than in most European countries. An editorial in the *British Medical Journal* in 1944 showed a new awareness of these national and even regional variations (later called 'postcode' differences), and made an early identification of Scotland as heading towards being the 'sick man of Europe'.

> Cool analysis of the problem [IMR] sticks to the facts . . . Looking at Glasgow's rate of 99 against England's 50 and Edinburgh's 66, we cannot help feeling that something is sadly wrong with our present day society that such disparities are allowed.

During the war, there was fresh concern about the important infectious diseases, notably after an initial wartime rise in diphtheria deaths. Uptake of the vaccine had been poor, resulting from the local authorities' lack of funds and enthusiasm plus residual anti-vaccination attitudes held by the public. Surprisingly, tuberculosis cases also rose steadily at this time, perhaps as the result of further spread of the disease after transfer of the tuberculosis sanatoria beds to other wartime uses. Childhood TB rose after children evacuated to rural areas were exposed to milk from untested, infected cows in this, the pre-pasteurisation era. Venereal disease increased during the war, and legislation in Defence Regulation 33B allowed tracing and compulsory treatment of contacts, authoritarian actions which were only acceptable in wartime.

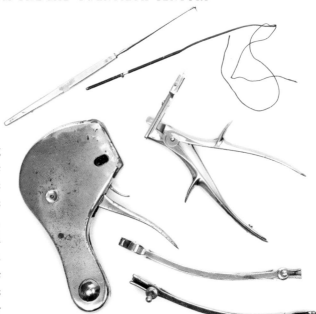

Wartime Hospitals

One wartime initiative meant that Scotland had a lasting and important boost to the hospital sector and health care expenditure in Scotland. In 1940 the fear of air raids meant that more hospital beds were required, and it was also agreed that if there was a southern invasion of Britain, a defensive military and government fall-back to Scotland was likely. A Scottish Emergency Medical Scheme with 16,000 extra beds was authorised, giving a 60% increase overall, and these were housed in rapidly erected hospitals built outside of centres of population, safe from enemy bombs. These temporary structures were constructed at Raigmore (Inverness), Bridge of Earn, Bangour (West Lothian), Stracathro (near Aberdeen), Killearn near Glasgow, Law (Lanarkshire), Ballochmyle (Ayrshire) and at Peel in the Borders. Other suitable buildings were also converted to hospital use, including the elegant Gleneagles Hotel, which had welcomed the German Foreign Minister Ribbentrop in the 1930s.

Making skilful political use of this opportunity was Tom Johnston, the Scottish Labour party's home rule sympathiser, surprisingly chosen by Churchill to be Scotland's Secretary of State in the wartime cabinet. Johnston, reluctant to accept, successfully obtained considerable freedom of action from Churchill.

With many casualties likely, an innovative step was taken in Scotland to encourage specialism. Unusually for the times, in addition to the consultants appointed in orthopaedics, psychiatry and eye disease, posts in plastic surgery and neurosurgery were added. These positions hardly existed in civilian practice, since surgeons usually favoured general surgery to optimise their private income. In Edinburgh, Norman Dott took the military brain surgery post. In the west, Jack Tough took charge of plastic surgery, based initially at Ballochmyle Hospital in Ayrshire, after training with England's only such specialist, Sir Harold Gillies, the veteran World War One surgeon. But trench warfare was not a feature of WW2, and any mutilating facial injury or skin loss was instead caused by burns.

Change of Use

The German air raids largely ceased in Scotland in summer 1941 when Hitler turned his forces against Russia.

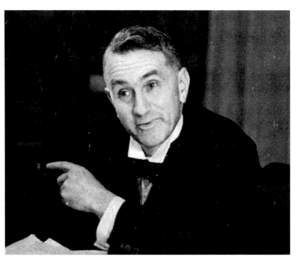

5.7 *Top*. Wartime injuries encouraged the emergence of specialty surgery. In Scotland units devoted to plastic surgery were set up, which led to new techniques and instrumentation such as these surgical instruments devised by Norman Dott (*photograph by Allan Shedlock of instruments in RCSEd*).

5.8 *Above*. Wartime politics. Among Tom Johnston's achievements as Secretary of State was the imaginative use of his Emergency Medical Service hospitals, which had lasting consequences for Scottish public expenditure (*Getty Images*).

Accordingly, Tom Johnston decided to open up the reserve unused EMS beds to treat civilian waiting-list cases, easing the burden on the hard-pressed charity-based city hospitals. Among his other initiatives, he set up a Council of State comprising all the surviving Scottish Secretaries, and they met to plan Scottish post-war strategy. Though mainly concerned with industrial development, one committee did consider the health services. With his EMS beds now available, Johnston also brought in his imagi-

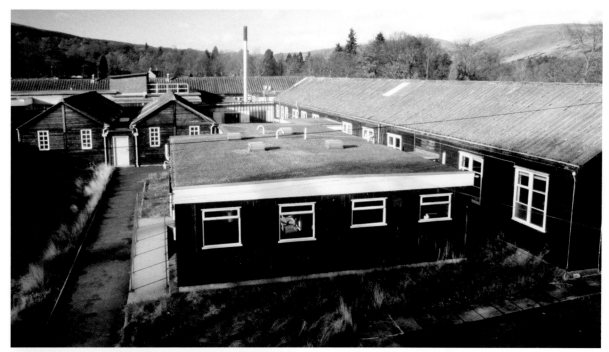

5.9 Peel Hospital. Large numbers of new hospital beds were made available in Scotland in the Emergency Medical Scheme. Built outside the cities, these temporary hospitals were retained in use for many decades (*Walter Baxter*).

native Clyde Basin experiment in January 1942, which gave a pioneering service for any workers in the important heavy industries in the West of Scotland who showed early signs of disability. The goal for this unusual scheme, familiar in the Soviet Union, was to anticipate further decline and restore health.

The EMS hospitals returned briefly to their original purpose in June 1944, when they dealt with the casualties resulting from the D-Day landings in Europe. Arriving by train in Scotland, after initial assessment, about 13,000 Allied casualties were admitted to the EMS hospitals, and nearly 3,000 injured German prisoners of war were also treated. Soon after, in Europe, the retreating Germans managed to resume the bombing of London with rocket-propelled V-bombs, and about 5,000 injured Londoners were sent for treatment in the Scottish EMS hospitals.

The EMS hospitals meant that Scotland had proportionately more doctors and nurses than the rest of the UK, and with 15% more beds, there was higher relative expenditure in Scotland in wartime. The unintended consequence was that, since these hospitals were not closed after the war, the finances of the new Scottish NHS hospital sector were off to a good start. More than fifty years later, at the end of the century, Scotland still had 2.4 doctors/1,000 population, while England had 1.9/1,000.

POST-WAR CHANGES

After the war, with a Labour government surprisingly in power instead of Churchill's Conservative Party, the wartime sacrifices had led to political pressure for a better life, as a reward not only for the military effort but also for the privations undergone by civilians. The new socialist government was determined that a Welfare State would be their gift, based on the Beveridge Report, and that within it, a health service was a priority.

Enacting this in the harsh post-war economic situation was not easy, although Britain was assisted by American Marshall Plan loans. There were other urgent national problems, particularly in housing, and in Scotland, Glasgow had some of the worst housing in Britain. It was well-known to planners and analysts that health in general was heavily influenced by housing, nutrition and the environment, and nowhere had this been made clearer than in Boyd Orr's earlier Scottish studies on health, food and income. But in 1948 the mood was that spending on more visible services like health care, rather than on hidden determinants of health such as housing, was the priority. Better housing had to wait until a council-house building drive under Harold Macmillan as Conservative housing minister from 1951.

HEALTH SERVICE NEEDS

In health care, the fundamental post-war defects were a patchy provision in general practice (primary care, as it was called later) and in financing the hospitals. The old 'voluntary' hospital system, largely paid for by charitable funding, was in terminal decline. Hospital treatment was free for low-income patients, and the hospital lady 'almoner' – the hospitals' early social worker – could also obtain payments from those who could afford it, but seldom did so in Scotland. The hospital fabric was old, and all the buildings dated from the great Victorian (even Georgian) hospital expansion. Maintenance had been neglected during the war, and modern new equipment was needed, since new technology was offering expensive and essential items, notably for radiotherapy and radiology. The chairman of the Edinburgh Royal Infirmary Board of Management was obviously relieved as the likely takeover of his and other hospitals approached after the war:

> Sooner or later we should have had to press for State assistance and even those whose heart has been with the voluntary system feel it is best to hand it over with good grace and wish them Godspeed.

Tax-payers had not hitherto paid for these hospitals, but were now not opposed to doing so.

Enter Bevan

At Westminster, the collectivist post-war mood meant the time was right for Bevan and the newly-elected Labour Party to act, particularly as expectations had been irreversibly raised. It was to be a hard and famous fight for Bevan, a young minister without cabinet rank at that time. Bevan had some links with Scotland. He lionised John Wheatley, the Scottish left-wing activist who was Minister of Health in 1924, and Bevan married fellow Labour politician Jenny Lee, from Fife, who had been a student at Edinburgh University. Bevan was a close colleague of George Buchanan, member of parliament for the Gorbals, Glasgow's famous area of deprivation, and Buchanan later became Under-Secretary of State for Scotland with health care responsibilities, until his retirement in 1948.

Bevan's plans were simple and comprehensive. Health care would be 'free at the point of use'. Paid for out of general taxation, it was progressive in nature, taking from the well-off to help the poor. Even the name was an inspired choice, since although it was primarily a curative service, the name implied much more, hinting that good health was also sought. All the hospitals would be taken

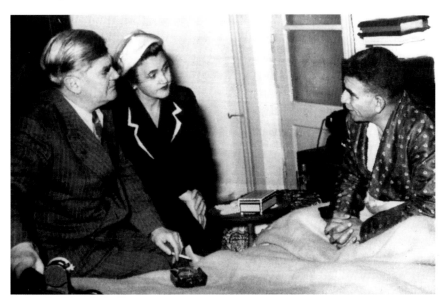

5.10 Bevan's NHS. Minister of Health Aneurin Bevan, provided with an ash tray, visiting an NHS hospital in 1950 with his wife Jenny Lee (*Getty Images*).

over, and their 'visiting' consultants, who had usually been unpaid (gaining hospital status and hence private practice in return) would now have a salary. All citizens could have a general practitioner of their choice, who was paid an annual fee for each patient joining their practice. Added to this 'capitation fee', a mileage allowance was paid, depending on the geographical area covered by the doctor, a reminder now that home visits were a prominent feature of general practice at that time. No other government support was given and the general practitioners were proud to be 'independent contractors', rather than salaried staff, accepting that they had to pay for their own practice premises and their other expenses from this single sum. For the patients, medicines on prescription were to be supplied free of charge, and some little luxuries were proposed for the new service. Patients could obtain in their own homes 'domiciliary visits' by hospital consultants, and there was a little-used provision for patients to obtain a 'second opinion' from other doctors.

Bevan was clear about the way ahead, and it was to be a national one-size-fits-all plan. As an international socialist, and still influenced by wartime centralism, he declared (of the coal industry) that 'there is no separate Welsh problem'. It meant fitting Scotland's health service into the national mould with convergence rather than divergence, and the earlier separate Scottish thinking was not on the agenda. But the *de jure* need for separate Scottish legislation on the NHS did leave some leeway for differences, although when the plans for the Scottish NHS legislation emerged, some senior Scottish figures were disappointed that the Scottish experience, and particularly the Cathcart Report, had been ignored, and a 'whiff of Harley Street' was instead detected.

However, the Scottish legislation did manage to incorporate some important concessions, notably that Cathcart-type health centres would be set up, and, with private practice at low levels in Scotland, and not highly regarded, no private pay-beds would be allocated to the Scottish hospitals, unlike in England. Importantly, the Scottish teaching hospitals were to join up with the large local municipal hospitals in single, large regional hospital boards. These Scottish differences were quite sensitive politically, and to avoid defeats by Bevan's critics during

the tense debates on the England and Wales NHS Bill, the Scottish Bill was delayed until he was safe. Bevan got his English Health Service legislation through Parliament, and the Scottish Bill with its nuances tip-toed in the following year as the National Health Service (Scotland) Act 1947.

NHS Negotiations

Though these Acts were passed in 1946 and 1947, the NHS could not start until Bevan had the support of the doctors. At first this did not seem likely. A quick vote by British Medical Association (BMA) members came down heavily against joining, and the *Glasgow Herald* suggested that Bevan should resign and *The Scotsman* warned that there would be serious difficulties in such a state-run scheme. For the next year, the BMA, then largely representing the general practitioners, opposed Bevan's proposals, as did an informal group of powerful London-based hospital consultants. The Conservative party, now in opposition, joined in and opposed the scheme during the parliamentary debates.

Under pressure, Bevan had to negotiate on the detail. He firstly shelved proposals that the health services be run by local authorities, a traditional tenet of Labour Party policy. Further concessions were made by Bevan to the London consultants' leaders, adding a confidential extra merit award scheme which would enhance senior consultant's salaries. The hospital doctors warmed to the idea of an NHS, thus splitting the profession. The BMA organised a further vote at local meetings on joining and in England, 10,909 doctors voted for joining the NHS, with 12,550 against. In Scotland attitudes were different, with 1893 voting for and 1341 against. With the doctors' opposition weakened in this way, the BMA gave in, and virtually all the doctors entered the new Service.

Scottish Differences

The Scottish administrative differences, though apparently arcane, had considerable significance. All the Scottish hospitals – voluntary, EMS and municipal – were now brought together under regional hospital boards, and the resulting upgrading of the status and the fabric of the municipal hospitals meant that all vestiges of their older

Poor Law role were steadily removed. They not only gave better quality care but also assisted the local medical schools with student teaching. The municipal hospitals could offer much-needed space for new units with innovative staff, and with so many patients to treat in the region, powerful support existed for developing specialist expertise. Glasgow's huge municipal Stobhill Hospital soon obtained an important academic unit which, among other initiatives, established geriatric medicine as a new specialty. Also in Glasgow, the former Govan Poor Law Hospital, now renamed the Southern General Hospital, was to house an internationally-famous neurosurgery unit. Financial support for innovation was also available. Each large Board could also afford specialist support units such as regional physics departments. When the Scottish voluntary hospitals were taken over by the NHS, though their reserves had dwindled, considerable endowment funds remained. These were amalgamated, and one-fifth of this fund top-sliced and moved into a £2 million Scottish Hospital Endowment Research Trust.

Four of the five Scottish hospital board areas had a university medical faculty, and Glasgow and Edinburgh also had their ancient royal colleges of physicians and surgeons. The colleges and the universities were to be closely involved with the work of the new NHS boards, and the linkage of these three organisations was unique in Britain. Though these bodies had different agendas, co-operation by them within each Board area was noticeable thereafter.

The contrast between Scotland and the situation in England, particularly London, was considerable. London's five small medical schools did not enter any new groupings and, with considerable financial endowments, were determined to remain detached and independent. Without other hospital links, notably with municipal hospitals, bed numbers for treatment and teaching remained small and specialism was seldom favoured. Lacking close university ties, teaching on subjects beyond clinical care was not readily at hand.

The Service

The NHS owed nothing to national experiments elsewhere. The unique national salaried service and free

prescriptions meant that all choices in medical care were made free of any cash nexus. There was no support for the unnecessary treatment, particularly surgical, which could be rewarding in fee-for-service systems, and the NHS doctors had no financial stake in increasing consumer demand. In particular, in Britain, routine tonsil removal steadily fell to a tenth of the pre-NHS level. Administrative costs were low, and in particular, paperwork and invoicing was minimal. The NHS was a huge public service used by virtually all of the population, and large amounts of useful data on health and health care emerged, though exploiting this opportunity was initially delayed by the view that generating paperwork on the NHS, notably hospital activity and stay, was an optional extra. National schemes for vaccination or screening, or obtaining advice for rational therapy, was easily organised. There was in consequence a continuous government interest in health care theory, central planning and 'reform'. The NHS attracted continuous attention and comment from politicians, doctors, administrators, academics, controversialists, columnists and pressure groups, all of whom offered comment, criticism and prescription to the government of the day. Verdicts on the service often depended on the writer's own viewpoint, and ranged from the NHS as 'the envy of the world' to regular statements that the NHS was 'on the point of collapse'.

Patients could be critical, yet were deeply attached to the NHS, and as a result, no political party entered any election thereafter proposing to dismantle the NHS. Nor did the British Medical Association make any sustained move to weaken or leave the new service. The reasons for the popularity of the NHS were not far to seek. The 'free' service was comprehensive and belonged to the users. At first the patients showed endless patience, and if there were queues, it was worth the wait. Crucially, there were no fears for the financial cost of treatment for ill-health. These fears continued to exist in other countries, particularly in America, where any proposals for a comparable health care system were opposed by doctors and conservative politicians who, from the start, demonised the NHS as 'socialised medicine'. The much-needed appearance of comprehensive health care in America had to await President Obama's reforms in the early twenty-first century.

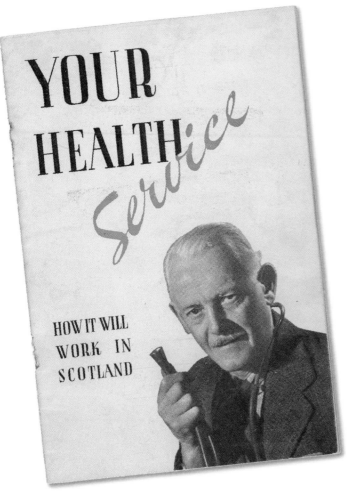

5.11 The New Service. This introduction to the Scottish NHS was widely distributed in 1948 (*Lothian Health Service Archives*).

The Launch

The 'appointed day' for the start of the NHS in Scotland was 5th July 1948, and it was an overnight change of some magnitude. Among the NHS staff, the consultants were now paid well for the first time. Since all consultants had similar pay, consultants could be found for remote hospitals or unfashionable specialties which lacked private practice. A pay rise for nurses helped reverse the wartime depletion of their numbers. All NHS staff had generous pension schemes, and other backing came from occupational health support. The NHS had one of the world's largest payrolls (exceeded only by the Chinese Red Army and the Indian Railways) and it was the biggest organisation in Scotland. It was a kindly employer, and jobs were usually for life. It encouraged altruism in the staff and morale in the new NHS was high.

Non-medical staff had the backing of powerful trade unions which had experience in negotiating nationally-agreed pay schemes. From 1971 the doctors and dentists had the support of their important Review Body on Doctors' and Dentists' Remuneration. By the 1970s it proved crucial, since inflation averaged 13% throughout the decade, peaking at 25% in 1975. During this difficult time, the doctors' earnings were maintained and even enhanced by the Review Body, and salaries rose steadily to exceed those of other professionals, notably university academics, whose salaries had been comparable in the past. Late in the day, these other professions sought the benefits of a trade union. Ministers of religion, traditionally as well paid in Scotland as doctors, suffered serious erosion of income and status at this time.

For the patient, prior to the NHS, only those in work were insured under National Insurance and hence entitled to health care from a 'panel' general practitioner. Cover for their dependents had increased pre-war partly via economical local personal insurance schemes, and hospital and dispensary care was free. Dental treatment had been largely private, and was seldom sought by those in most need. Now all treatment, including medicines and necessary appliances, was free. A striking example of the new era soon appeared, namely spectacles for the Scots requiring them, and half a million were issued in the first six months, partly because of fears that the BMA might still wreck the scheme.

Though hospital waiting lists had grown before the war, now they were coming down. A remarkable number of hernias and prolapses were operated on in the first months of the NHS in the big city hospitals. Dental treatment was also free, and with the dentists well paid by government for each procedure, there was plenty of work and the dentists were content. In spite of this, neglect of dental decay was still highly prevalent in Scotland, probably from the enduring fondness for sugary drinks and lack of oral hygiene. Many young persons had all their rotten teeth extracted from their rotten gums, often in one session, known sadly as their '21st birthday present'. Dentures were then fitted free of charge. Dental students from other dental schools in Scotland, and Newcastle, visited Glasgow to view a display of mass dental decay and gum disease. Later, in Glasgow in 1975, a survey of those aged over 65 showed that only 1 in 7 had their own teeth.

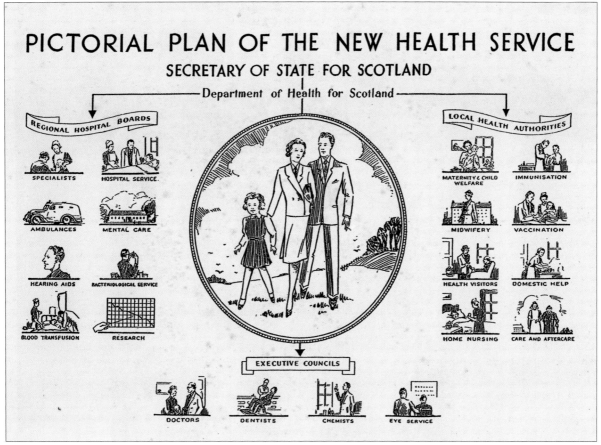

5.12 At its inception the 'tripartite' administrative structure of the NHS was thought to be of interest to the patients, and the relationship between hospital, general practice and local authority services is shown in this pamphlet. This structure was to last until unification of the three branches in 1974 (*Lothian Health Service Archives*).

Funding the NHS

In retrospect, there was some naivety on the part of government in their view that the new availability of comprehensive medical care would reduce disease and ill-health and hence that spending on health care would fall. Allied to this, the post-war government showed remarkably little concern for talking about money. There was a finite job to be done in health care, it was thought, and this would be paid for. But in the first year of the NHS, the cost of prescription drugs, still rather limited in range and often paid for before by the patient, increased sharply, and total costs were 50% higher. Bevan's original estimate of £145 million for the annual cost of the NHS more than doubled in its second year. 'Too bottle-minded' was the Scottish Secretary of State's conclusion about his flock's attitude to medication. A not-unrelated mood existed in the hospitals. The consultants, formerly used to the parsimony of their financially-stretched charitable institutions,

were now aware that their budgets were open-ended and that penny-pinching was over. They spent freely on supplies and equipment and added new costly items, notably the improved X-ray equipment.

The Treasury simply picked up all existing NHS expenditure, notably on hospitals. Payment for Scotland's additional wartime EMS hospital beds was allowed to continue when they were taken into the NHS. Since health care took about a third of Scotland's budget, this extra funding was a large element in making Scotland's public expenditure proportionately higher than in England. Later this largesse became increasingly noted and was watched closely outside Scotland in harder times.

Although there was no finite NHS budget, costs were partly contained by delays in building new hospitals. The best was made of the sturdy old famous buildings, though the long high-ceilinged 'Nightingale' wards, some still with central coal fires, were increasingly out-dated and unsuitable. Little had changed from the Glasgow hospital wards described in James Barke's 1936 novel *Major Operation*. The fabric was upgraded as best as possible, with dividers eventually giving some privacy within the large wards. Hospital stay was somewhat cheered by local hospital broadcasting via earphones fitted at the bedside, and these first appeared in the mid-1950s, offering entertainment and local news, including football commentaries.

The only new hospital to be built in Scotland at this time was at the Vale of Leven in 1955 in the west of Scotland, and it was unique since it emerged later that it was paid for from defence funds. The hospital's spacious design and broad corridors had another agenda, namely to house any mass casualties should Glasgow and nearby industrial Clydeside be attacked in a nuclear war. The next hospital building was not until the late 1960s, and in the meantime the Vale of Leven had many visits from interested administrators from elsewhere.

The large NHS hospitals were increasingly seen as central to the provision of health care, and pressure to close smaller ones mounted. Bevan, the moderniser, said he would rather 'survive in the cold altruism of a large hospital than expire in a gush of sympathy in a small one.' The small private nursing homes were also increasingly considered to be old-fashioned in comparison to the NHS hospitals, and these little organisations, often grouped together in Scottish 'Harley Streets' steadily closed. The large national medical insurance schemes which later would fund and equip the expansion of bigger private hospitals were still to come. Meanwhile, sophisticated laboratory tests, expensive radiological investigation and costly surgical equipment were only available in the NHS, and those patients who formerly favoured private treatment were now increasingly using the NHS, albeit putting up with less comfort.

Nursing at this time had some now-forgotten features. It was accepted that ward nurses were to be unmarried, and on marriage they would move to other roles in outpatient departments or elsewhere. The unmarried nurses were expected to live in the hospital and large nurses' homes were a feature of the main hospitals. These were usually reached only by traversing a spacious conservatory which allowed any visitors to be monitored. But no charges for residence were made, and for the nurses, it was an economical way of living. By 1959, Edinburgh had set up a university-based degree in nursing, and Europe's first university nursing degree followed, with a professiorial chair of nursing established in 1973.

NHS Concerns

There were some discontents within the service. Some grumbles came from local government, notably from medical officers of health and local politicians who had earlier run their large organisations including the municipal hospitals and other services, which were now lost to the NHS. A loss of democratic control had resulted, since local elections had given some accountability. Some prominent Labour Party politicians, notably Herbert Morrison, had campaigned to keep health under local government control, but this had been anathema to the doctors' leaders, who had unpleasant memories of being employees of the local authorities. Bevan had given way on this issue. The NHS continued to be heavily centralised thereafter, and this issue of a lack of local accountability was to resurface regularly.

One loss mourned at the time was the disappearance of the little mutual aid societies which were part of working class self-reliant culture. Sick clubs, Co-operative Society schemes and trade unions had given this self-help. Also involved were the friendly societies such as The Independent Order of Oddfellows, the largest friendly society in the world, and smaller ones like the Loyal Order of Ancient Shepherds, which had 39 lodges in the Lothians and Fife in 1910 and 6,000 adult members, giving cover for sickness, unemployment and burial expenses. Though such cover could not be comprehensive, it added to the pre-NHS state insurance schemes, and could help the dependents of those in work and even those out of work.

General Practice

The biggest discontent was soon shown by the general practitioners. The NHS gave them a regular, predictable income from the annual sum paid per patient, and they had no longer any need to collect fees or chase bad debts. This method of payment did not encourage adding new staff or equipment, nor was government keen to offer

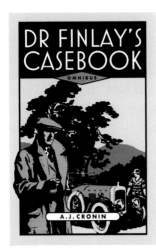

5.13 *Above.* Rural practice. *Dr Finlay's Casebook*, based on A. J. Cronin's autobiography, was screened by the BBC from 1962–71 with Cronin's help initially; a radio series followed from 1970 to 1978, with an ITV revival in 1993–96 (*Birlinn Ltd*).

5.14 *Right.* City surgeries. Converted city shops were often used for single-handed general practice, as here in central Glasgow. In the window, the doctor displays his consulting times plus a symbolic glass pharmacy jar (*Glasgow City Archives*).

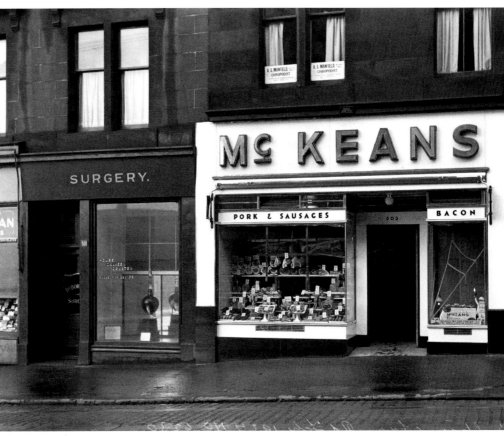

extra money for this purpose, citing the GPs' wish to be independent contractors. To add to this, with the arrival of the NHS, attendance at surgeries had increased markedly, as had out-of-hours calls. Also, the GPs were steadily excluded from admitting patients to local hospitals. Previously they had done so, doing some operative surgery there, but this was now frowned upon, as was surgery in the home, notably tonsil removal on the kitchen table. Midwifery was also moving away from general practice and routine hospital delivery was favoured, particularly in Scotland. In the towns, the GP's consulting took place, at best, in a comfortable room in a suburban house, with the doctor's wife as receptionist and telephone-answerer. At worst, single-handed GPs worked in the city centres using tiny sparsely-furnished former shops as consulting rooms. To add to the professional divide, the hospitals were now run as one service and general practice remained as another, run by the local

Executive Councils surviving from National Insurance administration days. With less time for patients and fewer facilities, the GPs felt that they were now merely a form-filling intermediary in the patient-chemist-hospital triangle. Perhaps recalling their opposition to the NHS, they felt restive as a result of their marginalisation.

In 1958 the *Scottish Medical Journal* rather patronisingly noted these concerns:

> We wonder if we are wrong in thinking that the general practitioner is the least happy of our colleagues. His financial reward at the end of the year is simply measured solely by the number of his patients and his mileage allowance. Many practitioners find themselves overworked and without the time to discuss the world and its ways with the patient. Gone are the opportunities to go to the local hospital and discuss matters with

a known consultant. The pressures of scientific medicine impel him to refer more and more of his cases to a hospital of which he no longer feels an integral part. If the health service is to prosper, we cannot be too tender in our regard for the conditions of general practice.

Rural practice, as romanticised in Cronin's *Dr Finlay's Casebook,* had also declined. The cottage hospitals, disliked by Bevan, had been a focus of local medical activity, one where the GPs treated acute illness and did some surgery, but these were disappearing.

The GPs became politically stronger when a College of General Practitioners was established in 1952. Later, they made serious threats to leave the NHS. The revolt was headed off when the government listened, not least because the clinical and economic importance of the GPs had been realised, since they saw and treated 90% of ills with 30% of the NHS budget. An added dimension was that the GPs were aware of the psycho-social background to their patients' ills, and they held the patients' lifelong clinical notes. In other health care systems, this sensible and efficient use of primary care was not fostered, and in

the US and Europe, immediate and unnecessary resort with simple ailments to costly specialists was, and is, widely made.

This pressure on the government succeeded, and the 'Doctor's Charter' of 1966 met many of the sources of discontent. The GPs' sturdy financial independence was partly given up when money was offered for practice staff and premises, although setting up the national network of health centres would still have to wait. The changes meant new scope and standards in primary care and the patients benefited. Teaching of general practice to students also started in the 1960s, and postgraduate training of doctors to prepare for general practice came in later.

In the sparsely populated Highlands, conditions were different. GPs' salaries were augmented by financial inducements given to compensate for small patient lists. At this time of dominance of the city hospital sector, the small hospitals in the Highlands also steadily closed. The air ambulance service to the Highlands and Islands still had a high profile, but otherwise there were no Scottish experiments in health care in remote areas, as of old. Later, helicopter transport and telemedicine were slow to appear.

The Broons

The Brown family have featured since 1936 in Dundee's popular national newspaper *The Sunday Post.* The family of nine live in a tenement flat with few rooms typical of Scottish industrial cities in the mid-twentieth century. Money is tight and they have no car. The older Broon men smoke and are short of stature, unlike the better-fed seven Broon children. The matriarch Maw 'Maggie' Broon is plump, as is daughter Daphne. The tales derive from life in a simple extended family and mealtimes are a feature. Doctors, nurses and illness are notably absent from the series, perhaps reflecting past stoicism in dealing with ill health. But the *Sunday Post's* weekly column 'The Doc Replies' had such influence that Scottish doctors were wise to be aware of the topics covered each Sunday, ready for their patients' questions on Monday morning.

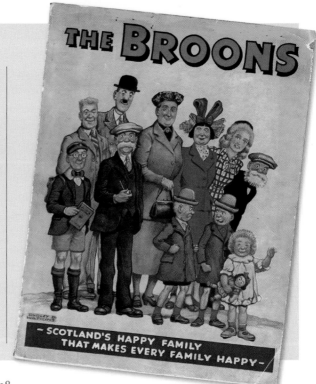

THE BROONS

~ SCOTLAND'S HAPPY FAMILY THAT MAKES EVERY FAMILY HAPPY ~

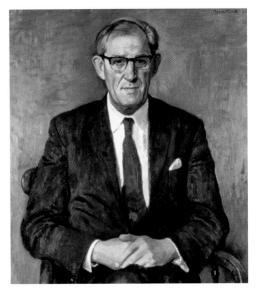

5.15 Obstetric care. Sir Dugald Baird (1899–1986), raised in Greenock, was a Glasgow University graduate, and, training at Glasgow's Royal Maternity Hospital, was well aware of the effects of adverse social conditions on the health of mother and child. Moving to Aberdeen, he set up and used his Aberdeen Maternity and Neonatal Databank from 1951 to study this relationship in the local well-defined area. He also hoped to add a 'fifth freedom' to Beveridge's list, namely of freedom from excess fertility, and to this end, he set up a free family planning clinic in Aberdeen. He was an important advisor to David Steel in framing the Abortion Act of 1967, notably in the wording of the socio-medical permission clause. Baird was given the Freedom the City of Aberdeen in 1965. His son David in Edinburgh led the team which introduced mifegyne (RU-486), the 'morning-after pill', to the UK (*Aberdeen Medico-Chirurgical Society*).

Later Costs

By the early 1950s, NHS finances were increasingly tight and costs rose steeply. National austerity resulted in devaluation of the pound, and prescription charges had been proposed in 1949. In 1951, the added burden of Korean War expenditure meant that Gaitskell, as Chancellor, introduced charges for spectacles and dentures, poignantly the iconic first items to be 'free' in the new NHS. Bevan and Harold Wilson resigned in protest and the Labour government was condemned by the Scottish Trades Union Conference. The Labour Party lost the election shortly afterwards, and in the incoming Conservative government, Chancellor Rab Butler's austerity budget added prescription charges and a dental consultation fee.

These concerns over rising NHS spending meant that the Conservative government took the opportunity to review the system. The Guillebaud Committee was asked to investigate the cost of the NHS, and it was thought that an alternative to the NHS might result. The Committee took three years to report, and there was surprise when they concluded that not only did the NHS give value for money, but that NHS expenditure should increase from its level at 3.5% of GDP.

Housing also rose in the political priorities since Britain's deteriorating housing stock was now notorious for overcrowding and lack of amenities. In 1951, 56 % of Scots families had no fixed bath, and 37% had no internal toilet, with Glasgow worst off. Further analysis later produced 'deprivation' data judged by a scoring system of adverse social factors, which again highlighted Glasgow's problems.

Slum clearance started, notably in Glasgow, together with an 'overspill' policy in which almost 200,000 of the population were moved out, and many young families left, attracted by the prospect of work in the new industries in the new towns growing up beyond the cities. Others were housed in new but disliked housing estates on the edge of the city, and the Castlemilk scheme, in particular, which took in Glasgow slum-dwellers, gained a reputation for poor planning and absence of the usual amenities of town life. The absence of public houses was a deliberate policy. Life in Castlemilk's high rise buildings was satirised by folk singers. *The Jeelie Piece Song* caught the mood, mourning that the move from the slum houses to high-rise buildings meant that children could no longer be given pieces (sandwich snacks) directly from the windows, as was the custom in the lower-level slum houses.

Study of the effect of these social influences on health, now identified as 'social medicine', continued to build on Boyd Orr's early lead in the 1930s, and from 1965 to 1985 further notable contributions again came from the Rowett Research Institute in Aberdeen. There in the north-east, the obstetrician Dugald Baird's research studies added to knowledge of the effect of housing, nutrition and social conditions on child and maternal health.

New Buildings

Early pioneering health centres for general practitioners were built at Sighthill in 1953 and Stranraer in 1955, but none thereafter for ten years. From 1965 health centres were at last appearing in numbers, and by 1983, 170 such centres existed. They housed many independent general

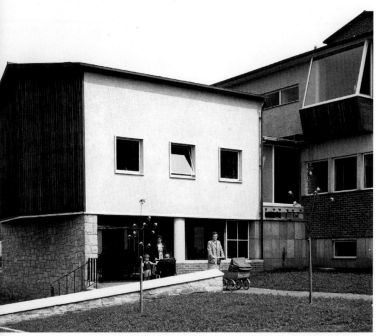

5.16 Health centres. In 1953, Sighthill in Edinburgh gained Scotland's first health centre (*Alexis Burnett*).

HEALTH: INFECTIOUS DISEASE

The post-war period saw steady improvements in the indicators of health. Infant mortality rates, always an indicator of general healthiness, fell steadily and expectation of life lengthened, but the biggest change in the pattern of disease in the post-war period was that infectious disease incidence fell rapidly. In 1900, these caused 50% of all deaths, and this was to fall to below 1% by the end of the century. The success came from a mix of influences, including improved social conditions, better nutrition, and the ever-lengthening list of antibacterial therapies, which ranged from chemotherapy for tuberculosis to multiple uses of penicillin, including prevention of the serious heart and kidney complications of streptococcal throat infections. But above all, there was a range of new immunisations.

In the mid-twentieth century some lethal, now forgotten, diseases were still about. Diphtheria was still a killer, and there were about 6,000 cases and 200 deaths annually in Scotland at this time. Poliomyelitis was a common summer disease, and in 1947 an epidemic caused 131 deaths in Scotland and also left a legacy of limb damage. Even smallpox outbreaks occurred, with 25 cases in Glasgow in 1942; the last incident, originating from a seaman, affected a similar number in 1950, but without any deaths. Other less dangerous infectious diseases like measles, mumps and whooping cough were just part of childhood experience, and were accepted with stoicism.

Immunisation

Prevention became steadily possible. At the end of the war, although an effective diphtheria vaccine had been available much earlier, only one third of children were covered by immunisation, in spite of a wartime drive to vaccinate. Acceptance of prevention had not been firmly established, and there was lingering public opposition to such mass schemes. Anti-vaccination sentiment derived from controversies earlier in the century, notably over vaccine effectiveness and the use of animals in their preparation. But by the mid-1950s, with the prevention strategy generally accepted, effective uptake by the public of the vaccine resulted and diphtheria became a disease of the past. The

practices, and their size enabled the appointment of nurses, physiotherapists and social workers. Other facilities such as X-ray equipment were available, and hospital consultants were encouraged to hold clinics in the centres in an attempt to bring the two services closer together.

In 1962 the ambitious Hospital Plan was announced, proposing to replace Britain's older institutions and also to add new ones. Major rebuilding of teaching hospitals started on site, or close by, in Glasgow and Edinburgh, and there were new district general hospital developments at Dumfries, Inverness, Dunfermline, Kirkcaldy, Ayr, Kilmarnock, Coatbridge, Motherwell, Greenock and Paisley. The larger projects were shrewdly phased, in case of economic downturns, and these did indeed occur.

last outbreak was in Motherwell in 1968, with six cases and two deaths. Tetanus and pertussis (whooping cough) immunisation joined diphtheria prevention by the early 1960s. In 1956, the Salk polio vaccine followed, and from 1962 the more acceptable oral Sabin version was available and polio also became a disease of the past.

Thus encouraged, the next group of infectious diseases to receive attention were not mass killers. Mumps was usually a mild childhood disease and measles might cause unpleasant secondary chest infections, but German measles (rubella), though usually running a benign course, could damage an unborn child. Immunisation was introduced for these diseases. Further vaccines appeared later against influenza and some forms of meningitis.

Latent concerns over vaccine use and safety re-emerged in February 1976, when Gordon Stewart, Glasgow's controversialist Professor of Public Health, publicised data showing occasional serious side effects of the whooping cough vaccine, including 36 alleged cases of brain damage. He claimed that the risks of the now rare disease were outweighed by the dangers of the vaccine. Extended press coverage resulted, and although it was pointed out that the disease was rare because of the vaccine, uptake of all vaccines fell. Cases of whooping cough did rise again. Some slight risk was admitted and the government introduced a Vaccine Damage scheme in 1979, giving a one-off payment in proven cases.

Tuberculosis

Earlier called 'consumption' or 'phthisis', tuberculosis was always of national concern and from 1900 special philanthropic and government schemes appeared to deal with it. Tuberculosis wards and sanatoria for rest and 'fresh air' treatment were available, and other initiatives of the time were surgical – using various lung collapse strategies. (The latter involved letting air into the chest and collapsing the lung, which could allow a large TB cavity to heal.) TB incidence in Britain was at its highest in Glasgow, being double the Scottish rate, and the Glasgow incidence was 50% higher than that of comparable industrial cities in England.

In 1946 one of many sufferers in Scotland was a visitor – London's Eric Blair (George Orwell) – who took

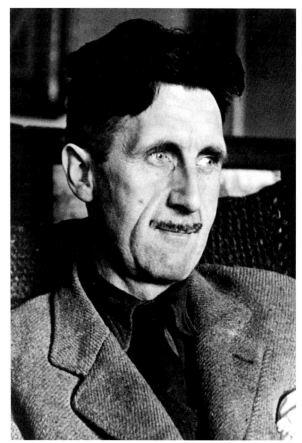

5.17 TB treatment. George Orwell, the novelist, was given the first supplies of streptomycin in Scotland in 1946 (*Getty Images*).

medical advice to go and live in a remote farmhouse on the island of Jura for the traditional open-air treatment. There he worked on his novel *1984*, and when his condition worsened, he moved to Hairmyres Hospital sanatorium near Glasgow, and to assist with rest, his typewriter was taken away. To treat the disease, streptomycin was newly available in America, but not in Britain. With the help of Orwell's influential friends, including Aneurin Bevan who had been Orwell's editor at the magazine *Tribune*, he was given the drug, which he paid for in America with the dollar royalties from his novel *Animal Farm*. He was the first to receive streptomycin in Scotland, but soon proved to be allergic to it. Before returning to London, he gifted the unused streptomycin to the hospital, and two other patients received it. He died shortly afterwards in 1950.

With the appearance of this anti-tuberculous therapy from the late 1940s onwards, one of Scotland's ancient scourges was on the wane. The success of streptomycin

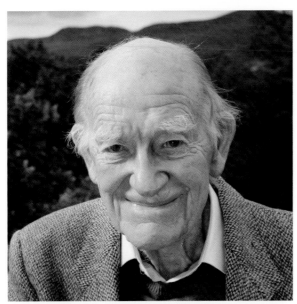

5.18 Lung disease. Sir John Crofton (1912–2009) devised a lasting and successful strategy for treating tuberculosis. Later he was an activist in the ASH campaign – Action on Smoking and Health – which highlighted smoking's effects on health and urged Government action (*Murdo Macleod*).

was followed and added to by newer agents like PAS, isoniazid and rifampicin. With these available as choices, it was a team led by Edinburgh's John Crofton which pioneered a combination of them, to prevent resistance developing, which established the routine success of anti-tuberculous therapy, and opened the way for the multi-drug strategies used in other situations later. His study was one of the first-ever randomised controlled trials of the kind which were soon to be essential in assessing any novel form of therapy.

BCG immunisation against the disease began to be used in 1950 for at-risk groups. This was extended steadily to all the population in the mid-1950s, after testing for pre-existing immunity, which proved to be surprisingly common, revealing in individuals an unsuspected earlier brush with the disease. The role of overcrowding in spreading tuberculosis was acknowledged and patients were re-housed to better accommodation under a special scheme.

In 1950, Hector McNeil, the Scottish Secretary, learned that the famous Swiss tuberculosis sanatoria had

spare capacity emerging as a result of the growing success of medical treatment. McNeil announced that his patients deserved the best of treatment, and persuaded the reluctant Ministry of Health to pay for the costs of sending some Scottish patients to Switzerland. The first group left Glasgow for Davos in June 1951, with press coverage arranged, and, as others were flown out in monthly groups, Scottish Red Cross officials looked after their welfare on arrival. This scheme had a high profile, and it ceased, not without protests in the west of Scotland, in 1957 when sanatorium treatment was no longer favoured. 1,043 patients had been treated.

In 1900, TB had been responsible for 155 deaths per 1,000. This fell to 1 per 100,000 by the end of the century. Until the 1950s, having the notorious disease was seldom admitted, but when chemotherapy proved successful, many let it be known that they had indeed been affected, but had been cured.

Latent Disease

With success in treating established cases of TB, the time was right to look for undetected disease. Though 'screening' was to be a routine strategy later, it was a novelty then. The matter had been considered before, but officials were gloomy about the uptake by the public of screening for TB, and assumed that the cost/benefit ratio would be unfavourable. It was also thought that the worst cases might not come forward, especially as hospitalisation for treatment should follow. Nevertheless, a Scotland-wide campaign started in February 1957, using the new economical miniature chest X-ray films, and the campaign was well-planned and energetic. Volunteers distributed leaflets to all houses, and following press briefings, there were special films for cinema use and celebrity endorsements were obtained. There were two campaign songs, planes flew banners over the cities and large companies donated space for the campaign's publicity on billboards.

The organisers were rewarded by an uptake of twice their expectation. Half the adult population of Scotland were screened within five weeks, picking up 2.5 new cases of TB per 1,000 population, plus some other hidden lung disease. It was a particularly important event in Glasgow's history. The city took some pride in the community spirit

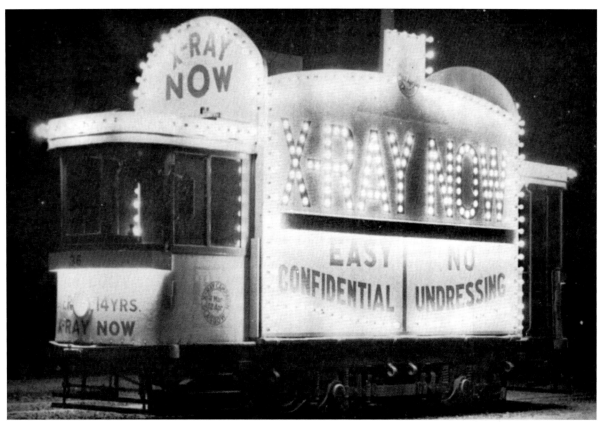

5.19 TB detection. Glasgow had a prominent part in the X-ray Campaign of 1957 against tuberculosis and, as part of the drive, this illuminated car toured the streets on the city's tramway system (*Glasgow District Council*).

Unpasteurised Milk

Pasteurisation of milk is considered to diminish the flavour of cheeses, and some makers continue to use untreated milk, notably Brie and Roquefort.

In 1995, the newly-marketed Lanark Blue cheese – 'Scotland's Roquefort' – made on a small scale south of Glasgow using untreated ewes' milk, had allegedly high levels of listeria bacteria. Though human infection was not known to have occurred, action was taken, and a costly, celebrated 19-day court action followed. The farmer's defence was funded by the cheese-making community and libertarian supporters, and the prosecution failed. The maker, compensated for loss of sales, was hailed as 'the man who saved Scottish cheeses'. No further concerns have emerged regarding unpasteurised milk.

that had emerged, and it assisted the city in starting to deal with its negative image. The Conservative Party then in power also gained credit from the campaign, particularly through the support of Lord Home, a former tuberculosis sufferer, then leader of the party in the Lords and a future Prime Minister.

Milk was known to pass on the bovine strain of TB to children, and with herds being increasingly tested, milk was graded according to risk. By the 1970s, all milk for public distribution was 'pasteurised', by using moderate heat for a short time to kill bacteria, notably salmonella and coliform strains. But this also destroyed some vitamins, useful enzymes and immunoglobulins; untreated milk is still therefore available in bottles, closed with a green top and bearing a suitable warning.

Later Epidemics

Infectious disease outbreaks could still occur and were newsworthy. The Aberdeen outbreak of typhoid in 1964 was a surprise, and was a reminder to the public, now accustomed to the decline in infectious disease, that

233

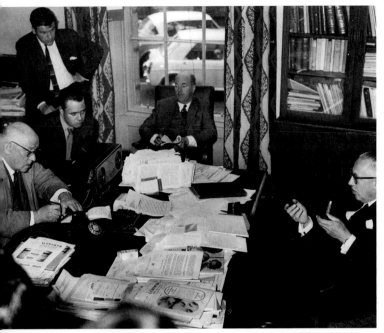

5.20 Typhoid epidemic. Dr Ian McQueen, the Medical Officer of Health, briefing journalists during the 1964 Aberdeen epidemic (*Press and Journal*).

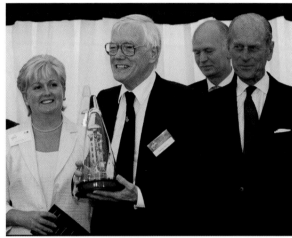

5.21 Hepatitis B. Sir Kenneth Murray (b. 1930) started as a laboratory technician and, graduating in Birmingham, moved to Edinburgh's Department of Molecular Biology in 1967. Influenced by the Hepatitis B outbreak in Edinburgh he used his knowledge of DNA sequencing to produce a vaccine in 1978. He donates the considerable resulting royalties to the Darwin Trust and its scientific studies (*University of Edinburgh*).

epidemics were still possible. There were over 500 admissions to the Aberdeen hospitals, which had to function for a while as typhoid hospitals. Those who had improved were detained to prevent further spread, and there was restriction of movement of the townspeople. Dr Ian MacQueen, the local Medical Officer of Health, took on an unusually high profile, and as a former journalist, he made himself available with daily press conferences; his nightly television appearances reported developments and advised the citizens. His detective work was a reminder of a past era in public health work, and he traced the infection to a contaminated corned beef tin imported from the Argentine.

It was some time before the city returned to normal. Tourism was badly affected, and Aberdonians travelling outside the city were sometimes shunned. The Milne Committee of Inquiry later suggested that, by sensationalising the events, MacQueen had stimulated undue public concern over food safety. Others defended his role in taking food safety issues away from the usual confidential management by government. The debate on how to handle such incidents continued, and with further national controversy over salmonella in eggs, E-coli in meat and the major issue of BSE in the late 1990s, trans-

parency over food safety was accepted, and the Food Standards Agency emerged.

Other Infections

An ever-present fear was of viral epidemics, and the ever-changing influenza virus always had potential for serious spread, unchecked by treatment or vaccines. Bird 'flu was feared in 2008 and swine 'flu arrived in 2009, causing 66 deaths in Scotland. As international travel increased, so did the potential for spread of better-controlled diseases like malaria, but also the lethal Ebola Fever. Hepatitis B virus infection is endemic in many parts of the world, and many carry the virus in their blood. In developed nations it had been known to cause infection after blood transfusion – called serum hepatitis. In the mid-1960s, contact with blood was commoner in hospitals, particularly in the new kidney dialysis units, and many hospitals throughout the world with these units were afflicted with hepatitis. An Edinburgh hospital was seriously affected from 1969, with four staff and seven patient deaths out of 40 cases. Anyone handling blood throughout the world was considered at risk and a vaccine was urgently required: this was made by a scientist in Edinburgh, Ken Murray.

OTHER HEALTH ISSUES

Though free dental care from 1948 slowly encouraged some in Scotland to take new pride in retaining teeth into adult life, dental decay and loss was still prominent in some regions of Scotland, and there was a possible solution. The benefits for dental health from natural fluoride in water was known, and water fluoridation was a logical way to improve Scotland's poor dental health. A fluoridation experiment was a success in Kilmarnock, giving better dental health there than in the non-fluorided areas in Ayr nearby. Chlorination of water had been routine in Scotland from 1939 to reduce survival of bacteria, and the flouride strategy seemed acceptable. It was on the verge of being introduced throughout Scotland when determined opposition appeared. In 1983, an edentulous Glasgow pensioner, put forward by opponents of 'mass medication', brought a Court of Session case against fluoridation by her local council. Her case was based on these general grounds, plus alleged fears that fluoride caused cancer. The judge was critical of some of the evidence, notably some 'junk science' presented to him, but he declined to give full support to fluoridation and all the schemes were reluctantly dropped. The proposal came up regularly thereafter, particularly as fluoride has been successfully introduced elsewhere outside of Scotland.

The Environment

A major public health issue was the polluted environment of British cities, notably that of heavily-industrialised Glasgow. It was a daunting challenge, since the attitudes and needs of industry clashed with health reform. Visibility and air quality in British cities was bad at most times, but the notable winter 'smogs' of 1952 led to the 1956 Clean Air Act, a classic and successful piece of public health legislation. The costly switch away from coal use could not be done overnight and came in sector by sector, and the first smoke-free zone to be established in Scotland was in 1956 at Sighthill in Edinburgh. Not until 1969 was there a smoke-free town – Coatbridge near Glasgow. The costs were considerable, and since 70% of Glasgow housing was owned by the city, assistance had to be given with the costs of installing alternative heating. But many

benefited, and winter deaths from respiratory causes declined markedly.

Other environmental and occupational hazards were steadily dealt with, often by low-key health and safety measures. Asbestos was widely used in industrial Glasgow, notably in shipbuilding, and to add to its known unpleasant effects, a link with mesothelioma – an uncommon form of lung cancer – was established in 1960. In the legal battles which followed, the activists in Clydeside Action on Asbestosis led to wider acknowledgment of the hazard and compensation resulted, even for its non-cancerous effects.

Road traffic accidents steadily fell, as did injuries from them, assisted by doctor-led advice to introduce compulsory use of helmets for motorcycle users and to place seat belts in cars. Safety in the shrinking coalmining industry continued to improve. Glasgow's crowded dockland warehouses were prone to spectacular fires, giving it the title of 'tinderbox city', and tighter controls followed. Public venue safety was again an issue after a second Ibrox

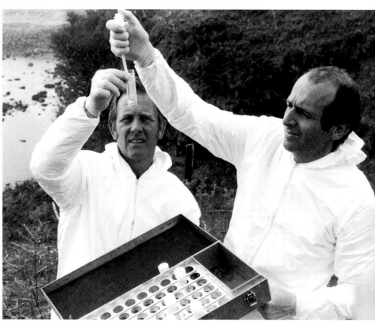

5.22 Porton Down biological weapons research staff removing soil samples from Gruinard Island in 1986 to test for residual anthrax spores (*Scotsman Publications*).

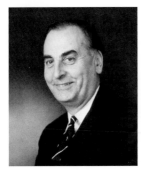

5.23 Geriatric care. Sir Ferguson Anderson (1914–2001) in Glasgow in the 1960s identified the deficiencies in managing ill-health in old age. He successfully introduced the specialty of geriatrics, in which rehabilitation and social adjustment is added to curative care. He was appointed in 1965 to the world's first chair of geriatrics in Glasgow, and then became an advisor to the World Health Organisation. In Glasgow he hosted the first international conference on the subject (*Glasgow University Archives*).

Stadium disaster in 1971 when 66 deaths resulted from surges in the crowd. Though 25 spectators had died earlier at Ibrox in 1902, no immediate national action was taken until the similar Heysel and Hillsborough stadium deaths in the late 1980s prompted legislation.

Though the purity of Glasgow's drinking water was a source of civic pride ever since the supply from Loch Katrine was obtained a century earlier, it came under suspicion in the 1970s. Being slightly acid, it was slowly removing lead from the old water pipes of the city, particularly in the slum areas. A temporary scare arose that mass sub-clinical lead poisoning was taking place, causing subtle brain damage and lowered intelligence. Lead paint, then widely used in children's cots, was also implicated. These claims were only gradually refuted.

In 1990, Scotland's most dangerous place was, at last, rendered safe. Britain's biological warfare studies in WW2 led to a successful trial in 1942 of anthrax spores on Gruinard Island off the west coast of Scotland. When the spores were released from a bomb, a flock of sheep was killed. But the spores persisted in the soil. The nature of the experiment had to be admitted and the island put under long-term quarantine. In 1986, after activists' protests, expensive decontamination of the soil was carried out, and sheep grazing and human visits were permitted four years later.

Care of the Elderly

When the municipal hospitals were integrated into the NHS under the new large regional hospital boards, these hospitals' former Poor Law role was noticed, since many wards still housed 'aged' indigent inmates. At Stobhill Hospital in Glasgow, a former municipal hospital, Dr Ferguson Anderson encountered these long-stay citizens and rejected nihilistic management, substituting active treatment plus social intervention and support. With a slogan of 'we are all geriatricians now', he enthused others, and with geriatric medicine (later changed to 'diseases of

the elderly') emerging as a specialty, many of his staff and students took important posts elsewhere. Later, the Scottish Office policy from 1980 onwards made care of the elderly a priority.

Health Education

Health education had always been given by doctors in an individual way, adding holistic lifestyle advice to any specific therapy. Health education by central authorities had been envisaged in the Cathcart Report of 1934, but acceptance that this was a task for government was slow to emerge. The Scottish Health Education Unit appeared in 1968, and its first project was the necessary negative advice on smoking. Slowly its work changed from negative campaigning to positive health promotion on a broad front. The Unit seemed to have some freedom of action and its marketing skills were admired, particularly in its attempts to counter the view that drinking and smoking was a mark of maturity and virility in the young. In the drive against smoking, they faced the power of the tobacco companies, but the national ban on televised advertisements for cigarettes in the 1960s was helpful. Using celebrities, and linking physical fitness with non-smoking, the unit also made inventive use of the claim that the Scottish 1982 World Cup football team was a 'no-smoking squad'. The Edinburgh Commonwealth Games athletes in 1986 carried 'Smoking is for Losers' logos. Later, in 1991, one of the Unit's songs briefly reached the top 10 in Scotland's pop charts.

These efforts in Scotland were linked to some other specific campaigns, notably the ones mounted by the national Action on Smoking and Health (ASH), established by London's Royal College of Physicians in 1971 as a response to the Conservative government's failure to accept proposals from the College for legislation to curb smoking. Edinburgh's Sir John Crofton was an activist in the ASH campaign and his wife Eileen chaired its Scottish Committee. Anti-smoking legislation steadily emerged.

MEDICAL TEACHING

Graduates from Scotland's medical schools were always produced in greater numbers than Scottish needs, and export of newly-qualified doctors was still prominent in the second half of the century. For slightly older 'junior' doctors there were periods when unregulated competitive training within the Scottish hospital sector led to bottle-necks in promotion, and some emigrated a few years after qualification. At the end of the 1960s in particular, there was marked migration of young doctors from the Scottish hospitals, notably to the growing opportunities in Canada, adding another element to the Scottish medical diaspora of old.

The proportion of women medical students in Scotland steadily rose and passed 50% in the 1990s, and this figure continued to rise. Scotland's first woman professor was Margaret Fairlie, appointed in 1940 to the chair of midwifery at Dundee.

Scotland's medical schools flourished in the post-war era, with the proportion of students to population being almost 50% higher than in England. Training in medicine involved a long six-year course, starting with three years of science studies before hospital teaching was reached, followed until 1960 by conscription for male students as National Service army doctors. The Scottish medical schools had a continuing advantage from the large number of hospitals and patients available in the new extensive hospital regions, and most of the new NHS consultants in the region taught students and were granted honorary university staff status. The main teaching hospitals were linked with other university departments on the campus and these offered facilities for joint biomedical research ventures. The link with the universities was seen in other ways, bringing in teaching from other faculties. Teaching of public health had always been a feature in Scotland, and this was broadened to include contributions from others such as sociologists. With a growing awareness of the complexity of health care, input was also at hand from the new cadre of medical ethicists.

Teaching of general practice had started in 1948 in Edinburgh as a student elective, and was based on a general practice situated in the building which, in the eighteenth century, housed Andrew Duncan's famous Royal Public Dispensary. Rockefeller Foundation grant money assisted expansion of the unit in 1952, and in 1959 it offered diagnostic services to local doctors. Then, with the growing importance of general practice, it evolved into the world's first academic unit in 1963, headed by the James MacKenzie Chair of Medicine in Relation to General Practice. Teaching of general practice elsewhere in Britain's medical schools was strengthened by the recommendations of the Royal Commission on Medical Education of 1968.

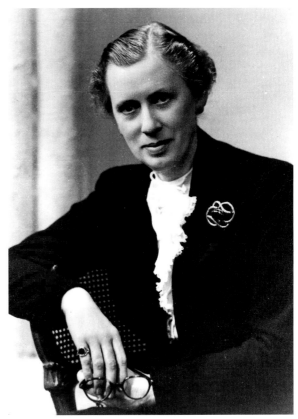

5.24 Women doctors. Margaret Fairlie (1891–1963) was the first woman to hold a professorial chair in Scotland. She graduated from St Andrews University in 1915, then worked in Dundee, Edinburgh and elsewhere as a gynaecologist before returning to Dundee in 1919 as a consultant. After a visit to the Curie Clinic in Paris, she became a pioneer user of radiation therapy in Scotland. In 1936 she was made Head of Obstetrics and Gynaecology at Dundee Royal Infirmary and was appointed to the chair in 1940 (*Dundee University Archives*).

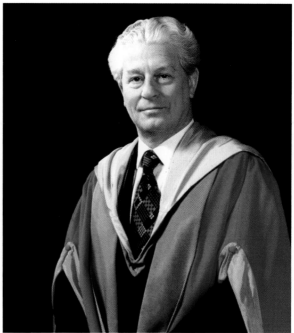

5.25 Specialist medicine. Specialism flourished in Scotland in the post-World War Two era, and the large Regional Plastic Surgery Unit at Canniesburn Hospital in Glasgow was headed by Tom Gibson (1915–1993), who was known for his early studies on tissue transplant rejection (*RCPSG*).

RESEARCH AND DEVELOPMENT

In the post-war period, Scottish medical research and scholarship showed considerable vitality: indeed the period might be seen as a second medical Enlightenment. As in the earlier Scottish Enlightenment, this vitality did not appear at a time of economic strength, but at a time of post-WW2 hardship. Just as the Scottish Enlightenment flourished when patronage of the aristocracy and government was removed by their move to London, post-war Scottish medicine turned to scholarship at a time when private medicine had declined. In this time of collective confidence, Scotland made significant contributions to world clinical medicine as well as bringing significant insights into basic medical sciences. As in the earlier Enlightenment, the evidence of success was that students and doctors from other countries were attracted into Scotland, and there was also the export of talent to play a part in medical care and teaching elsewhere. As in the earlier Enlightenment, a remarkable number of new medical texts emerged; many became the standard works in their subject and held this dominant role after many editions. The *Scottish Medical Journal* was born from an amalgamation of two proud and ancient Glasgow and Edinburgh periodicals, and it gave a united response to the new health service. In fiction, Colin Currie's novels, written under the pseudonym Colin Douglas, starting with *The Houseman's Tale,* gave insights into Edinburgh medicine of the day.

To help explain these interesting developments in Scotland, which amplified an ever-present Scottish tradition in medical research and development, some supportive factors can be noted. One was the size of the new university-associated Scottish hospital system, and the acceptance of specialism, which together encouraged the culture of innovation. Glasgow's famous busy Burns Unit attracted Nobel-prize winner Peter Medawar during WW2 to carry out a famous study of skin grafting with surgeon Thomas Gibson. Scottish plastic surgery, neurosurgery and cardiology in particular also flourished, based on large specialised units.

The importance of research in Scotland had been signalled by health service funding from the outset via the Scottish Hospital Endowments Research Trust (SHERT). The large hospital boards had support from niche forward-looking units like regional physics departments, and Glasgow's local unit gave input to Ian Donald's celebrated ultrasound work, which was also assisted by SHERT money.

In the 1960s competition for academic and NHS consultant posts was intense in Scotland, and research output and achievement was seen as important for promotion. Scotland had been first in the UK to have the benefits of full-time salaried professorial chairs in academic clinical departments, and junior academic posts were highly regarded at the time. Plenty of local talent emerged to fill these chairs in the post-war period, particularly as private practice had little attraction. Within Scotland, Glasgow's academic surgery thrived under the leadership of Sir Charles Illingworth, whose department favoured scientific physiological studies of relevance to surgery, and from his department came all the heads of university surgery departments in Scotland at the time, while others took such posts in England, where suitable applicants were lacking. Many other academic staff also moved out of Scotland to head university clinical and laboratory departments in England. To deal with the low level of research

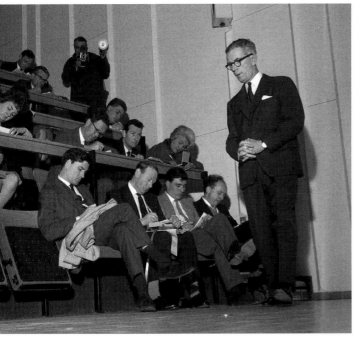

5.26 Ian Aird (1905–1962) was one of the many Scots surgeons who took their new approach into England and helped establish London's Post-graduate Medical School as a world famous medical centre. He gained public acclaim for his separation of conjoint 'Siamese' twins, and his textbook of surgery of 1949 was the standard work of the day (*Press Association*).

activity in London, the Royal Post-Graduate Medical School at Hammersmith had been set up in 1935, and from 1939 onwards, the Scot Sir John McMichael, as head of medicine, set out to create 'a little Edinburgh in the west of London'. By the 1950s, largely staffed by Scots, this small ex-Poor Law hospital had been transformed into an internationally famous research and teaching institution. The Scottish staff were full-time and uninvolved in London's private practice sector. McMichael was a committed socialist, as was Jim Dempster, the hospital's Scottish pioneering transplant surgeon, and this caused them difficulties in obtaining US visas. Ian Aird, from Edinburgh, head of the surgical unit, was a fluent Russian speaker, and hence the hospital was a favourite venue for the few Russian medical visitors who reached the West during this Cold War era.

The favourable milieu in Scotland also drew in medical talent from outside to take senior posts, attracted by the hospital links with the universities, the higher status of academic versus private medicine in Scotland, the large clinical departments with their research facilities and the culture of innovation. Notable in this influx were men like Ian Donald, Michael Woodruff, the surgeon, and Sir John Crofton the physician.

SHARED ATTITUDES

In this period, the traditional Scottish doctors' concern for collective as well as individual health was again seen in the interest they took well beyond their own clinical spheres. The physician Douglas Black's famous report raised lasting concern for inequality in health between the classes, an interest continued by Scottish studies on social deprivation using Aberdeen's Carstairs Index. The obstetrician Dugald Baird sought maternal health for all, as did Ian Donald in his new Queen Mother's Hospital where, he said, 'every mother is a duchess'. Even Archie Cochrane's emphasis (described later) on the results of group studies rather than individual responses might arise from this attitude, and even in brain surgery, Glasgow's famous Coma Scale can be seen as seeking an improvement in the management of all cases, rather than in niche neurological areas. Lord Sutherland's report later advocating free personal care for the elderly also fits with this Scottish concern for society as a whole.

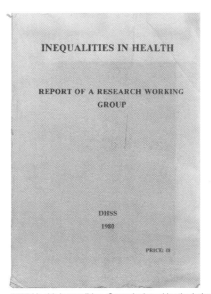

5.27 Health inequalities. Commissioned by the Labour government in 1977, Sir Douglas Black's famous Report in 1980 identified serious inequalities in health according to social class. It was not delivered until after the election and the incoming Conservative government distanced themselves from its recommendations, releasing only these 260 cheaply-printed copies over a bank holiday week-end. In spite of this, the content quickly aroused huge and lasting interest. Black (1913–2002), a St Andrews University graduate, was the government's Chief Scientist at the time (*HMSO*).

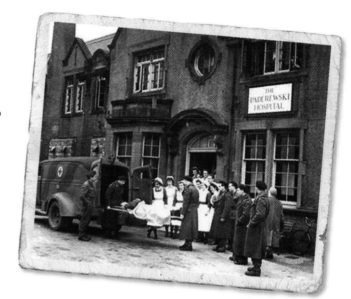

5.28 Polish émigrés. The Polish Medical School in Edinburgh, set up in 1941, was given a building in the Western General Hospital complex. Renamed the Paderewski Hospital, it was also used for student teaching (*1st Mac.com*).

THE COLLEGES' EXAMS

From earliest times, the Scottish Colleges' diplomas in surgery and medicine could serve as the medical students' final degree, but steadily, after the Medical Act of 1858, the universities' own degrees gained greater status and acceptance. In response the three Colleges' diplomas were combined as the 'Triple Qualification' from 1884, and this was used for graduation and medical registration mainly by the students of the small extramural medical schools. University medical students also often sat this Triple Qualification, which was held prior to the university final examinations, as an insurance policy. If happily both were passed, an impressive array of qualifications resulted to put on a doctor's otherwise bleak brass plate. The use of the Triple Qualification dwindled, but had occasional use, until it was discontinued in 1993.

The best known extramural schools were Anderson's College and St Mungo's College in Glasgow, and the School of Medicine of the Royal Colleges in Edinburgh. These had added to the production of Scottish doctors by the universities, often enabling those without funds, or otherwise unable to enter university, to train in medicine. But in the post-war centralising climate, these small schools were seen as oddities at a time of rising standards, and the Goodenough Report on Medical Schools of 1944, which had many criticisms of aspects of medical education throughout Britain, declined to support these little colleges. In the Report, Edinburgh and Glasgow university medical schools had escaped censure, unlike those in London, and, perhaps relieved, the Scottish universities were not unhappy to see their local extramural schools disappear.

Also closing down with the extramural schools was the Polish Medical School in Edinburgh. Set up in 1941

by Polish doctors who had escaped from the invasion of their country by the Germans, they were later joined by other doctors and students fleeing from the Russians. With instruction in Polish, they planned to have staff ready to restore that country's health care system after the war, but when the communist takeover prevented this, many of the doctors instead stayed on in Scotland. It closed in 1949 after 227 students had passed through, having gained qualifications suitable for both Britain and Poland.

Postgraduates

There was increasing concern over the old assumption that, after medical training, the newly-qualified doctor was ready to deal with all the ills of mankind. The colleges stepped in to arrange further training, and their diplomas now evolved into postgraduate qualifications. Obtaining them was essential to promotion, and part of the journey through practical vocational training. With Glasgow's Faculty changing to 'Royal College' status by 1952, its status was enhanced and all three Scottish Colleges now had fellowships and memberships available.

These two-part examinations proved attractive to overseas doctors who were not on the NHS payroll, and the three Colleges' finances prospered as a result of the examination fees charged and tuition courses run. With increasingly healthy finances, the Scottish Colleges expanded their teaching and advisory roles, taking added responsibility for postgraduate training. A specialist Fellowship brought in later by the Edinburgh College of Surgeons for senior junior doctors was used to signal fitness for a consultant post.

INFLUENCE ABROAD

Scotland still shared the values of the David Livingstone tradition, namely that Scotland could, or even should, give help abroad, and an early instance was when Sir J.D.S. Cameron, President of the Royal College of Physicians of Edinburgh, went to Dacca to teach after retirement in 1965. There he set up their Institute for Postgraduate Medicine and Research. Thereafter, more formal Scottish support was organised elsewhere abroad, often seconding NHS or university staff to assist teaching there and to support early health services. Periods of training in Scotland for some of these nations' talented doctors was also arranged. Edinburgh University was linked with Baroda in a World Health Organisation scheme in the 1960s, while Glasgow assisted medical schools in Nairobi, Kenya and Makerere, Uganda, from 1964. Later, Glasgow sent staff to Oman from the late 1970s, and Omani doctors returned for training in Glasgow.

In connection with this, the Scottish Colleges started to hold at least the first part of their diploma examinations in distant locations, which was not only convenient for those sitting the examinations, but helped to stimulate local interest in postgraduate activity. The first move was made by the Edinburgh College of Surgeons, setting up an examination in Hong Kong in 1966, which was soon followed by Bangladesh, Pakistan, Malaysia, Singapore, Saudi Arabia, Sri Lanka, Myanmar, Nepal and India.

SCOTTISH CONTRIBUTIONS

Life sciences

Alexander Todd was born in Glasgow and graduated from Glasgow University in 1928. After chemistry research posts in London, and elsewhere, he returned to Edinburgh University in 1934, settling in Manchester in 1938. There he started his major work, notably synthesising adenosine triphosphate (ATP) and in 1955 he unravelled the structure of vitamin B_{12}, gaining the Nobel Prize for chemistry in 1957. He was the long-serving chairman from 1952 to 1964 of the British Government's advisory committee on scientific policy and was Chancellor of Glasgow's University of Strathclyde from 1975. Knighted in 1954, he was created Baron Todd in 1962.

Hans Kosterlitz, the German biochemist, was attracted to Aberdeen in 1934 through the research interests of Nobel prize winner J.J.R.Macleod, the local professor of physiology. After a long career, and of retirement age, Kosterlitz identified the central nervous system transmitter called endorphin (encephalin or 'endogenous morphine') which can block pain pathways by occupying receptors. Released from the pituitary and hypothalamus it allegedly has systemic effects, including the 'endorphin rush' of exercise. Aberdeen University's research Kosterlitz Centre opened in 2010.

Sir David Lane (born 1952) studied and worked at University College London, and was appointed to

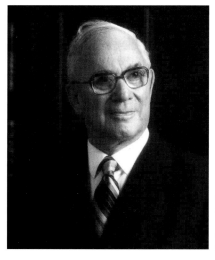

5.29 *Far left*. Lord Todd (1907–1997) (*Michael Noakes*).

5.30 *Left*. Hans Kosterlitz (1903–1996) (*Aberdeen University Archives*).

Post-war Life Sciences

Physiology continued to give insights of value to clinical medicine. The isolation of the adrenal corticosteroids was important, and identification of the variety of cell receptors in the smooth muscle of arteries and in the stomach led to development of important new drugs. In gastroenterology, an understanding of the role of hormones and nerve supply to the stomach assisted rational surgical treatments. Increasingly clinicians developed their own physiological studies, notably in cardiology and respiratory physiology. Biochemistry soon became the pacesetter in understanding the body. Successful unravelling of the structure of large molecules like haemoglobin and adenosine triphosphate led to the triumph of understanding DNA. The double helix molecule was clearly not a static part of a cellular soup, and molecular biology was born. Major insights into genetic influences on disease followed, and further success with insertion of genetic material into cells meant that cloning was possible. In immunology, the mechanism of rejection of tissue and organ grafts was understood, and ways to make grafts survive emerged. Cell death (apoptosis) turned out to be an orderly mechanism of significance.

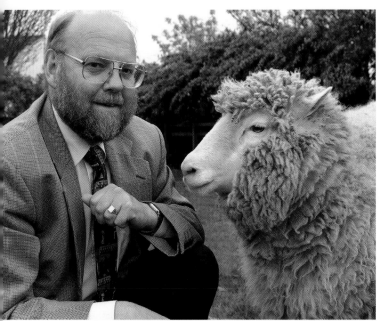

5.31 Cloning. Sir Ian Wilmut is shown with Dolly, the world's first cloned mammal, preserved, after death, in the National Museum of Scotland (*Photo courtesy of the Roslin Institute, The University of Edinburgh*).

Dundee University in 1990. In 1979 he identified the tumour suppressor gene p53, known as the 'guardian of the genome', since its mutations can cause failure of tumour regulation. He was Chief Scientist at the Cancer UK organisation from 1997 and brought in important biotechnology developments to Dundee.

Sir Ian Wilmut (born 1944) studied at Nottingham, then trained in the techniques of cell preservation at Cambridge. In 1996, at the Roslin Institute near Edinburgh, working with Keith Campbell, they cloned a mammal from mature cells for the first time. Adult sheep nuclei were moved to de-nucleated ova, and one of the twenty-nine hybrid embryos thus created survived to be the cloned lamb Dolly. Adult cloning was not thought possible until this time and the discovery immediately opened up major possibilities.

Andrew Wylie and John F. R. Kerr joined Alistair Currie in studies in the University of Aberdeen which firmly established the concept of 'apoptosis' in 1972. The word was suggested to them by Aberdeen's professor of Greek, and apoptosis refers to the normal orderly self-destruction of body cells necessary to allow cellular change of quality in the body. Interest in apoptosis spread rapidly after the Aberdeen work.

MEDICINE/THERAPEUTICS

Sir James Black (1924–2010), assisted by a scholarship, studied medicine at St Andrews University. He started his research career as a physiologist in the Glasgow University Veterinary School, and moved to the pharmaceutical sector when he joined the ICI company in 1958. His approach was 'pharmaceutical engineering'. Instead of conventional random testing of compounds, he designed molecules whose structures were likely to be effective, notably in attaching to and blocking cell receptors. He first introduced the beta-blocker propranolol in 1964 to treat hypertension and heart disease, and it quickly became the world's bestselling drug. He succeeded again with a blocker of the stomach H_2 receptor, and via reduced acid secretion this healed ulcers without surgery. His Nobel Prize in 1988 was followed by an award of the Order of Merit in 2000.

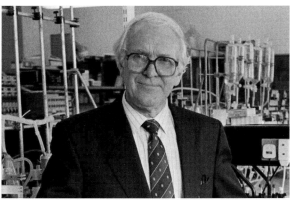

5.32 Sir James Black (*Getty*).

SURGICAL PRACTICE

Scottish brain surgery had developed in the 1930s under Norman Dott who established a department of neurosurgery in Edinburgh's Royal Infirmary in 1937. His contributions included the first identification of aneurysms in the brain arteries by X-rays, and he was first to treat this cause of sub-arachnoid haemorrhage by dealing directly with the tiny aneurysms. He reported his 39 patients treated in this way from 1926 onwards. He developed the specialty and he was made a Freeman of the City of Edinburgh in 1962.

In Glasgow, the large neurosurgical unit had a special interest in head injuries, not only in dealing with the purely surgical challenge, but also seeking to achieve accurate assessment of all cases and speedy, safe transfer after injury. From this developed the famous Glasgow Coma Scale of 1974, drawn up by Professor Brian Jennett and Sir Graham Teasdale. The GCS is in worldwide use in identifying the severity of injury, and has entered popular culture via the language of medical television dramas. Jennett (1926–2008) trained in Liverpool and was appointed to the new chair of neurosurgery at Glasgow University in 1968, where he quickly assembled a world-class multidisciplinary department. He had a leading role in obtaining public acceptance of brain death, and his textbooks had international influence.

Sir Alfred Cuschieri (born 1938) was educated in Malta and after a surgical post in Liverpool was appointed to the chair of surgery in Dundee in 1976. In the late 1980s, he pioneered the new techniques to permit

Medical Treatment

In the immediate pre-WW2 period, pharmaceutical agents in use were few, hardly more than digitalis, sulpha drugs, morphine and simple antacids. Holistic management of disease by diet and regimen was prominent. The situation was transformed by the arrival of a series of powerful new drugs, notably an increasing range of antibiotics, plus steroids, anticoagulants and the beta- and H2-blockers. Investigation of disease was enhanced by biochemical and haematological tests and radiology gave important new information. New technology allowed interventions to treat coronary artery disease and made haemodialysis possible in kidney failure.

Surgical Advances

In the 1950s, surgery advanced in scope and quality and the pattern of surgical practice constantly evolved. Chest surgery emerged to meet the needs of tuberculosis, but lung cancer provided a new challenge and heart surgery for congenital and acquired valvular disease quickly followed. Coronary artery surgery emerged and direct surgery on diseased peripheral blood vessels became common. There was a rapid growth in complex heart, brain and transplant surgery and this was assisted by major advances in anaesthesia, radiology and intensive care. New technology, notably fibre optics, gave endoscopic examination and guided instrument surgery followed.

The quality of surgery as a service within the NHS was increasingly looked at through audit of outcomes. Shorter waiting times and speedy management, particularly of cancer, were sought, and screening measures found a place first in cancer of the cervix, then in early detection of breast and colon cancer.

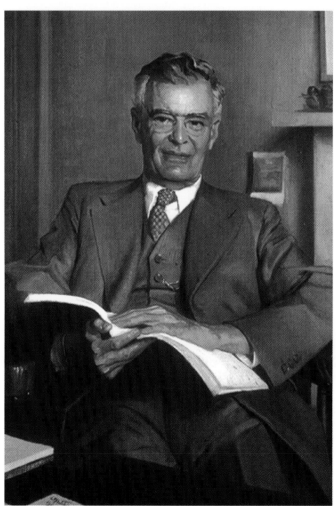

5.33 Professor Norman Dott (1897–1973) (*RCSEd*).

5.34 Part of the Glasgow Coma Scale.

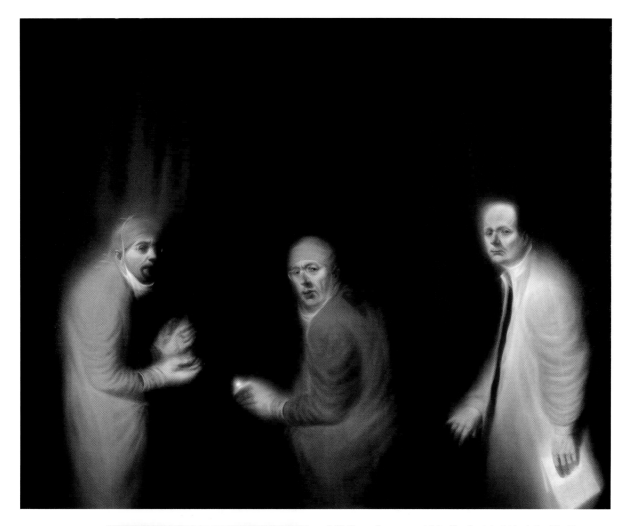

5.35 *Above*. Cancer specialists. Ken Currie's vivid painting *The Three Oncologists* shows the Dundee cancer experts Sir Alfred Cushieri, Sir David Lane and Bob Steele. It has appeared in lists of the world's 100 most important contemporary images (*National Galleries/Ken Currie*).

5.36 *Left*. Sir Michael Woodruff (*RCSEd*).

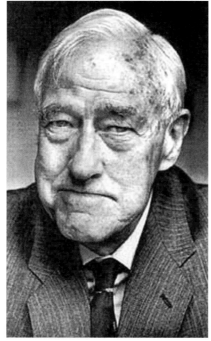

'keyhole' (minimally invasive) surgery, and in 1987 had been the first in the UK to use these methods in patients.

Sir Michael Woodruff (1911–2001) trained in surgery in Australia, moved to Aberdeen in 1948 and thereafter to the chair of surgical science in Edinburgh in 1957 as the only surgeon in Britain interested in experimental transplantation. In 1960 he carried out Britain's first kidney grafting between twins. Shortly after, he had one of the longest non-twin kidney graft survivors, and in 1964 introduced anti-lymphocyte serum to suppress the immune response. It found wider use as a biological agent, notably in the later monoclonal form. He also studied the immunological response to cancer, revealing important insights.

PSYCHIATRY

A pioneering move in Scotland came when Dr George Bell at the Dingleton Hospital in the Borders in 1949 decided to open up the wards in his institution, traditionally kept locked, as in all psychiatric institutions at the time, to prevent 'escapes'. Bell's open-door initiative, the first in Britain, was carefully planned in consultation with the apprehensive local community. This important and symbolic unlocking of the wards of the hospital which held 440 patients led to no significant incidents and can be seen as the first move in the later change to care in the community. With these changes, Dingleton was closed in 2001, and a 30-bed psychiatric in-patient unit sufficed instead.

In British psychiatry, Ronald D. Laing (1927–89) studied at Glasgow University and worked at the local Gartnavel Royal mental hospital as the youngest consultant psychiatrist in the UK. Moving to London's Tavistock Clinic in 1956, he joined the anti-psychiatry movement, denying the medical model of mental illness, and publishing *The Divided Self* (1960) which had international influence. He set up psychiatric therapeutic communities and offered 'rebirthing' workshops. He himself led a turbulent professional and private life. Although his ideas assisted the 'care in the community' movement, his opposition to drug treatment has not prevailed.

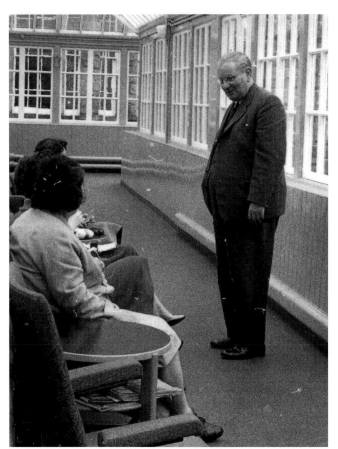

5.37 Psychiatric care. George Bell the psychiatrist was in charge of Dingleton Hospital near Melrose in the Borders from 1945 to 1962, and in 1949 was first to bring in an 'open door' policy in such institutions (*Keith Millar*).

Psychiatry

Post-World War Two psychiatry was still based on the large 'asylum' hospitals deliberately situated far from the main towns and cities. Compulsory admission, retention and loss of autonomy was still common and active treatment was rare, although electro-convulsive therapy (ECT) was used from 1939 in serious depression, as was insulin shock therapy. Brain-damaging lobotomy operations had a short vogue in the 1950s. These methods declined sharply after the arrival of chlorpromazine (Largactil) in 1951, which led to further success with other agents. National policy on the use of mental hospitals changed and large reductions in in-patient numbers followed. Those released were instead treated with care in the community assisted by the new community psychiatric nurses. A Scottish Health Advisory Service from 1970 inspected the facilities for mental illness or learning difficulties.

RADIOLOGY

Ian Donald (1910–87) was educated first in Edinburgh, then in South Africa, where he took his medical degree. He moved to London in 1937, and in 1954, attracted by the opportunities in Scotland, he was appointed to a chair of gynaecology and obstetrics in Glasgow. Transferring ultrasound techniques from local industrial use, in 1958 he published his famous paper 'On detection of abdominal masses by pulsed ultrasound' with J. MacVicar and T.G. Brown. Improved machines rapidly emerged, and the technique was of revolutionary importance in medicine. Donald was implacably opposed to the 1967 Abortion Act, and this taking a public stance on a contentious issue excluded him from major British public honours.

Radiology

In the post-war years, new radiological methods transformed medical diagnosis and treatment. Contrast media methods such as barium for visualising the stomach and intestines, and dyes to study the kidney improved, but it was ultrasound and CT scanning which gave new images and new insights in obstetrics, medicine and surgery. Scotland was a major innovator in ultrasound and MRI scanning.

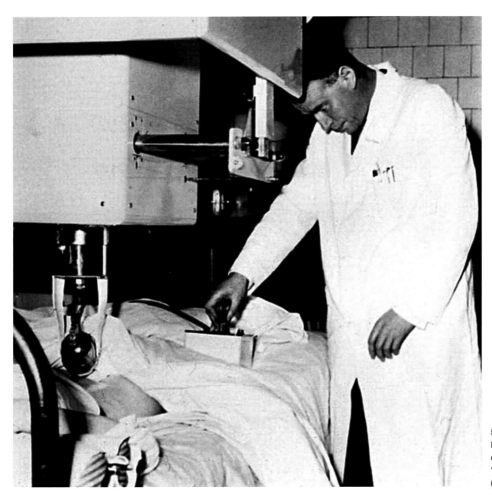

5.38 Ultrasound emerges. Ian Donald is shown with one of his cumbersome early 'sonar' scanners (*Craig Richardson*).

THE MID-1970S ONWARDS

After the 1960s, the mood changed and the year 1974 was a turning point. In that year's oil crisis, supplies to the West were cut off by OPEC, the Stock Market fell by 73% and a period of stagflation followed, with inflation running steadily in double figures. Some of the old certainties had gone and the pace of innovation slowed. For a public accustomed to new 'wonder drugs' regularly appearing, these launches became less frequent and those that did emerge were worryingly expensive and often had only marginal effects. Without new antibiotics, resistant organisms became common, and hospitals became increasingly seen as dangerous places. Demographic change meant, as the Cathcart Report had foretold, that 'diseases of later life would represent a larger proportion of the total sum'.

For the first time, there was acceptance that health spending had to be capped, and the NHS, accustomed to government steadily picking up the bills, was now constrained by cash limits. This now-familiar position was reached in 1976, but was unfamiliar then. Overall spending was later given a boost by Blair's 'expensive breakfast' in 2000, when he agreed that the NHS proportion of UK GNP would rise to European levels, though the Scottish level was already that. Charges crept in, notably in dentistry, and the NHS was no longer too proud to accept charitable gifts, notably of kidney dialysis machines and CT scanners.

The NHS had to look to costs and priorities, and it was concluded that tighter management and greater central control was needed. This appeared as a flurry of recommendations and reports, which soon tailgated each other, and it was noted wryly that 1975 was the only year free of a major review or implementation of the previous one. Acronyms for new administrative bodies came and went with regularity. A Royal Commission on the health services was set up but, reporting in 1979, made no major suggestions for change.

The patients, hitherto happy with their free NHS, were now restive and less tolerant than of old. Expectations regarding treatment had risen and patients sought improvements; private health care and alternative medicine also gained support. Planners realised that the patient had perhaps been forgotten in the continuous political and academic introspection on the NHS, and that the time had come for the service to be more consumer-orientated.

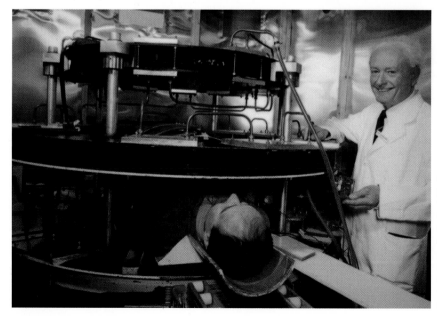

5.39 New scanners. John Mallard was professor of Medical Physics at Aberdeen from 1965 to 1992 and pioneered construction of the first isotope scanning device and a three-dimensional scanner. Shortly after he introduced some of the major techniques which allowed MRI (magnetic resonance imaging) scanning to develop, and Aberdeen had the world's first total body scanner in clinical use. (*Aberdeen University Archives*).

GP SERVICE

The importance of the NHS general practitioner in dealing with most of the NHS contacts between patient and doctor was increasingly supported for its many benefits. The role of the GP as controller of the first or only part of the patients' journey was realised, and that costs at this stage were crucial. Day-to-day changes in primary care appeared, notably new appointments systems, and support staff were greatly increased in the enlarging health centres. In the 1950s, up to one quarter of GP consultations had been home visits, but this old style of practice almost disappeared, and general practice night work was taken over by agencies, plus telephone advice systems such as NHS24. Health care in the Highlands and Islands had some attention and began to gain the support of telemedicine and routine helicopter emergency evacuation.

The Nation's Health
Scotland's population structure changed steadily and declined overall, and in 1997 deaths exceeded births for the first time. Though all measures of health were improving, and people were living longer, national comparisons were increasingly unfavourable, and in Europe, only the Portuguese had shorter life spans. There was a puzzling rise in disability and illness as judged by the steep rise in benefit payments for disability and ill-health: 'getting better but feeling worse' was the verdict. The 'new' diseases to hit Scotland hard were notably obesity, late-onset diabetes and alcohol and smoking-related disease, which gave the highest rate of lung cancer in the world. These problems seemed paradoxical in the presence of a strong NHS, but there was a new realisation that higher spending, after all, could buy better health in some instances of 'amenable mortality'. Those aged over 65 were growing in numbers, and the increasing size of the over-85 group had important consequences for health care, notably dementia.

Inequalities in health between social classes in Britain persisted in spite of the recognition of its extent after the challenging Black Report in 1980. The problem was vividly seen in Scotland, and even the beginnings of an

approach to equity proved elusive. By 2000 there was still a seven-year difference in life span between those in central Glasgow and those in the suburbs. Social deprivation also meant childhood poverty, low immunisation rates, low uptake of health services and a failure to heed health education.

To add to smoking-related disease, alcohol took an increasing toll, and other new challenges appeared, included drug addiction. Heroin use emerged as a problem in 1968 first in Glasgow, and injection-related HIV started in 1982. AIDS followed, and the culture surrounding drugs is described in Irving Welsh's novel *Trainspotting* (1993). A pioneering but controversial needle-exchange was brought in successfully in Edinburgh and helped contain the spread of disease.

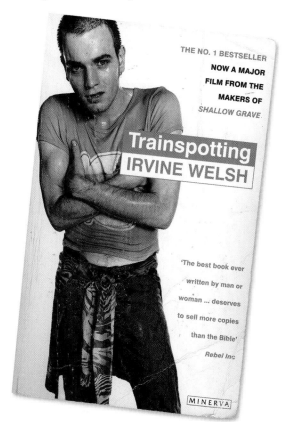

5.40 *Trainspotting* was Irvine Welsh's first novel and became a cult work, with a film version following in 1996. The language of the book offended many, including the Booker Prize judges (*Getty*).

THE SERVICE

The huge centrally-run health service was regularly criticised for alleged inefficiency and waste, in spite of the repeated confirmation that administrative costs were much lower than in other health care systems. With a Conservative government in power from 1979, Thatcherite free-market ideas for the NHS were aired. Though the Conservatives retained power until 1997, and moved to deregulate state industries, they hesitated to bring in major changes in health care, and although under increasing scrutiny, as a result of its popularity the NHS survived largely intact. The alleged benefits of competition were sought by complex internal markets from 1989, and hospitals in some Scottish areas were asked to compete against each other, without much enthusiasm. In rural Scotland where single hospitals covered large areas, the idea of internal competition was quite inappropriate. General practice fundholding was tried from 1991, but these schemes were modified or abolished later.

Complex hospital management changes, always seeking efficiency and economy, continued apace. Hospital Trusts were encouraged, but in Scotland there was opposition to the English foundation hospital schemes, which gave more financial freedom, but no more money, to individual hospitals. Compulsory tendering was introduced, and franchising of space in the hospital lobbies was encouraged for retail outlets and snack bars. Private Finance Initiatives proved attractive in getting hospitals and schools built quickly, and though this kept the capital cost off the national debt, large interest payments were needed from local NHS budgets, and the schemes were more expensive in the longer term than using public funds. In Scotland, the first hospitals built with these contracts were at Hairmyres and Law.

ADMINISTRATION

In 1962, Lord Craigton, the Conservative Minister of State for health, speaking to doctors in Glasgow, recalled that the limited remit of hospital management before the war was to provide

> an efficient, heated, clean, wholesome sickhouse, equipped with the necessary furniture and fittings for the reception of patients; and to provide the necessary medicine and food.

He hinted that changes were coming and that powerful lay managers would emerge, replacing the medical superintendent and the matron. By 1966, hospital managers with financial and administrative powers were reluctantly accepted by the doctors. By 1983 an NHS Chief Executive was in place in Edinburgh, and local health board general managers followed shortly afterwards.

Economic pressure meant faster through-put of hospital patients, and after surgery or childbirth, the norm was no longer a week in bed. In the past, patients were often admitted for leisurely investigation, which assisted student teaching, but instead preliminary out-patient investigation was now used. Bed numbers in Scotland contracted from about 60,000 in 1980 to 35,000 two decades later, and in-patient stay fell from 23 days to 5 days; the rise of hospital infection later also encouraged a speedy exit. Day surgery, pioneered by James Nicoll in Glasgow much earlier, now found managerial support, if not patient approval, and slowly the hospital was losing its ancient dominant role in health care. More hospital closures also proceeded apace, not only in rural areas, but also in the cities, and scattered casualty departments were replaced by central Accident and Emergency units. But communities could show support for their older or small hospital, and public protests often succeeded in the short term. The most notable incident was when the iconic Bruntsfield Hospital for Women in Edinburgh was threatened. Its tradition of women-only staff and notable lineage back to the pioneers of women's education and women's health in Edinburgh roused opposition from patients, and this managed to delay closure for some years.

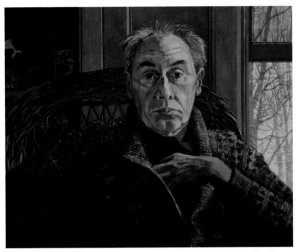

5.45 R. D. Laing (1927–1989) wrote pioneering and controversial books on psychiatry, including *The Divided Self: An Existential Study in Sanity and Madness* (1960) (*National Galleries of Scotland*).

Regulations
regarding the
Visiting of Patients.

1. Patients may be visited on Wednesdays and Saturdays and public holidays, from two till five o'clock, by not more than two friends at a time. In cases of serious illness special permission to visit may be given. On their first visit relatives should see one of the doctors to give information regarding the patient.

2. In conversing with patients visitors should be cheerful, and should not refer to anything that might cause the patient to be discontented.

3. Knives, scissors, needles, and all instruments with which personal injury could be done, are not to be given to patients, neither must letters from patients be taken by visitors to be posted.

4. Visitors are positively prohibited from bringing matches, wine, beer, or spirits into the Institution, or giving same to patients; but visitors may bring or send to their friends fruit, sweets, or cakes, and also newspapers and books. Such should, however, be given to the nurse or attendant, who will afterwards give them to the patient. Permission to give any other article than those mentioned must be obtained from the doctor.

5. Under no circumstances are visitors permitted to give money to patients, or gratuities to nurses or attendants.

6. The special consent of the Superintendent shall be required in the case of visits to patients by persons in connection with business transactions.

7. These regulations are framed in the best interests of the patients, whose welfare is the sole object of the Institution, and infringement of these rules will lead to permission to visit being afterwards refused.

5.42 Institutional attitudes. Glasgow's huge Lennox Castle housed those with 'mental sub-normality' and had these stern regulations for visitors still in force in the 1950s. By 1982 Lennox Castle was closed and all those in it had returned to community care (*GGHB Archives*).

Psychiatric care

The biggest change was for psychiatric patients when the new 'care in the community', also known less graciously as 'disincarceration', started in 1980. The new view was that many patients could leave the ancient asylums, and eventually half the 17,000 in-patients did move out of these large psychiatric institutions and many were shut. For those with learning difficulties (earlier called 'mental subnormality') the change was even more marked. Lennox Castle, Britain's largest institution of this kind, deliberately placed 10 miles from Glasgow, was also closed. At its peak 1,620 individuals with subnormality lived there, but by 2002 it was found possible to close it completely. With care in the community as a replacement, small care units took over, uncertainly at first.

Another deficiency in the large city hospitals was a reluctance to deal with the limitations of curative medicine in the care of advanced cancer patients. First to help with this role were the hospices, often run by religious organisations, like the Marie Curie Hospice in Glasgow,

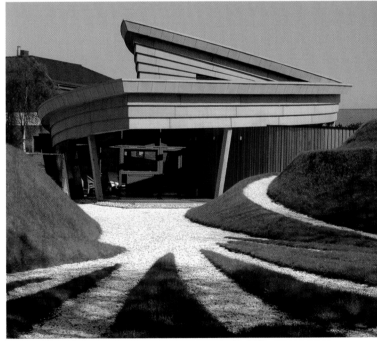

5.43 Holistic care. Maggie's Centre in Inverness shows the inspired architectural design typical of the Centres (*Maggie's Cancer Caring Centres*).

one of nine in the UK, and Edinburgh's St Columba's Hospice. These gave only in-patient care, and some time later, out-patient support from Maggie's Centres emerged, with the first of these appearing in Edinburgh. Maggie Jencks, who died in 1995, sought to establish a half-way house between the hospice and hospital, one in which a cheerful ambience, with an absence of uniforms, badges and reception desks, offered holistic care assisted by a new openness about a diagnosis of cancer. Starting with an inspired design for a new building close to the Western General Hospital in Edinburgh, the format was soon copied elsewhere in Scotland, then in England, and soon after in Barcelona and Hong Kong.

PATIENTS' ATTITUDES

By the 1970s, the patients were better informed and more assertive than before. More information came from the media, and television's *Your Life in their Hands* from 1958 dispelled some of health care's mystique and controversially screened a surgical operation for the first time. Massive briefing on health matters from the internet came in later. Increasingly well-informed 'customers' (or even 'clients' – words which replaced 'patient') wished better involvement. Hospital staff now asked in-patients if they would assist with students' teaching, and detailed requests and explanation of any proposed research studies were provided and detailed informed consent obtained. Other customers made their concerns known in other ways, ranging from political pressure, local grumbles to the new lay management or to the General Medical Council, or by major litigation. The NHS doctors were now glad to be covered by government indemnity, and thus spared costly insurance at a time when medico-legal actions were steadily increasing in all countries. Scotland had a curious role in this rise of litigation, since a Scottish case, *Donoghue v Stevenson* of 1928 – the 'snail in the soft drink' case – has international celebrity. It was a claim for damages from a contaminated bottle of ginger beer served in a Paisley café; the case reached the House of Lords, where it was upheld. This established the worldwide doctrine of a 'duty of care' on the part of manufacturers and providers, even when no contract existed.

Though the NHS was not short of worthy planning reports and analysis, it was now realised that the patient had perhaps been forgotten. Commentators in the 1970s noted that the patients until then had treated the revered NHS 'like a church', but now regarded it as more of 'a garage'. The patient's new view was that repairs should be prompt and skilled, with some checks on quality. But ironically, the perception of the human body in health and disease was now changing, and it was seen less like a machine with faults from time to time. The ill-*person* had returned in this new holistic view.

An attempt to have a patient's voice in the NHS had been made with the Community Health Councils, set up in 1974, but these lacked powers and contented themselves

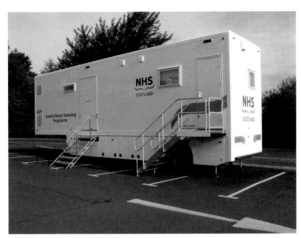

5.44 Screening. Scottish experience and advice led to the UK's breast cancer screening programme, the world's first, starting in 1988 (*NHS National Services Scotland*).

with local, peripheral issues. The Councils lasted only until 2003. More overt were the aspirations in the Patients' Charter of 1991, which perhaps only restated the obvious goals of any such health service as the NHS. Lay input rose in many health care activities, local and national, notably in the General Medical Council membership. Helpful support groups devoted to individual diseases steadily emerged.

The shortcoming most noticed by the customers were long waiting lists, and there was increasing success in driving them down. 'One-stop clinics', for example dealing with breast disease, gave prompt assessment, with consultation, radiology and biopsy if necessary, at one session. Screening for some diseases, notably by mammography for breast cancer, as advocated by Edinburgh's Sir Pat Forrest, met approval. He was invited by the Minister of Health in 1985 to convene an expert group, and following their advice, the NHS Breast Screening Programme was established, the world's first national scheme, and was operational from 1988. National bowel cancer screening was thereafter organised by Professor Bob Steele at Dundee.

By mid-century there was a steady rise in the private health care sector, though it remained smaller in size in Scotland than in England. The growth in the financial power of the private health insurance companies had meant that there was capital available for investment in private hospitals and their facilities. With the cost recouped by insurance premiums, new technology, notably expensive scanners, quickly paid for themselves. These facilities added to the traditional attractions of private care.

ALTERNATIVE MEDICINE

One paradox was that in spite of the earlier rapid progress in scientific medicine, from the 1970s there was a steadily rising recourse to alternative medicine. This counter-culture was perhaps a response to the slowing of general medical advance, or as the result of the failure of conventional medicine to deal satisfactorily with the commoner aches and pains or the new wave of degenerative disease. Added to this, scientific medicine's reductionism, technical expertise and the niceties of controlled trials had perhaps discouraged the art of healing.

One interesting Scottish survivor was the Napiers group of herbalist shops which had almost disappeared in the 'scientific sixties', but now made a strong recovery. They were also an interesting reminder of the ancient debt of conventional medicine to plant lore. To keep a place in the medical market place, Napiers had reluctantly to reconsider their traditional methods of extraction to meet the precision demanded of the orthodox pharmaceutical sector. Acupuncture and other treatments, notably chiropraxy, flourished, and High Street shops offering these services appeared, often adding extra 'natural' therapies. Disliking the 'alternative' label, this sector gained more status when adopting the 'Complementary' title and the group were increasingly known as CAM – Complementary and Alternative Medicine. Sceptical but tolerant general practitioners might recommend these alternative therapies, well aware that powerful placebos had their place in the therapeutic skills. Health foods sold well, and the advice of the new nutritionists, particularly those with a high profile in the media, was listened to.

Homeopathy had been a puzzling but inconspicuous addition to the NHS from the start and the NHS service included a Homeopathic Hospital in Glasgow. But homeopathy alone failed to attract the tolerance shown to other CAM offerings and was increasingly marginalised.

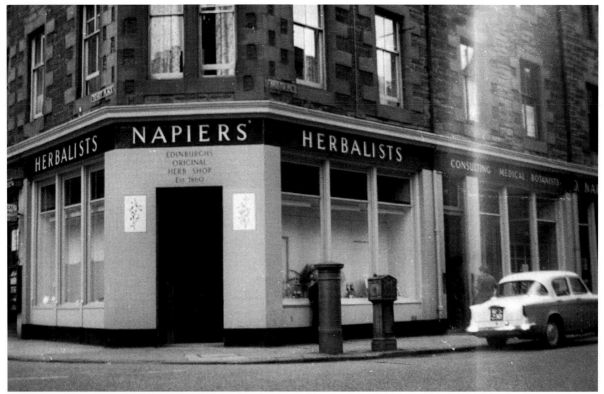

5.45 Complementary medicine. Napiers herbalist shops survived in Edinburgh from 1860 and revived strongly with the increasing use of alternative medicine (*Napiers*).

THERAPY

In the past, new therapy usually became established when it reached self-evident efficacy. However, many of the new agents appearing later in the century seemed of modest or disputed benefit, and also were costly. Helping assessment, the Cochrane Library's database of 'good science' studies was available, named after the Scot, Archie Cochrane, whose early advocacy of controlled trials and evidence-based medicine was widely accepted. In England, the National Institute for Clinical Excellence (NICE) emerged to approve new drugs for NHS use and they also had to consider value for money. But the Scottish equivalent, SIGN, run by the Scottish Colleges, dealt with effectiveness only, leaving it to another body to judge value for money.

The refusal to provide marginally effective but costly drugs met opposition, and led to public pleading for named individual lives, particularly of cancer patients. To defend withholding drugs on statistical grounds seemed heartless, as the media were not slow to point out, and debate continued case by case.

QUALITY OF CARE

The Lothian Surgical Audit started in 1946, and it anticipated by decades the routine audits of later. It confidentially reviewed any death after surgery in the region. Though reporting by individual surgeons was voluntary, it was well-supported, and as it evolved, it was increasingly seen as a model of its kind. Other similar surveys followed slowly and, eventually finding general favour, audit was formally built into the NHS by the white paper *Working for Patients* of 1989. The early acceptance of the Lothian scheme, and the resulting concern of the profession for quality, is thought in Scotland to have prevented the situation which occurred at Bristol Royal Infirmary, where a major investigation confirmed that unacceptable cardiac surgery death rates there had continued unchecked and unnoticed.

SCOTTISH DEVOLUTION

From the 1970s onwards, there had been pressure to strengthen political powers within Scotland, without clear public support for independence, and after prolonged political debate, one false start and an inconclusive referendum in 1979, in May 1999 a Scottish Parliament was set up. The health service got its new name – NHS Scotland – in 2000, having been renamed as the Scottish Health Service in a Conservative government report on the eve of its national defeat in 1997. The ruling party in the parliament was called the Scottish Executive, though this was changed to 'Scottish Government' promptly after the Scottish Nationalist Party became the ruling minority in 2007.

Some Westminster powers were devolved to Edinburgh, notably control of the NHS, and some were retained, including regulation of the medical profession and legislation on abortion. The powers gained in Scotland were less than a full federal arrangement, since tax-raising, though possible, was initially left to Westminster, and the new Parliament's funds were given in one block grant from the Treasury, within which priorities could be adjusted. A fine new Parliament building was slowly erected in Edinburgh.

The transfer to Scotland of political power over health matters was assisted by the existence of other already devolved institutions. The Scottish legal system had always been independent, and hence was ready to take on the expansion of legislation on health. The doctors' Scottish Colleges had been sturdily 'devolved' from their inception centuries ago, and remained proudly independent. There was already administrative devolution, with increasing numbers of civil servants at St Andrews House in Edinburgh from 1939. Indeed, all that was required for devolution was the political layer.

The changes in Scottish Health Service politics were immediate. Full debates and regular questions to the First Minister on health matters were routine, and the Scottish Parliament had 50 such debates in its first 18 months, as against four in the last two pre-devolution years at Westminster. After devolution, Scottish health matters had a higher and more informed profile in the media. On routine issues, Scottish civil servants could deal with matters quickly, having their own minister at hand, rather than having to go through London for approval of any Scottish action.

Until devolution, all Scottish legislation on health had been versions of the Westminster equivalent. But now the way was open for separate thinking and action – 'local solutions to local problems' had been the devolutionist's mantra. As each part of Britain went its own way, commentators looked with interest for any differences, and characterised England's NHS as 'market managerial' and Wales' as 'localist'. Scotland was concluded to have 'co-operative medical professionalism', a compliment to the Scottish staff who had from, the first, been supportive of the NHS.

The first health care legislation after devolution was a low key event. A legal nicety was uncovered about the status of high-risk, incarcerated mentally-ill criminals, which meant they might be freed. Speedy action via the Mental Health (Public Safety and Appeals) (Scotland) Act 1999 closed the exit. The next, and less rushed, legislation was the much-needed Adults with Incapacity (Scotland) Act 2000. Bigger cross-border differences soon emerged. With a turn of speed, Scotland successfully introduced a smoking ban in public places on 11 March 2006, while England hesitated, and it had remarkable and immediate support in Scotland. More controversial was the Scottish parliament's response to the issue of free personal care for the elderly. The Aberdeen-born former Stirling academic Lord Sutherland, Principal and Vice-Chancellor of Edinburgh University from 1994–2002, chaired the Royal Commission on Long-term Care of the Elderly, reporting in 1999. Now known as the Sutherland Report, it proposed that all domiciliary care for the elderly should be free. This was rejected as unrealistic by the Westminster government on grounds of cost, but the report was accepted in Scotland, and costly free personal care, provided by local authorities, not without concern, started in 2002.

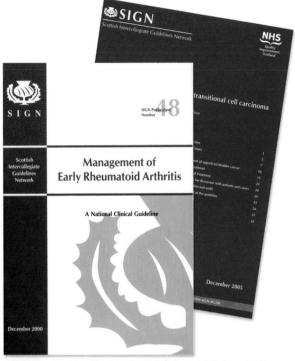

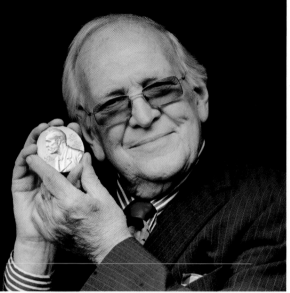

5.46 National policies. The three Scottish Colleges jointly issued guidelines which gave guidance on best practice, starting in 1995 and usually dealt with contentious or developing therapies (*SIGN*).

5.47 Nobel prize medal. Sir James Black was awarded the Prize in 1988 for Physiology of Medicine (*National Museum of Scotland*).

Funding

In 1979 in the run-up to expected devolution of political power to Scotland, Joel Barnett, a civil servant at the Treasury, proposed a formula to prevent cross-border post-devolution argument about allocation of funding to Scotland and Wales. Previous spending was based on the older Goschen Formula which gave 11% to Scotland, based on the earlier larger population. Barnett proposed that this level of existing expenditure would remain, but any *new* money would be allocated on the up-to-date population proportion, which had reduced to about 10% of the UK total. This formula was designed to lead to convergence of expenditure over decades. However, the higher spending in Scotland continued in the short term, and continued to be watched closely from outside.

Envoi

The Scots are living longer and patterns of disease constantly change. Skilled health care is freely available, and new forms of therapy, some of them costly, steadily arrive to challenge all involved. As part of global development, Scottish health care draws on international experience, but has regularly given back insights to assist the rest of the world. It is a profound and ancient tradition.

THEMATIC BIBLIOGRAPHY
AND FURTHER READING

———

This list contains both the items used in the preparation of the various chapters in the book, and also suggestions for further reading for each thematic section. The latter have been added to enable more detailed study of specific topics or themes which may not be covered in depth in the book. It is not an exhaustive list, but bibliographies within these listed items will also point to further relevant reading. The sections are divided and subdivided thematically to assist with finding relevant works. Some key works are listed in several sections.

1. General Works – Historical and Social Background

1.1 General Histories

Brown, D., Finlay, R. and Lynch, M. (eds), *Image and Identity. The Making and Remaking of Scotland Through the Ages* (Edinburgh, John Donald, 1998)

Devine, T. M., *The Scottish Nation* (London, Penguin Press, 1999)

Flinn, M. W., *Scottish Population History from the 17th Century to the 1930s* (Cambridge, Cambridge University Press, 1977)

Houston, R. A. and Knox, W., *The New Penguin History of Scotland* (London, Penguin Press, 2001)

Lynch, M., *Scotland, A New History* (London, Croom Helm, 1991)

Lindesay, R., *The History of Scotland* (Edinburgh, Baskett & Co., 1928)

McKeown, T., *The Modern Rise of Population* (London, Edward Arnold, 1976)

Tabraham, C. and Baxter, C., *The Illustrated History of Scotland* (Broxburn, Lomond Books, 2003)

Webster, A., Kyd, J. K. et al, *Scottish Population Statistics: Including Webster's Analysis of Population, 1755* (Edinburgh, Scottish Academic Press for The Scottish History Society, 1975)

1.2 Early Peoples

Armit, A., *Celtic Scotland* (London, Batsford, 2005)

Ashmore, P. J., *Neolithic and Bronze Age Scotland* (London, Batsford, 2000)

Benton, S., 'Excavation of the Sculptor's Cave, Covesea', *Proceedings of the Society of Antiquaries of Scotland*, 12 January (1931), pp.177–216

Bryce, T., 'On the Cairns and Tumuli of the Island of Bute. A Record of Explorations during the Season of 1903', *Proceedings of the Society of Antiquaries of Scotland* 38, 14 December 1931, pp.17–81.

Hardy, K. & Wickham-Jones, C.R., 'Scotland's First Settlers: the Mesolithic Seascape of the Inner Sound, Skye and its contribution to the early prehistory of Scotland', *Antiquity* 2002, pp.825–33.

MacLennan, W.J., 'Stature in Scotland over the Centuries'. *Journal of the Royal College of Physicians of Edinburgh*, 33 (2003), pp.46–53.

Mithen, S., et al., 'Plant Use in the Mesolithic: Evidence from Staosnaig, Isle of Colonsay, Scotland,' *Journal of Archaeological Science*, 28 (3) (2001), pp.223–234.

Ritchie, G. J. N. and Ritchie, A., *Scotland. Archaeology and Early History* (Edinburgh, Edinburgh University Press, 1991)

1.3 Romans

Breeze, D., *Roman Scotland: Frontier Country* (London, Batsford, 2006)

Herodian, *History of the Roman Empire since the Death of Marcus Aurelius.* Book III. Section 14 (235AD)

Keppie, L., *The Legacy of Rome – Scotland's Roman Remains* (Edinburgh, John Donald, 2004)

Maxwell, G. S., *The Romans in Scotland* (Edinburgh, Mercat Press,1989)

1.4 Dark Ages and Medieval

Bannerman, J., *Studies in the History of Dalriada* (Edinburgh, Scottish Academic Press, 1974)

Barrell, A. D. M., *Medieval Scotland* (Cambridge, Cambridge University Press, 2000)

Bede, *The Life of St Cuthbert* (723)

Brotherstone, T. and Ditchburn, D. (eds.), *Freedom and Authority. Historical and Historiographical Essays Presented to Grant G. Simpson* (East Linton, Tuckwell Press, 2000)

Brown, M., *The Wars of Scotland, 1214–1371* (Edinburgh, Edinburgh University Press, 2004)

Cowan, E. G. and Macdonald, R. A. (eds) *Alba. Celtic Scotland in the Medieval Era* (East Linton, Tuckwell Press, 2000)

Ditchburn, D., *Scotland and Europe. The Medieval Kingdom and its Contacts with Christendom* (East Linton, Tuckwell Press, 2001)

Fraser, J. E., *From Caledonia to Pictland. Scotland to 795* (Edinburgh, Edinburgh University Press, 2009)

Woolf, A., *From Pictland to Alba 789–1070* (Edinburgh, Edinburgh University Press, 2007)

1.5 Early Modern

Devine, T. M. and Jackson, G. (eds), *Glasgow. Vol 1. Beginnings to 1830* (Manchester, Manchester University Press, 1995)

Bannerman, John, *The Beatons. A Medical Kindred in the Classic Gaelic Tradition* (Edinburgh, John Donald, 1986)

Dawson, J., *Scotland Reformed, 1488–1587* (Edinburgh, Edinburgh University Press, 2007)

Ewen, E., and Meikle, M. (eds) *Women in Scotland c1100–c1750* (East Linton, Tuckwell, Press, 1999)

Lynch, M. and Dingwall, H. M., 'Elite society in town and country', in Dennison, E. P., Ditchburn, D. and Lynch, M. (eds), *Aberdeen before 1800. A New History* (East Linton, 2002)

Mitchison, R., *Lordship to Patronage. Scotland 1603–1745* (Edinburgh, Edinburgh University Press, 1990)

Rorie, D., *The Book of Aberdeen* (Aberdeen, Executive Committee of the Aberdeen Division of the British Medical Association, 1939)

Short, A. I., Lennard, T. W. J. et al, *James IV of Scotland: Sovereign and Surgeon,* Durham Thomas Harriot Seminar Occasional Paper 7 (London, Historical Association, 1992)

1.6 Enlightenment

Broadie, A., *The Cambridge Companion to the Scottish Enlightenment* (Cambridge, Cambridge University Press, 2003)

Carter, J. and Pittock-Wesson, J. (eds), *Aberdeen and the Enlightenment* (Aberdeen, Aberdeen University Press, 1987)

Daiches, D., Jones, P., et al., (eds), *The Scottish Enlightenment 1730–1790; A Hotbed of Genius* (Edinburgh, Edinburgh University Press, 1986)

Dickson, A. and Treble, J. H. (eds), *People and Society in Scotland Vol. 3 1914–1990* (Edinburgh, John Donald, 1992)

Fraser, W. H., and Morris, R. J. (eds), *People and Society in Scotland Vol.2 1830–1914* (Edinburgh, John Donald, 1990)

Hook, A. and Sher, R. (eds), *The Glasgow Enlightenment* (East Linton, Tuckwell Press, 1995)

1.7 Modern

Breitenbach, E. and Gordon, E. (eds), *Out of Bounds: Women in Scottish Society 1800–1945* (Edinburgh, Edinburgh University Press, 1992)

Devine, T. M. and Orr, W. *The Great Highland Famine: Hunger, Emigration and the Scottish Highlands in the Nineteenth Century* (Edinburgh, John Donald, 1988)

Devine, T. M. and Finlay, R. J. (eds), *Scotland in the Twentieth Century* (Edinburgh, Edinburgh University Press,1996)

Fry, M.W., *Patronage and Principle: A Political History of Modern Scotland* (Aberdeen, Aberdeen University Press, 1987)

Fry, M., *The Dundas Despotism* (Edinburgh, John Donald, 2004)

Cameron, E. A., *Impaled upon a Thistle. Scotland since 1800* (Edinburgh, Edinburgh University Press, 2010)

Checkland, S. and Checkland, O., *Industry and Ethos. Scotland 1832–1914* (Edinburgh, Edinburgh University Press, 1984)

Gordon, J. (ed.), *The New Statistical Account of Scotland by the Ministers of the Respective Parishes, under the Superintendence of a Committee of the Society for the Benefit of the Sons and Daughters of the Clergy* (Edinburgh & London, W. Blackwood & Sons, 1845)

Harvie, C., *No Gods and Precious Few Heroes. Scotland 1914–1980* (Edinburgh, Edinburgh University Press, 1981)

Hilton, B., *A Bad and Dangerous People? England 1783–1846* (Oxford, Clarendon Press, 2006)

Hoppen, K. T., *The Mid-Victorian Generation. England 1783–1846* (Oxford, Oxford University Press, 1998)

Porter, R., *Enlightenment. Britain and the Creation of the Modern World* (London, Penguin Press, 2000)

Searle, G. R., *Morality and the Market in Victorian Britain* (Oxford, Clarendon Press, 1998)

Searle, G. R., *A New England? Peace and War. England 1886–1918* (Oxford, Clarendon Press, 2004)

Sinclair, J. (ed.), *The Statistical Account of Scotland, 1791–1799* (Wakefield, EP Publishing, 1982)

Szatkowski, S. (ed.), *Capital Caricatures. A Selection of Etchings by John Kay* (Edinburgh, Birlinn, 2007)

Woodham-Smith, C., *The Great Hunger* (London, Hamish Hamilton, 1962)

2. General Works on the History of Medicine

Boyd, D. H. A., *Amulets to Isotopes. A History of Medicine in Caithness* (John Donald, Edinburgh, 1998)

Brunton, D., *Medicine Transformed: Health, Disease and Society in Europe, 1800–1930* (Manchester, Manchester University Press in association with the Open University, 2004)

Burnett, J., *The Scots in Sickness and Health* (National Museums of Scotland, 1997)

Comrie, J. D., *History of Scottish Medicine, Two Vols* (London, Baillière, Tyndall and Cox, 1932)

Conrad, L. L. et al, *The Western Medical Tradition 800BC–1800AD* (Cambridge, Cambridge University Press, 1995)

Dingwall, H. M., *A History of Scottish Medicine. Themes and Influences* (Edinburgh, Edinburgh University Press, 2003)

Guthrie, D. *A History of Medicine.* (London, Thomas Nelson and Sons, 1945)

Hamilton, D., *The Healers. A History of Medicine in Scotland* (Edinburgh, Canongate, 2003)

Porter, R. (ed.), *The Cambridge Illustrated History of Medicine* (Cambridge, Cambridge University Press, 2001)

Porter, R., *The Greatest Benefit to Mankind. A Medical History of Humanity from Antiquity to the Present* (London, Harper Collins, 1997)

Lane, J., *A Social History of Medicine* (London, Routledge, 2001)

Lawrence, C., *Medicine in the Making of Modern Britain, 1700–1920* (London, Routledge, 1994)

Lloyd, O. L., Williams, R. R., Berry, W. G. and Florey, C. V. (eds), *An Atlas of Mortality in Scotland* (London, Croom Helm, 1987)

Loudon, I., *Western Medicine. An Illustrated History* (Oxford, Oxford University Press, 1997)

3. Medicine and Medical Practice in Scotland
(General Works – see also Medical Education, Medical Theories, Lay Medical Practice, Hospitals, Institutions, Plants and Medicine)

3.1 Greek and Roman medicine

Celsus, A. C., *De Medicina.* Vol. VII (25BC)

Comrie, J. D., *History of Scottish Medicine.* Two Vols (London, Baillière, Tyndall and Cox, 1932)

Pliny, *Natural History*, Book XXX, Section 13 (77–79 AD)

Sprengell, C. (ed.), *The Aphorisms of Hippocrates and the Sentences of Celsus, with Explanations and References to the Most Considerable Writers in Physick and Philosophy* (London, printed for R. Bonwick, 1708)

3.2 Epidemics, Plague, Leprosy, Syphilis

Creighton, C., *A History of Epidemics in Britain*, Vol. 1 (Cambridge, The University Press, 1894)

Hudson, E., 'Diagnosing a case of venereal disease in fifteenth century Scotland', *British Journal of Venereal Diseases*, 48 (1972), pp.146-153.

Jillings, K., *Scotland's Black Death* (Stroud, Tempus, 2003)

Kaufman, M. H. and MacLennan, W. J., 'Robert the Bruce and leprosy'. *Proceedings of the Royal College of Physicians of Edinburgh*, 30 (1) (2000), pp.75–80.

Marwick, J. D. et al (eds), *Extracts from the Records of the Burgh of Edinburgh 1528–1557* (Edinburgh, Scottish Records Society, 1869–82)

Mullett, C. F., 'Plague Policy in Scotland in the 16th and 17th Centuries', *Osiris* 9 (1950) pp.435–456

Rawcliffe, C., *Leprosy in Medieval England* (Boydell Press, Woodbridge, 2006)

Simpson, J. Y. (ed. Stuart, J., *On Leprosy and Leper Hospitals in Scotland and England, Archaeological Essays Volume II* (Edinburgh, Edmonston & Douglas, 1882)

Singer, D., 'Some Plague Tractates: Fourteenth and Fifteenth Century', *Proceedings of the Royal Society of Medicine* 9 (1916), pp.159–212

Taylor, M. et al, 'A Mediaeval Case of Lepromatous Leprosy from 13–14th Century Orkney, Scotland', *Journal of Archaeological Science* 27 (2000), pp.1133–1138

3.3 Medicine to c1500

Bannerman, John, *The Beatons. A Medical Kindred in the Classic Gaelic Tradition* (Edinburgh, John Donald, 1986)

Comrie, J. D., *History of Scottish Medicine, Two Vols* (London, Baillière, Tyndall and Cox, 1932)

Cockayne, T., *Saxon Leechdoms, Vol II, The Leech Book of Bald Book 1* (London, Longman, Green, Longman, Roberts and Green, 1865)

Grattan, J. H. G. and Singer, C., *Anglo-Saxon Magic and Medicine* (London, Oxford University Press, 1952)

Dingwall, H. M., *A History of Scottish Medicine. Themes and Influences* (Edinburgh, Edinburgh University Press, 2003)

Holmes, N. M. McQ., *Trinity College Church, Hospital and Apse* (Edinburgh, City of Edinburgh Museums and Art Galleries, 1988)

Kerr, N. W., 'The Prevalence and Pattern of Distribution of Root Caries in a Scottish Medieval Population'. *Journal of Dental Research,* 69 (1990), 857–60

Moffatt, B., *Reports into Researches at the Medieval Hospital at Soutra* (Soutra Hospital Archaeoethnopharmacological Research Project, 1988–1992)

MacLennan, W. J., 'Medieval Hospitals in Scotland: a cure for body or soul', *Journal of the Royal College of Physicians of Edinburgh* 22 (Suppl. 12) (2003), pp.36–41

Yeoman, P., *Pilgrimage in Medieval Scotland* (Edinburgh, Historic Scotland, 1999)

3.4 Medicine c1500–c1750

Bannerman, John, *The Beatons. A Medical Kindred in the Classic Gaelic Tradition* (Edinburgh, John Donald, 1986)

Comrie, J. D., *History of Scottish Medicine, Two Vols* (London, Baillière, Tyndall and Cox, 1932)

Dingwall, H. M., *Physicians, Surgeons and Apothecaries. Medical Practice in Seventeenth Century Edinburgh* (East Linton, Tuckwell Press, 1995)

Dingwall, H. M., '"To be insert in the *Mercury*": Medical practitioners and the press in eighteenth-century Edinburgh', *Social History of Medicine* 12 (1) (2000), pp.23–44

Dingwall, H. M., 'Illness, disease and pain', in Foyster, E. A. and Whatley, C. (eds), *A History of Everyday Life from 1600–1800 in Scotland* (Edinburgh, Edinburgh University Press, 2010), pp.108–36

Mackinnon, D., *A Descriptive Catalogue of Gaelic Manuscripts in the Advocates' Library, Edinburgh and Elsewhere in Scotland* (Edinburgh, W. Brown, 1912)

3.5 Medicine and Enlightenment c1750–1850

Berkeley, E. and Berkeley, D. S., *Dr Alexander Garden of Charles Town* (Chapel Hill, University of North Carolina Press, 1969)

Brock, W. R., *Scotus Americanus. A Survey of the Sources for Links Between Scotland and America in the Eighteenth Century* (Edinburgh, Edinburgh University Press, 1982)

Brunton, D. 'Smallpox inoculation and demographic trends in eighteenth-century Scotland.' *Medical History* 36 (4) (1992), pp.403–29

Buchan, W., *Domestic Medicine; or, the Family Physician: . . . Chiefly Calculated to Recommend a Proper Attention to Regimen and Simple Medicines* (Edinburgh, Balfour, Auld and Smellie, 1769)

Buchan, W., *Domestic Medicine; a Treatise on the Prevention and Cure of Diseases, by Regimen and Simple Medicines, with the Latest Corrections and Improvements* (Manchester, S. Johnson & Son, 1876)

Bynum, W. F. and Porter, R., *Medical Fringe and Medical Orthodoxy 1750–1850* (London, Croom Helm, 1987)

Bynum, W. F., *Science and the Practice of Medicine in the Nineteenth Century* (Cambridge, Cambridge University Press, 1994)

Bynum, W. F. and Porter, R., *William Hunter and the Eighteenth-Century Medical World* (Cambridge, Cambridge University Press, 1985)

French R. K., *Robert Whytt. The Soul and Medicine* (London, Wellcome Institute, 1969)

Jacyna, L. S., *Philosophic Whigs. Medicine, Science and Citizenship in Edinburgh 1789–1848* (London, 1994)

Lawrence, C., *Medicine as Culture: Edinburgh and the Scottish Enlightenment* (London, University College. Ph.D. thesis, 1984)

Lobban, R. D., *Edinburgh and the Medical Revolution* (Cambridge, Cambridge University Press, 1980)

Moore, J. C., *The History of the Small-pox* (London, Longman, 1815)

Mortimer, B. E., 'The Nurse in Edinburgh c.1760-1860: the Impact of Commerce and Professionalisation' (Edinburgh, University of Edinburgh Ph.D. thesis, 2002)

Rae, I., *The Strange Story of Dr James Barry* (London, Longmans, Green and Co., 1958)

Risse, G. B., *New Medical Challenges During the Scottish Enlightenment* (Amsterdam, Rodopi, 2005)

Withers, C. W. J. and Wood, P. B. (eds), *Science and Medicine in the Scottish Enlightenment* (East Linton, Tuckwell Press, 2002)

3.6 Medicine c1850–1950

Crockett R., *Leaves from the Life of a Country Doctor (Clement Bryce Gunn M.D., J.P.)* (Edinburgh, Ettrick Press, 1935)

Digby, A., *The Evolution of British General Practice* (Oxford, Oxford University Press, 1999)

Hooper, M. and Gormley, G., *Bodies for Sale* (New York, London, Franklin Watts, 1999)

Loudon, I., *Medical Care and the General Practitioner, 1750–1850* (Oxford, Oxford University Press, 1986)

Patrizio, A. and Kemp, D., *Anatomy Acts: How We Come to Know Ourselves* (Edinburgh, Birlinn, 2006)

Tuchman, A. M., *Science, Medicine and the State in Germany 1815–1871* (Oxford, Oxford University Press, 1993)

3.7 Medicine 1950–2010

Berridge, V., *Health and Society in Britain since 1939* (Cambridge, Cambridge University Press, 1999)

Bliss, M., *The Discovery of Insulin* (Chicago, Chicago University Press, 2007)

Calder, J. F., *History of Radiology in Scotland 1896–2000* (Edinburgh, Dunedin Academic Press, 2001)

Loudon, I., Horder, J. and Webster, C. (eds), *General Practice under the National Health Service 1948–1997* (London, Clarendon Press, 1999)

Taylor, H. P., *A Shetland Parish Doctor* (Lerwick, Manson, 1948)

4. Lay Medicine and Healing

Beith, M., *Healing Threads. Traditional Medicines of the Highlands and Islands* (Edinburgh, Polygon, 1995)

Black, F., 'Scottish charms and amulets' *Proceedings of the Royal Society of Antiquaries of Scotland*, Series 3 No. 3 (1893) pp.433–526

Bradley, J., Dupree, M. and Durie, A., 'Taking the Water Cure. The Hydropathic Movement in Scotland 1840–1940', *Business and Economic History* 26 (2) (1997), pp.426–37.

Buchan. D. (ed.), *Folk Tradition and Folk Medicine in Scotland. The Writings of David Rorie* (Edinburgh, Canongate Academic, 1994)

Carmichael, A. (ed) *Carmina Gadelica. Hymns and Incantations Collected in the Highlands and Islands of Scotland in the Last Century* (Edinburgh, Floris Books, 2006)

Davidson, T., *Rowan Tree and Red Thread: A Scottish Witchcraft Miscellany of Tales, Legends and Ballads* (Edinburgh, Oliver & Boyd, 1947)

Gillies, H. C. (ed.), *Regimen Sanitatis. The Rule of Health. A Gaelic Medical Manuscript of the Early Sixteenth Century or Perhaps Older: from the Vade Mecum of the Famous Macbeaths, Physicians to the Lords of the Isles and the Kings of Scotland for Several Centuries.* (Glasgow, Maclehose, 1911)

Kirkpatrick, E. M., *The Little Book of Scottish Grannies' Remedies* (London, Michael O'Mara, 2001)

Henderson, L., 'Charmers, spells and Holy Wells. The repackaging of belief', *Review of Scottish Culture* 19 (2007), pp.10–26

Martin, M., *A Description of the Western Islands of Scotland circa 1695* (Edinburgh, Birlinn, 1999)

Miller, J., 'Devices and directions. Folk healing aspects of witchcraft practice in seventeenth-century Scotland', in Goodare, J. (ed.), *The Scottish Witch-Hunt in Context* (Manchester, Manchester University Press, 2002), pp.234–51

Morris, R. and Morris, F., *Scottish Healing Wells: Healing, Holy, Wishing and Fairy Wells of the Mainland of Scotland* (Sandy, Alethea Press, 1982)

Thin, R., 'Medical quacks in Edinburgh in the Seventeenth and Eighteenth centuries', *Book of the Old Edinburgh Club*, 22 (1939), pp.132–60

Sharma, U., *Complementary Medicine Today. Practitioners and Patients* (London, Tavistock/Routledge, 1991)

5. Plants and Medicine

Allen, D. E., and Hatfield, G., *Medicinal Plants in Folk Tradition. An Ethnobotany of Britain and Ireland* (Cambridge, Timber Press, 2004)

Atkinson, T., *Napier's History of Herbal Healing, Ancient and Modern* (Edinburgh, Luath Press, 2003)

Darwin, T., *The Scots Herbal. The Plant Lore of Scotland* (Edinburgh, Mercat Press, 1997)

Dickson, C. and Dickson, J., *Plants and People in Ancient Scotland* (Stroud, Tempus, 2000)

Fleming, L. W., 'A medical bouquet. Poppies, cinchona and willow', *Scottish Medical Journal* 44, (6) (1999), pp.176–179.

Hatfield, G., *Memory, Wisdom and Healing. The History of Domestic Plant Medicine* (Stroud, Sutton, 2005)

Milliken, W. and Bridgewater, S., *Flora Celtica. Plants and People in Scotland* (Edinburgh, Birlinn, 2004)

Porter, R. and Teich, M. (eds), *Drugs and Narcotics in History* (Cambridge, Cambridge University Press, 1995)

Walker, A., *A Garden of Herbs. Traditional Uses of Herbs in Scotland* (Glendaruel, Argyll Publishing, 2004)

6. Medical Theories

Brown, J., *The Elements of Medicine; Or, A Translation of the Elementa Medicinæ Brunonis. With Large Notes,*

Illustrations, and Comments. By the Author of the Original Work. (London, J. Johnson, 1788)

Bynum, W. F., Porter, R. et al., *Brunonianism in Britain and Europe* (London, Wellcome Institute for the History of Medicine, 1988)

Cullen, W., *Synopsis Nosologiae Methodicae: In Usum Studiosorum. Editio Altera. In Quarta Parte Emendata; et Adjectis Morborum Speciebus Aucta* (Edinburgh, A. Kincaid & W. Creech, 1772)

Currie, J., *Medical Reports on the Effects of Water, Cold and Warm, as a Remedy in Fever and Other Diseases* (London, printed for T. Cadell and W. Davies; and W. Creech, Edinburgh, 1805)

Gordon, A., *Treatise on the Epidemic of Puerperal Fever of Aberdeen* (London, printed for G. G. and J. Robinson, 1795)

Gregory, J., *Lectures on the Duties and Qualifications of a Physician* (London, printed for W. Strahan and T. Cadell, 1772)

Gregory, J. and McCullough, L. B., *John Gregory's Writings on Medical Ethics and Philosophy of Medicine* (Boston, Academic Publishers, 1998)

Jacyna, L. S., *Philosophic Whigs: Medicine, Science, and Citizenship in Edinburgh, 1789–1848* (London, Routledge, 1994)

McCullough, L. B., *John Gregory and the Invention of Professional Medical Ethics and the Profession of Medicine* (Boston, Kluwer Academic, 1995)

Monro, A., *An Account of the Inoculation of Small Pox in Scotland. By Alexander Monro Senior* (Edinburgh, printed for Drummond and Balfour, 1765)

7. Medical Education

Baillie, M., *The Morbid Anatomy of Some of the Most Important Parts of the Human Body* (London, for Johnson and Nicol, 1793)

Calman, K. C., *Hospital Doctors. Training for the Future* [The Calman Report] (Heywood, Heywood Health Publications, 1993)

Calman, K. C., *Medical Education: Past, Present and Future* (Churchill Livingstone and Elsevier, Edinburgh, 2007)

Collins, K., *Go and Learn. The International Story of Jews and Medicine in Scotland* (Aberdeen, Aberdeen University Press, 1988)

Corner, B. C., *William Shippen Jr. Pioneer in American Medical Education* (Philadelphia, American Philosophical Society, 1951)

Kaufman, M. H., *The Regius Chair of Military Surgery in the University of Edinburgh, 1806–55.* (Amsterdam, Rodopi, 2003)

Kaufman, M. H., *Edinburgh Phrenological Society: A History* (Edinburgh, William Ramsay Henderson Trust, 2005)

Kaufman, M. H., *Medical Teaching in Edinburgh During the 18th and 19th Centuries* (Edinburgh, Royal College of Surgeons of Edinburgh, 2003)

McLachlan, G. (ed), *Medical Education and Medical Care. A Scottish-American Symposium* (London, Oxford University Press, 1977)

Miles, A., *The Edinburgh School of Surgery before Lister* (London, A. & C. Black Ltd., 1918)

Modernising Medical Careers (London, Department of Health, 2003)

Nutton, V. and Porter, R., *The History of Medical Education in Britain* (Amsterdam, Rodopi, 1995)

Pennington, C., *The Modernisation of Medical Teaching at Aberdeen in the Nineteenth Century* (Aberdeen, Aberdeen University Press, 1994)

Rosner, L., *Medical Education in the Age of Improvement. Edinburgh Students and Apprentices 1760–1826* (Edinburgh, Edinburgh University Press, 1991)

Shaw, G., *Staffing the Service. The Next Decade. Report to the Scottish Joint Consultative Committee and the Scottish Home and Health Department Following Review of Hospital Medical Staffing Estimates in Scotland* [The Shaw Report] (Edinburgh, Scottish Home and Health Department, 1987)

Todd, A. R., *Report of the Royal Commission on Medical Education 1965–68* [The Todd Report](London, HMSO, 1968)

Tomaszewski, W., *The University of Edinburgh and Poland* (Edinburgh, private publication, 1968)

8. Institutions

(Universities, Medical Schools and Medical and Surgical Colleges)

Adam, A., Smith, D. and Watson, F. (eds) '*To the Greit Support and Advancement of Helth'. Papers on the History of Medicine in Aberdeen arising from a conference held during the Quincentenary Year of Aberdeen University,* (Aberdeen, Aberdeen History of Medicine Publications, 1996)

Anderson, R. G. W., Simpson, A. D. C. et al, *Edinburgh and Medicine: a Commemorative Catalogue of the Exhibition Held at the Royal Scottish Museum, Edinburgh, June 1976–January 1977 to Mark the 250th Anniversary of the*

Foundation of the Faculty of Medicine of the University of Edinburgh, 1726–1976 (Edinburgh, Royal Scottish Museum, 1976)

Anderson, R. G. W., Simpson, A. D. C. et al, *The Early Years of the Edinburgh Medical School: A Symposium Jointly Organised by the Royal Scottish Museum and the Scottish Society of the History of Medicine in Connection with the Special Exhibition Edinburgh and Medicine and the 250th Anniversary of the Foundation of the Faculty of Medicine of the University of Edinburgh, Held in the Royal Scottish Museum, Chambers Street, Edinburgh, on 26th June 1976* (Edinburgh, Royal Scottish Museum, 1976)

Barfoot, M., *'To Ask the suffrages of the Patrons': Thomas Laycock and the Edinburgh Chair of Medicine, 1855* (London, Wellcome Institute for the History of Medicine, 1995)

Blair, J. S. G., *History of Medicine in the University of St Andrews* (Edinburgh, Scottish Academic Press, 1987)

Blair, J. S. G., *History of Medicine in Dundee University* (Dundee, John S. G. Blair, 2007)

Carter, J. and Withrington, D. (eds), *Scottish Universities: Distinctiveness and Diversity* (Edinburgh, John Donald, 1992)

Craig, W. S., *History of the Royal College of Physicians of Edinburgh* (Oxford, Blackwell Scientific Publications, 1976)

Creswell, C. H., *The Royal College of Surgeons of Edinburgh: Historical Notes from 1505 to 1905* (Edinburgh, Oliver and Boyd, 1926)

Dingwall, H. M., *A Famous and Flourishing Society. The History of the Royal College of Surgeons of Edinburgh, 1505–2005* (Edinburgh, Edinburgh University Press, 2005)

Dingwall, H. M., 'The emergence of an elite craft: the Incorporation of Surgeons of Edinburgh, 1505–c1600', in Goodare, J. and MacDonald, A. A. (eds), *Sixteenth-Century Scotland. Essays in Honour of Michael Lynch* (Leiden, Brill, 2008), pp.189–210

Dingwall, H. M., 'The importance of being Edinburgh. The rise and fall of the Edinburgh Medical School in the eighteenth century', in Cunningham, A., Grell, O. P. and Arrizabalaga, J. (eds), *Centres of Excellence? Medical Travel and Education 1500–1789* (Aldershot, Ashgate, 2010), pp.305–24

Dow, D. A. and Calman K. C., *The Royal Medico-Chirurgical Society of Glasgow: a History, 1814–1989* (Glasgow, The Royal Medico-Chirurgical Society of Glasgow, 1989)

Duncan, A., *Memorials of the Faculty of Physicians and Surgeons of Glasgow 1599–1850* (Glasgow, Glasgow University, 1896)

Gairdner, J., *Sketch of the Early History of the Medical Profession in Edinburgh* (Edinburgh, Oliver and Boyd, 1864)

Geyer-Kordesch, J. and Macdonald, F, *Physicians and Surgeons in Glasgow. The History of the Royal College of Physicians and Surgeons of Glasgow 1599–1858* (Oxford, Clarendon Press, 1999)

Gibson, T., *The Royal College of Physicians and Surgeons of Glasgow* (Midlothian, Macdonald, 1983)

Gray, J., *History of the Royal Medical Society 1737–1937* (Edinburgh, Edinburgh University Press, 1952)

Guthrie, D., *Extramural Medical Education in Edinburgh and the School of Medicine of the Royal Colleges* (Edinburgh, E. & S. Livingstone, 1965)

Hull, A. and Geyer-Kordesch, J., *The Shaping of the Medical Profession: the History of the Royal College of Physicians and Surgeons of Glasgow, 1858–1999* (London, Hambledon, 1999)

Jenkinson, J., *Scottish Medical Societies, 1731–1939: Their History and Records* (Edinburgh, Edinburgh University Press, 1993)

Kaufman, M. H., *The Regius Chair of Military Surgery in the University of Edinburgh, 1806–55.* (Amsterdam, Rodopi, 2003)

Macintyre, I. M. C. and MacLaren, I. (eds), *Surgeons' Lives: An Anthology of College Fellows over 500 Years* (Edinburgh, Royal College of Surgeons of Edinburgh, 2005)

McCrae, M., *Physicians and Society. A Social History of the Royal College of Physicians of Edinburgh* (Edinburgh, John Donald, 2007)

Rodger, E. H. B., *Aberdeen Doctors at Home and Abroad: the Narrative of a Medical School* (Edinburgh, Blackwood, 1893)

Royal College of Physicians of Edinburgh, *Historical Sketch and Laws of the Royal College of Physicians of Edinburgh from its Institution to August 1891* (Edinburgh, Printed for the Royal College of Physicians, 1891)

Smith, C. J. and Collee, J. G., *Edinburgh's Contribution to Medical Microbiology* (Glasgow, Wellcome Trust Unit for the History of Medicine, 1994)

Underwood, E. A., *Boerhaave's Men at Leyden and After* (Edinburgh, Edinburgh University Press, 1977)

Pitcairne, A., *The works of Dr. Archibald Pitcairn: Wherein are Discovered the True Foundation and Principles of the Art of Physic* (London, printed for E. Curll, 1715)

Trèohler, U. and Royal College of Physicians of Edinburgh, ' 'To Improve the Evidence of Medicine': the 18th Century British Origins of a Critical Approach* (Edinburgh, Royal College of Physicians of Edinburgh, 2000)

9. Individuals of note

Bates, A. W., *The Anatomy of Robert Knox. Murder, Mad Science and Medical Regulation in Nineteenth Century Edinburgh* (Brighton, Sussex Academic, 2010)

Brown, K., *Penicillin Man. Alexander Fleming and the Antibiotic Revolution* (Stroud, Sutton Publishing, 2004)

Bowman, A. K., *The Life and Teaching of Sir William Macewen* (Glasgow, William Hodge and Co, 1942)

Chalmers, J., *Andrew Duncan Senior. Physician of the Enlightenment* (Edinburgh, National Museums of Scotland Enterprises Ltd., 2010)

Cheyne, W. W., *Lister and His Achievement* (London, Longmans, 1925)

Doig, A., *William Cullen and the Eighteenth Century Medical World: A Bicentenary Exhibition and Symposium Arranged by the Royal College of Physicians of Edinburgh in 1990* (Edinburgh, Edinburgh University Press, 1993)

Eastwood J. and Eastwood M., *E. B. Jamieson, Anatomist and Shetlander* (Lerwick, The Shetland Times Ltd., 1999)

Finer, S. E., *Life and Times of Sir Edwin Chadwick* (London, Methuen, 1952)

Godlee, R. J., *Lord Lister* (Oxford, Clarendon Press, 1924)

Gordon-Taylor, G. and Walls, E. W., *Sir Charles Bell: His Life and Times* (Edinburgh, Livingstone, 1958)

Illingworth, C. F. W., *There is a History in All Men's Lives* (Blanefield, Heatherbank Press, 1988)

Jeal, T., *Livingstone* (Newhaven and London, Yale University Press, 2001)

Kaufman, M. H., *Dr John Barclay (1758–1826): Extramural Teacher of Human and Comparative Anatomy in Edinburgh* (Edinburgh, RCSEd, 2007)

Kaufman, M. H, *Robert Liston, Surgery's Hero* (Edinburgh, RCSEd, 2009)

Lawrence, M., *Shadow of Swords: A Biography of Elsie Inglis* (London, Joseph, 1971)

Leneman, L., *In the Service of Life: The Story of Elsie Inglis and the Scottish Women's Hospitals* (Edinburgh, Mercat Press, 1994)

McGirr, E. M., *Cullen in Context: William Cullen, MD (1710–1790)* (Glasgow, University of Glasgow Press, 1990)

McCrae, M., *Simpson. The Turbulent Life of a Medical Pioneer* (Edinburgh, Birlinn, 2010)

Manson-Bahr, P. E. C., *Patrick Manson. The Father of Tropical Medicine* (London, Nelson, 1962)

Moore, W., *The Knife Man* (London, Bantam, 2006)

Nye, E. R. and Gibson, M. E., *Ronald Ross: Malariologist and Polymath* (Basingstoke, Macmillan, 1997)

Richards, R. L., *Rae, John* (Toronto, University of Toronto Press)

Robertson, E., *Glasgow's Doctor: James Burn Russell* (East Linton, Tuckwell Press, 1998)

Rosner, L. M. and University of Edinburgh History of Medicine and Science Unit, *Andrew Duncan M.D., F.R.S.E. (1744–1828)* (Edinburgh, Scotland's Cultural Heritage, 1981)

Rush C. and Shaw J. F., *With Sharp Compassion. Norman Dott, Freeman Surgeon of Edinburgh* (Aberdeen, Aberdeen University Press, 1990)

Thomson, J. (with new introduction by Mike Barfoot), *An Account of the Life, Lectures and Writings of William Cullen* (Bristol, Thoemmes Press, 1997)

Wrench, G. T., *Lord Lister. His Life and Work* (London, Unwin, 1913)

Woodruff, M. F. A., *Nothing Venture, Nothing Win* (Edinburgh, Scottish Academic Press, 1996)

Wright-St. Clair, R. E., *Doctors Monro: A Medical Saga* (London, Wellcome Historical Medical Library, 1964)

10. Hospitals

Austin, T., *The Story of Peel Hospital, Galashiels* (Selkirk, Bordersprint, 1996)

Birrell, G., *A Most Perfect Hospital. The Centenary of the Royal Hospital for Sick Children at Sciennes* (Edinburgh, Royal Hospital for Sick Children NHS Trust, 1995)

Boog Watson, W. N., *A Short History of Chalmers Hospital* (Edinburgh, Livingstone, 1964)

Boyd, D. H. A., *Leith Hospital, 1848–1988* (Edinburgh, Scottish Academic Press, 1990)

Browne, W. G., *Old Raigmore Hospital 1941–85. A Fragment of History* (Nairn, W. G. Browne, 1990)

Catford, E. F., *The Royal Infirmary of Edinburgh 1929–1979* (Edinburgh, Scottish Academic Press, 1984)

Craig, R. J., *'Up By': A History of Rosslynlee Hospital* (Midlothian, R. J. Craig, 2008)

Dow, D., *The Rottenrow. The History of the Glasgow Royal Maternity Hospital 1834–1984* (Carnforth, Parthenon Press, 1984)

Dow, D. D., Leitch, M. M. and MacLean, A. F., *From Almoner to Social Worker. Social Work at Glasgow Royal Infirmary 1932–1982* (Glasgow, Glasgow Royal Infirmary, 1982)

Eastwood, M. and Jenkinson, A., *A History of the Western General Hospital* (Edinburgh, John Donald, 1995)

Gray, J. A., *The Edinburgh City Hospital* (East Linton, Tuckwell, 1999)

Gibson, H. J. C., *Dundee Royal Infirmary. The Story of the Old Infirmary with a Short Account of Recent Years* (Dundee, W. Kidd, 1948)

Hendrie, W. A. F. and Macleod, D. A. D., *The Bangour Story. A History of Bangour Village and General Hospitals* (Edinburgh, Mercat Press, 1992)

Irving, G., *Dumfries and Galloway Royal Infirmary. The First 200 Years 1776–1975* (Dumfries, Robert Dinwiddie & Co., 1975)

Levack, Ian D. and Dudley, H. A. F., *Aberdeen Infirmary. The People's Hospital of the North-East* (London, Baillière Tyndall, 1992)

Hay, D. F., *Lister at the Royal* (Glasgow, University of Glasgow Press, 1977)

Hoy, C., *A Beacon in Our Town. The Story of Leith Hospital* (Hoy, Edinburgh, 1988)

Jenkinson, J. L. M., Moss, M. and Russell, I., *The Royal. The History of Glasgow Royal Infirmary 1794–1994* (Glasgow, Glasgow Royal Infirmary NHS Trust, 1994)

McQueen, L. and Kerr, A. B., *The Western Infirmary 1874–1974. A Century of Service to Glasgow* (Glasgow, John Horn Ltd., 1974)

Macdonald, F. A, 'The Infirmary of the Glasgow Town's Hospital 1733–1800: A Case for Voluntarism', *Bulletin of the History of Medicine* 73 (1999), pp. 64–105

Risse, G. B., *Hospital Life in Enlightenment Scotland. Care and Teaching at the Royal Infirmary of Edinburgh* (Cambridge, Cambridge University Press, 1986)

Risse, G. B., *Mending Bodies, Saving Souls. A History of Hospitals* (New York, Oxford University Press, 1999)

Robertson, E., *The Yorkhill Story. The History of the Royal Hospital for Sick Children, Glasgow* (Glasgow, Yorkhill and Associated Hospitals Board of Management, 1972)

Slater S. D. and Dow D. A. *The Victoria Infirmary of Glasgow, 1890–1990. A Centenary History.* (Glasgow, Victoria Infirmary Centenary Committee, 1990)

Turner, A. Logan, *Story of a Great Hospital. The Royal Infirmary of Edinburgh 1729–1929* (Edinburgh, Oliver and Boyd, 1937)

Wright Thomson, A. M., *The History of the Glasgow Eye Infirmary 1824–1962* (Glasgow, John Smith, 1963)

Yule, B., *Matrons, Medics and Maladies: Inside Edinburgh Royal Infirmary in the 1840s* (East Linton, Tuckwell Press, 1999)

11. Medicine and War

Blair, J. S. G., *The Royal Army Medical Corps 1898–1998. Reflections of One Hundred Years of Service* (RAMC, 1998)

Cook, H. J., 'Practical medicine and the British armed forces after the "Glorious Revolution"', *Medical History* 34 (1990), pp.1–26.

McGrigor, M. (ed.), *Sir James McGrigor: the Scalpel and the Sword: the Autobiography of the Father of Army Medicine* (Dalkeith, Scottish Cultural Press, 2000)

Kaufman, M. H., *Surgeons at War. Medical Arrangements for the Treatment of the Sick and Wounded in the British Army during the Late Eighteenth and Nineteenth Centuries* (London, Greenwood Press, 2001)

Kaufman, M. H., *Musket-Ball and Sabre Injuries from the First Half of the Nineteenth Century* (Edinburgh, RCSEd, 2003)

Pringle, J., *Observations on the Diseases of the Army* (London, printed for A. Millar, D. Wilson and T. Payne, 1752)

Whitehead, I. R., *Doctors in the Great War* (London, Leo Cooper, 1999)

12. Mental Health, Psychiatry
(for psychiatric hospitals, see Hospitals)

Houston, R. A., *Madness and Society in Eighteenth Century Scotland* (Oxford, Clarendon Press, 2000)

Jones, K., *Asylums and After. A Revised History of the Mental Health Services From the Early 18th Century to the 1990s* (London, Athlone Press, 1993)

Rosner, L. M. and University of Edinburgh History of Medicine and Science Unit, *Andrew Duncan M.D., F.R.S.E. (1744–1828)* (Edinburgh, Scotland's Cultural Heritage, 1981)

Scull, A., Mackenzie, C., and Hervey, N., *Masters of Bedlam* (Princeton, Princeton University Press, 1996)

Shorter, E., *A History of Psychiatry* (London, John Wiley & Sons, 1997)

Thomson, C. (ed.), *The Origins of Modern Psychiatry* (Chichester, New York, Wiley, 1987)

Tuke, D. H., *The History of the Insane in the British Isles* (London, Kegan Paul, Trench, 1882)

13. Public and National Health

Alison, W. P., *Observations on the Management of the Poor in Scotland, and its Effects on the Health of the Great Towns* (Edinburgh, Blackwood, 1840)

Alison, W. P., 'On the Destitution and Mortality in Some of the Large Towns in Scotland', *Journal of the Statistical Society of London* 5 (3) (1842), pp.289–292

Alison, W. P., *Observations on the Famine of 1846–47* (Edinburgh, Blackwood & Sons, 1857)

Carlyle, T., *Past and Present* (London, Chapman and Hall, 1843)

Cowan, R., *Vital Statistics of Glasgow: I. Statistics of Fever and Small Pox Prior to 1837. II. Statistics of Fever for 1837. III. Remarks Suggested by the Mortality Bills* (Glasgow, David Robertson; Edinburgh, Adam and Charles Black, 1848)

Crowther, M. A. and White, B., *On Soul and Conscience: the Medical Expert and Crime: 150 Years of Forensic Medicine in Glasgow* (Aberdeen, Aberdeen University Press, 1988)

Ferguson, T., *Dawn of Scottish Social Welfare: A Survey from Medieval Times to 1863* (London, Nelson, 1948)

Health in Scotland (Scotland, Scottish Executive, 2002)

Jenkinson, J. L. M., *Scotland's Health 1919–1948* (Oxford, Peter Lang, 2002)

Levitt, I. (ed.), *Government and Social Conditions in Scotland 1845–1919* (Edinburgh, Scottish History Society, 1988)

Levitt, I., *Poverty and Welfare in Scotland 1890–1948* (Edinburgh, Edinburgh University Press, 1988)

Loudon, I., *The Tragedy of Childbed Fever* (Oxford, Oxford University Press, 2000)

McLachlan, G. (ed.), *Improving the Common Weal. Aspects of the Scottish Health Service* (Edinburgh, Edinburgh University Press, 1987)

McCrae, M., *The National Health Service in Scotland. Origins and Ideals* (East Linton, Tuckwell Press, 2003)

Nottingham, C. (ed.), *The First 50 Years of the NHS in Scotland* (Aldershot, Ashgate, 2000)

Roberton, J., *A Treatise on Medical Police, and on Diet, Regimen, &c* (Edinburgh, Printed by J. Moir, 1808)

Smith, C. J., *Edinburgh's Contribution to Medical Microbiology* (Wellcome Unit for the History of Medicine, Glasgow, 1994)

Tait, H. P., *A Doctor and Two Policemen* (Edinburgh, McKenzie & Storrie, 1974)

Watt, A., *The Glasgow Mortality Bill, for the Year Ending 31st December, 1840: Containing Tables of the Registered Births and Baptisms, Marriages, Burials, etc., etc., Within the City and Suburban Districts of Gorbals and Barony parishes* (Glasgow, W. G. Blackie & Co., 1841)

Watt, A., *The Glasgow Bills of Mortality for 1841 & 1842* (Glasgow, The Town Council, 1844)

Watt, A., *The Vital Statistics of Glasgow for 1843 and 1844* (Glasgow, David Robertson, 1846)

Webster, C., *The Health Services Since the War,* Vol. 1 *Problems of Health Care: The National Health Service before 1957* (London, HMSO, 1888)

Webster, C., *The Health Services Since the War,* Vol. 2 *Government and Health Care: The National Health Service 1958–1979* (London, The Stationery Office, 1996)

Wilson, T. S., 'Clearing the air', in Lenihan, J. and Fletcher, W. W. (eds), *Health and the Environment* (Glasgow, Blackie, 1976), pp.136–59

Wilson, T. S., 'The National Health Service 1948-80', in Checkland, O. and Lamb, M. (eds), *Health Care as Social History. The Glasgow Case* (Aberdeen, Aberdeen University Press, 1982)

14. History of Surgery

Jones, P., *A Surgical Revolution. Surgery in Scotland, 1837–1901* (Edinburgh, John Donald, 2007)

Kaufman, M. A., 'Caesarian operations performed in Edinburgh during the eighteenth century', *British Journal of Obstetrics and Gynaecology* 102, (1995), pp.186–91.

Lawrence, C., *Medical Theory, Surgical Practice: Studies in the History of Surgery* (London, Routledge, 1992)

Lowe, Peter, *The Whole Course of Chirurgerie: Wherein is Briefly Set Downe the Causes, Signes, Prognostications & Curations of All Sorts of Tumors, Wounds, Vlcers, Fractures, Dislocations & all Other Diseases, Vsually Practiced by Chirurgions, According to the Opinion of All Our Ancient Doctours in Chirurgerie* (London, printed by Thomas Purfoot, 1597)

Macintyre, I. and MacLaren, I., *Surgeons' Lives* (Edinburgh, Royal College of Surgeons of Edinburgh, 2005)

Stanley, P., *For Fear of Pain. British Surgery 1790–1850. Clio Medica* 70 (Amsterdam, New York, Rodopi, 2003)

15. Influence of Scottish Medicine abroad

Dow, D. A. (ed.), *The Influence of Scottish Medicine: an Historical Assessment of its International Impact* (Carnforth, Parthenon, 1988)

Rosner, L., 'Thistle on the Delaware. Edinburgh medical education and Philadelphia practice 1800–1825', *Social History of Medicine* 5(1) (1992), pp.19-42

McLeod, R. and Lewis, M. (eds), *Disease, Medicine and Empire* (London, Routledge, 1988)

Ross, A. C., *David Livingstone: Mission and Empire* (London, Hambledon, 2002)

16. Entry of Women into Medicine

Alexander, W., *First Ladies of Medicine: The Origins, Education and Destinations of Early Women Medical Graduates of Glasgow University* (University of Glasgow, Wellcome Unit for the History of Medicine, 1987)

Bonner, T. N., *To the Ends of the Earth. Women's Search for Education in Medicine* (Cambridge, Massachusetts, Harvard University Press, 1992)

Geyer-Kordesch, J. and Ferguson, R., *Blue Stockings, Black Gowns, White Coats. A Brief History of Women Entering the Medical Profession in Scotland in Celebration of One Hundred Years of Women Graduates at the University of Glasgow* (University of Glasgow, Wellcome Unit for the History of Medicine, 1994)

Hardy, A. and Conrad, L., *Women in Modern Medicine* (Amsterdam, Rodopi, 2001)

Roberts, S., *Sophia Jex-Blake: A Pioneer in Nineteenth Century Medical Reform* (London, Routledge, 1993)

Todd, M., *The Life of Sophia Jex-Blake* (London, Macmillan, 1918)

17. History of Dentistry

Dingwall, H. M., 'A pioneering history: dentistry and the Royal College of Surgeons of Edinburgh', *History of Dentistry Research Group Newsletter* (2004), pp.4–10

Henderson. T. B., *History of the Glasgow Dental Hospital and School 1879–1959* (Glasgow, C. L. Wright, 1963)

Marlborough, H. S., 'The emergence of a graduate dental profession, 1858–1957' (Glasgow, University of Glasgow Ph.D. Thesis, 1995)

Menzies Campbell, J., 'A brief history of dentistry in Scotland until 1951', reprinted from *Dental Magazine and Oral Topics* (London, 1957)

Menzies Campbell, J., *Dentistry Then and Now* (Glasgow, printed privately, 1981)

Merrill, H. W., 'Thoughts on the history of dentistry in Scotland', *Dental History* 23 (1992), 15–24

Meyer, R. M., 'The development of dentistry: A Scottish perspective c.1800–1921' (Glasgow, University of Glasgow Ph.D. Thesis, 1994)

Noble, H. W., 'Dental practice in Glasgow, 1790–99', *Dental Historian* 27 (1994), pp.3–7

18. Websites

18.1 Books/documents

Bede's life of St Cuthbert:http://www.fordham.edu/halsall/basis/bede-cuthbert.html

Comrie's *History of Scottish Medicine to 1860*: http://www.electricscotland.com/HISTORY/medical/scottish_medicinendx.htm

Edinburgh bookshelf: http://www.edinburghbookshelf.org

George Chalmers's *Caledonia or a Historical and Topographical Account of North Britain*: http://www.inkeeper.net/books/pdf/caledonia.htm

H. C. Gillies's *Regimen Sanitatis: A Gaelic Medical Manuscript of the Early Sixteenth Century or Perhaps Older* (Glasgow 1911. Robert Maclehose): http://www.archive.org

John of Fordun's *Chronicle of the Scottish Nation*, W. S. Skene (ed) Edinburgh 1871: http://www.archive.org

James Lind Library: http://www.jameslindlibrary.org

Leprosy and Leper Hospitals in Scotland and England. In J. Y. Simpson's *Archaeological Essays* Vol II (1882): http://www.archive.org

Mackinnon, D., *A Descriptive Catalogue of Gaelic Manuscripts in the Advocates' Library, Edinburgh and Elsewhere in Scotland* (1912): http://www.archive.org

Pliny's *Natural History*: http://old.perseus.tufts.edu

Tacitus's *Life of Agricola*: http://old.perseus.tufts.edu

The Leech Book of Bald (Cockayne's *Saxon Leechdoms*, Vol II): http://www.archive.org

The poems and fables of Robert Henryson: http://books.google.co.uk

The Trinity Hospital Fund: http://www.edinburgh.gov.uk/internet/council/council_tax_and_finance/council_finance/CEC_trinity_hospital_fund

William Camden's *Britain, or, a Chorographicall Description of the most flourishing Kingdomes, England, Scotland, and Ireland* (1610): http://www.philological.bham.ac.uk/cambrit

18.2 Organisations/Sources for Images

Historic Glasgow: http://www.historicglasgow.com

Lothian Health Service Archive: http://www.lhsa.lib.ed.ac.uk

National Archives of Scotland: http://www.nas.gov.uk

National Galleries of Scotland: http://www.nationalgalleries.org

National Galleries (London):
   http://www.nationalgallery.org.uk/
Northern Health Services Archives:
   http://www.nhsgrampian.org
National Library of Scotland:
   http://www.nls.uk
Records of the Parliaments of Scotland to 1707:
   http://www.rps.ac.uk
Royal Botanic Garden, Edinburgh:
   http://www.rbge.org.uk/
Royal College of Physicians of Edinburgh:
   http://www.rcpe.ac.uk
Royal College of Physicians and Surgeons of Glasgow:
   http://www.rcpsg.ac.uk
Royal College of Surgeons of Edinburgh:
   http://www.rcsed.ac.uk
Scotland and Medicine:
   http://www.scotlandandmedicine.com

Survey of Scottish Witchcraft database:
   http://webdb.ucs.ed.ac.uk/witches
University of Aberdeen Archives:
   http://www.abdn.ac.uk/historic/Manuscripts.shtml
University of Dundee Archives:
   http://www.dundee.ac.uk/archives/
University of Glasgow Archives:
   http://www.archives.gla.ac.uk
University of Edinburgh Special Collections:
   http://www.ed.ac.uk/schools-departments/information-services/ services/library-museum-gallery/crc/collections/special-collections/eua
Wellcome Images:
   http://images.wellcome.ac.uk
Wellcome Trust Library:
   http://library.wellcome.ac.uk

PICTURE CREDITS

——

Chapter One

1.1 Reconstruction of a scene at a hunter-gatherer site at Crail, Fife. Illustration by Mary Kemp Clarke (*from Caroline Wickham-Jones and Magnar Dalland 'A small Mesolithic site at Craighead Golf Course, Fife Ness, Fife', in* Tayside and Fife Archaeological Journal *No 4, November 1998*).

1.2 Skara Brae in Orkney. Photograph (© *Historic Scotland*).

1.3 Yellow Iris (also called Yellow Flag). Photograph (*Bron Wright*).

1.4 Bronze Age Skull. Drawing (*from Bryce TH,* Proc. of Soc of Antiquaries of Scotland, *1903, 38 (December 14) p. 67*).

1.5 Meadowsweet. Illustration by James Sowerby (1757–1822) (*Royal Botanic Garden, Edinburgh*).

1.6 Sphagnum. Illustration by James Sowerby (1757–1822) (*Royal Botanic Garden, Edinburgh*).

1.7 Huperzia selago (Fir Clubmoss). Photograph (*Kath and Richard Pryce*).

1.8 Samolus valerandi (Brookweed). Photograph (*Kath and Richard Pryce*).

1.9 Carved Roman Stone from the Antonine Wall, found at Bridgeness, West Lothian. Photograph (© *National Museums Scotland*).

1.10 Bronze forceps, dating from between 140 and 210 AD, found at Cramond, near Edinburgh. Photograph (© *National Museums Scotland*).

1.11 Knife handle, dating from between 140 and 210 AD, found at Cramond, near Edinburgh. Photograph (© *National Museums Scotland*).

1.12 and 1.13 Two sides of a steatite Roman prescription stamp, found at Tranent, East Lothian. Photographs (© *National Museums Scotland*).

1.14 The Drosten Stone. Ninth century carved stone, St Vigeans, Angus (© *RCAHMS*).

1.15 Ninth century carved stone, Aberlemno churchyard, Angus (© *RCAHMS*).

1.16 Hedge Woundwort. Photograph (*David Wright*).

1.17 A physician administering leeches to a patient. Colour reproduction of a lithograph by F-S. Delpech after L. Boiully, 1827 (*Wellcome Library, London*).

1.18 St Cuthbert's knee being healed by a stranger. Twelfth-century manuscript in the Bodleian Library, Oxford (*Wellcome Library, London*).

1.19 St Cuthbert healing a young man of plague. Twelfth-century manuscript in the Bodleian Library, Oxford (*Wellcome Library, London*).

1.20 St Cuthbert healing a child dying of plague. Twelfth-century manuscript in the Bodleian Library, Oxford (*Wellcome Library, London*).

1.21 The River Fillan, near Tyndrum, 2010. Photograph (*Peter Wright*).

1.22 Reconstruction of a scene at the Holy Pool of St Fillan, Strathfillan, Perthshire (*illustration by Susie Wright*).

1.23 Feverfew. Illustration by Kathryn Ball (*Wellcome Library, London*).

1.24 Collection of various recipes. Eleventh-century Anglo-Saxon manuscript (*Wellcome Library, London*).

1.25 Trade between Scotland and Northern Europe in the period 1000–1600 AD (*illustration by Susie Wright*).

1.26 Reconstruction of a scene in Glasgow of pilgrims at the tomb of St Kentigern. Illustration by David Simon (*from Peter Yeoman's Pilgrimage in Medieval Scotland, Historic Scotland*).

1.27 Wooden box, used for collecting money for those suffering from plague, depicting St Roch dressed as a pilgrim. Photograph (*Wellcome Library, London*).

1.28a Fourteenth-century pilgrim badge, showing image of St Andrew. Photograph (© *Fife Council Museums: St Andrews*).

1.28b Fourteenth-century pilgrim badge, showing image of St Andrew. Photograph (© *Perth Museum and Art Gallery, Perth & Kinross Council*).

1.29 Dance of death. Woodblock by Hans Holbein (1497–1593) (*Glasgow University Library, Special Collections*).

1.30 Gilbert Skeyne's *Ane Breve Descriptioun of the Pest.* Title page. Published in Edinburgh in 1568 by Robert Leprevik (*National Library of Scotland*).

1.31a and b The Bannatyne manuscript. Sixteenth century (*National Library of Scotland*).

1.31 Music manuscript, with a marginal illustration of a leper. Early fifteenth century (*British Library, Lansdown MS 541, f 127*).

1.32 Model taken from a plaster cast of the skull of Robert Bruce (© *Stirling Smith Art Gallery and Museum*).

1.33 Syphilis. Woodcut from Joseph Grunbeck's *Tractatus de pestilentiali Scorra sive mala de Franzos* (Augsberg) (*Wellcome Library, London*).

1.34 Provand's Lordship, Glasgow, in the nineteenth century. Photograph (*Glasgow University Library, Special Collections*).

1.35 Soutra Aisle. Drawing (*Wellcome Library, London*).

1.36 Consultation note of Michael Scot in 1221. Thirteenth-century manuscript from Gonville and Caius College, Cambridge (*Wellcome Library, London*).

1.37 Trinity Hospital, Edinburgh, view from Calton Hill. Photograph, D. O. Hill and R. Adamson. 1840s (*Glasgow University Library, Special Collections*).

1.38 Trinity Hospital, Edinburgh. Women's ward. Engraving by T. Stewart after D. Wilson, 1848 (*Wellcome Library, London*).

1.39 Pages 25 and 26 of Gaelic medical manuscript Adv. MS.72 (Gaelic MS.IV). Sixteenth century (*National Library of Scotland*).

1.40 Front cover of Gaelic medical manuscript Adv. MS.72 (Gaelic MS.IV). Sixteenth century (*National Library of Scotland*).

1.41 Page f130v from the Gaelic medical manuscript Adv 72.1.2. (*National Library of Scotland*)

1.42 Part of a manuscript, with William Schevez's name inscribed at the top. Fifteenth-century manuscript (*Glasgow University Library, Special Collections*).

1.43 Memorial brass to the memory of Duncan Liddell, Aberdeen (*Wellcome Library, London*).

1.44 Sculptured stone found in Mary King's Close, Edinburgh in 1859. Fifteenth century. Photograph (© *National Museums Scotland*).

1.45 Jerome Cardan. From Joannes Sambucus's *Veterum aliquot ac recentium medicorum philosophorumque Icones,* (Antwerp, 1574) (*Wellcome Library, London*).

1.46 Crystal ball charmstone, which belonged to the Stewarts of Ardsheal in Argyllshire (© *National Museums of Scotland*)

Chapter Two

2.1 Royal Infirmary of Edinburgh. Engraving of the Royal Infirmary of Edinburgh by John Elphinstone, *c*1750 (*LHSA*).

2.2 Oil painting of 'an incident from the rebellion of 1745', by David Morier *c*1745–50 (*The Royal Collection © 2011 Her Majesty Queen Elizabeth II*).

2.3 University of Leiden. Line engraving, seventeenth century (*Wellcome Library, London*).

2.4 Title page of Alexander Monro *primus, Anatomy of the Humane Bones* (Edinburgh, 1726) (*RCPE*).

2.5 Smallpox/cowpox. Watercolour painting of eighth-day smallpox by George Kirkland, 1802 (*Wellcome Library, London*).

2.6 Diagram of the humours and temperaments (*Susie Wright,* 2011).

2.7 Zodiac Man, folding almanac, vellum, late-fourteenth century (*Wellcome Library, London*).

2.8 Bloodletting instruments used by Dr Hugh McFarquhar, late-eighteenth century (*Courtesy of Tain Museum*).

2.9 Scurvy grass. Watercolour by James Sowerby, 1799 (© *Royal Botanic Garden, Edinburgh. Licensor www.scran.ac.uk*)

2.10 Scurvy grass sorrel. Photograph (© *Royal Botanic Gardens, Edinburgh*).

2.11 Conjoined twins. Illustration from F. Liceti and G. Blasius, *De Monstris* (Amsterdam, 1665) (*Wellcome Library, London*).

2.12 Alchemy. Representation of alchemy equipment, from collection of watercolour drawings, 1782 (*Wellcome Library, London*).

2.13 King James IV, portrait in oils by H.H.R. Woodford, 1955 (*RCSEd*).

2.14 Bloodletting. Oil painting, Jacob Toorenvliet, 1666 (*Wellcome Library, London*).

2.15 Andreas Vesalius. Engraving from Philippe Galle, *Vivorum Doctorum de Disciplinis Bene Merentium Effigies XLIII* (Antwerp, 1572) (*Wellcome Library, London*).

2.16 Image from Vesalius' *De Humani Corporis Fabrica* (Basel, 1543) (*Wellcome Library, London*).

2.17 Location of Curryhill House, from James Gordon of Rothiemay, *Edinudunensis Tabulam* (1647) *(By courtesy of the Trustees of the National Library of Scotland)*.

2.18 Old Surgeons' Hall, Edinburgh, watercolour, after Sandby, *c*1750 *(RCSEd)*.

2.19 Dissection. Pen drawing of anatomy theatre at Leiden by William Buytenwegh, seventeenth century *(Wellcome Library, London)*.

2.20. Page from William Harvey, *Exercitatio Anatomica de Motu Cordis* (Frankfurt, 1628) *(RCPE)*.

2.21 Mary, Queen of Scots, portrait in oils, unknown artist, *c*1610 *(National Galleries of Scotland)*.

2.22 Letter of Exemption granted to Edinburgh surgeons by Mary, Queen of Scots, in 1567 *(RCSEd)*.

2.23. Sir Robert Sibbald, portrait in oils *(RCPE)*.

2.24 Archibald Pitcairne. Portrait in oils by Sir John Medina, *c*1700 *(RCSEd)*.

2.25 *Scotia Illustrata*. Image from Sibbald's *Scotia Illustrata* (Edinburgh,1684) *(RCPE)*.

2.26 Location of physic garden at Holyrood, from from James Gordon of Rothiemay, *Edinudunensis Tabulam* (1647) *(By courtesy of the Trustees of the National Library of Scotland)*.

2.27 Hall of Royal College of Physicians, Edinburgh, line engraving by T. H. Shepherd, after J. Henshall and J. Craig, 1829 *(RCPE)*.

2.28 Horn for bloodletting or cupping, made of parchment or skin, eighteenth or nineteenth century *(National Museums of Scotland)*.

2.29 Painted china bleeding dish *(RCSEd)*.

2.30a Peter Lowe. Portrait in oils, copy of original, artist unknown, 1822 *(RCPSG)*.

2.30b Robert Hamilton. Portrait in oils, copy of original artist unknown, 1822 *(RCPSG)*.

2.31 Leather gloves owned by Peter Lowe *(RCPSG)*.

2.32 Title page of first edition of Peter Lowe, *The Whole Course of Chirurgerie. Wherein is Briefly Set Down the Causes, Signs, Prognostications & Curations of all Sorts of Tumors… of all Our Ancient Doctours in Chirurgerie* (London, 1597) *(RCPSG)*.

2.33a and 2.33b Images from 1634 edition of Lowe's *Discourse of the Whole Art of Chirurgerie* (title changed after 1597 edition) *(RCSEd)*.

2.34 Image from 1634 edition of Lowe's *Discourse* *(RCSEd)*.

2.35 Matthew Mackail. Portrait in oils, unknown artist, late seventeenth century *(University of Aberdeen)*.

2.36. Alexander Monro *primus*, portrait in oils, attributed to Allan Ramsay, 1860 *(RCSEd)*.

2.37a George Drummond. Portrait in oils by John Alexander, 1752 *(LHSA)*; 2.37b Herman Boerhaave. Line engraving by J. W. Kaiser after painting by C. Troost, *c*1735 *(Wellcome Library, London)*; 2.37c Earl of Islay. Archibald Campbell, portrait in oils by Allan Ramsay, *c*1759 *(National Galleries of Scotland)*; 2.37d John Monro. Portrait in oils by William Aikman, 1715 *(RCSEd)*.

2.38 Sir Stuart Threipland. Portrait of Sir Stuart Threipland, physician to the Young Pretender and member of the Royal Medical Society, by William Delacour *(in a private collection)*

2.39 Eighteenth-century consultation, drawing with water-colour, eighteenth century. *(Wellcome Library, London)*.

2.40 Hellebore *(Wellcome Library, London)*; Senna, drawing from P. A. Mattioli, *Commentaires sur ces Six Livres de Ped. Discoride Anazarbeen de la Materie Medicinale* (Lyons, 1572) *(RCPE)*; Blackthorn. Watercolour by James Sowerby (1801) *(©Royal Botanic Garden, Edinburgh. Licensor www.scran.ac.uk)*; Rhubarb. Photograph *(Wellcome Library, London)*.

2.41 Penicuik medicine chest. Photograph *(Courtesy of Sir Robert Clerk)*.

2.42 Threipland medicine Chest. Photograph *(RCPE)*.

2.43a Alexander Monro *secundus*. Portrait in oils by J.T. Seton *(RCSEd)*; 2.43b John Rutherford. Portrait in oils *(RCPE)*; 2.43c Robert Whytt. Portrait in oils by G. B. Bellucci, 1738 *(RCPE)*.

2.44 Foetus in Utero. Illustration from Alexander Hamilton, *Anatomical Tables with Explanations* (Edinburgh, 1787) *(Wellcome Library, London)*.

2.45 Notebook. Notes on bones from a notebook on surgery and anatomy compiled by Robert Whytt, *c*1731-2 *(Wellcome Library, London)*.

2.46 Bladder stones. Showing variety of size and shape of bladder stones *(Wellcome Library, London)*.

2.47 Post mortem report, 1702, *GD158/296 (National Archives of Scotland)*.

2.48 Amputation. Line engraving by J. Guillemeau (Paris, 1594) *(Wellcome Library, London)*.

2.49. Archibald Pitcairne's medical practice. Dc.1.62, Praxeos Pitcarnianae *(University of Edinburgh, Special Collections Department)*.

2.50 Accounts for surgeon employed to treat poor in Edinburgh, 1710. Moses Bundle 136/5321 *(Edinburgh City Archives)*.

2.51 Trepanning. Engraving from J. Guillemeau, *Le Chirvrgie Francoise Recueillie des Anciens Médecins* (Paris, 1594) *(Wellcome Library, London)*.

2.52 Eighteenth-century trepanning instruments, Stanton of London *(RCPSG)*.

2.53 Plate from Lowe, *Discourse* *(RCSEd)*.

3.16 The Royal College of Surgeons of Edinburgh. William Fulton, 1991 (*RCSEd*).

3.17 Surgeons' Hall Museum (*RCSEd*).

3.18 The Royal College of Physicians and Surgeons of Glasgow (*RCPSG*).

3.19 Physicians Hall, George Street, Edinburgh. Drawing by Thomas H Shepherd; engraving by J Henshall, *c*1829 (*RCPE*).

3.20 The hall of the Aberdeen Medico-Chirurgical Society in King Street, Aberdeen (*Aberdeen Medico-Chirurgical Society*).

3.21 Illustration from *Observations on the Fungus Haematodes* by James Wardrop.

3.22 Calves' heads and brains or a phrenological lecture. L Bump after J Bump, 1826 (*Wellcome Library, London*).

3.23 A bedridden, sick, young woman being examined by a doctor, accompanied by her anxious parents. Engraving by F. Engleheart, after Sir David Wilkie, 1838 (*Wellcome Library, London*).

3.24 Measles. Illustration from Buchan's *Domestic Medicine*.

3.25 Paisley cholera poster (*Renfrewshire Libraries*).

3.26 Hemlock (*Conium maculatum*). Coloured reproduction of a wood engraving by J. Johnstone (*Wellcome Library, London*)

3.27 Domestic medicine chest, Georgian House, Edinburgh (*National Trust for Scotland*).

3.28 Cinchona bark prepared as a roll for ease of shipment (*Science Museum, London*).

3.29 Opium poppy (*Papaver somniferum*). Print by M. A. Burnett after Gilbert T. Burnett, 1853 (*RCPE*).

3.30 Syringe used by Dr Andrew Wood (*RCSEd*).

3.31 Robert Penman. Painting by unknown artist, *c*1828 (*RCSEd*).

3.32 Robert Penman. Photograph, *c*1855 (*RCSEd*).

3.33 James and Rab grieving for Ailie. Illustration from *Rab and His Friends*.

3.34 John Bell. Oil on canvas. Unknown artist, *c*1801 (*National Portrait Gallery, London*).

3.35 Sir Charles Bell. Oil on canvas. John Stevens, *c*1821 (*National Portrait Gallery, London*).

3.36 Opisthotonos. Oil on canvas. Charles Bell, 1809 (*RCSEd*).

3.37 Malignant ulcer on the tongue. John Lizars, 1859. Illustration from *Practical Observations on the Uses and Abuses of Tobacco*.

3.38 Robert Liston. Calotype. David Octavius Hill and Robert Adamson, *c*1847 (*Wellcome Library, London*).

3.39 James Syme. Albumen print. John Adamson, *c*1855 (*Scottish National Portrait Gallery*).

3.40 Gregory family tree.

3.41 'The Cut Finger'. Engraving by Joly from an original painting by Sir David Wilkie (*Wellcome Library, London*).

3.42 William Buchan by an unknown artist (*Wellcome Library, London*).

3.43 Frontispiece of *Domestic Medicine* by William Buchan.

3.44 Edinburgh Royal Infirmary 1741–1889. Print of watercolour painting by J. Sanderson. 1885 (*Lothian Health Services Archive*).

3.45 Edinburgh University Old Quadrangle. William Playfair. Etching by W. H. Lizars, 1823 (*National Museum of Scotland*).

3.46 Four generations of the Monro family: John Monro by William Aikman, 1715; Alexander Monro *primus*, 1868, attributed to Allan Ramsay; Alexander Monro *secundus* by John T. Seton; Alexander Monro *tertius* by Kenneth Macleay (*all Royal College of Surgeons of Edinburgh*).

3.47 Robert Knox, From an original calotype by David Octavius Hill, *c*1843 (*Wellcome Library, London*).

3.48 Watching and warding. *Northern Looking Glass*, August 1825 (*University of Glasgow*).

3.49 Surgeon Square. Thomas Shepherd, *c*1829 (*RCSEd*).

3.50 Bell family tree. Benjamin Bell (1749–1806) by Sir Henry Raeburn, *c*1790 (*Bourne Fine Art, Edinburgh*); Benjamin Bell (1810–1883), photograph; Joseph Bell by George Fiddes Watt, 1896 (*RCSEd*).

3.51 Foulis Academy of Arts exhibition, 1761, Inner Quadrangle, Glasgow University. From an engraving by David Allan (*University of Glasgow*).

3.52 Joseph Black by David Martin. Oil on canvas, 1787 (*Royal Medical Society – on loan to National Galleries of Scotland*).

3.53 'The Alarm, or the Kirkyard in Danger'. *Northern Looking Glass*, 1825 (*University of Glasgow*).

3.54 The Lecture Room. *Northern Looking Glass*, 1825 (*University of Glasgow*).

3.55 James McCune Smith. Engraving by Patrick H. Reason (*New York Historical Society*).

3.56 King's College and Old Aberdeen. Francis Oliver Finch, *c*1820 (*University of Aberdeen*).

3.57 Marischal College, Aberdeen. James Giles, 1840 (*University of Aberdeen*).

3.58 William Smellie. Self-portrait. Oil on canvas (*RCSEd*).

3.59 William Cullen. Oil on canvas. Attributed to William Cochran, *c*1768 (*RCPE*).

3.60 Mathew Baillie. Attributed to Thomas Barber, *c*1805 (*Royal College of Physicians of London*).

3.61 John Hunter. Copy after original portrait by Joshua Reynolds, artist unknown. (*RCSEd*).

4.26 An ovarian cyst being drained. Drawing from *Diseases of the Ovaries: Their Diagnosis and Treatment* by Thomas Spenser Wells (*Wellcome Library, London*).

4.27 An ovarian cyst being removed. Drawing from *Diseases of the Ovaries: Their Diagnosis and Treatment* by Thomas Spenser Wells (*Wellcome Library, London*).

4.28 Thomas Keith (1827–1895). Painting (*RCSEd*).

4.29 Joseph Lister (1927–1912). Oil on canvas. Painting by Dorofield Hardy after the original by W. Ouless (*RCSEd*).

4.30 Sir William Sharpey, FRS (1802–1880). Photograph (*Wellcome Library, London*).

4.31 Sir Alexander Ogston (1844–1929). Painting (*Wellcome Library, London*); Ogston operating. Photograph (*Aberdeen City Library*).

4.32 Sir William Macewen. Photograph (*Wellcome Library, London*).

4.33 Murdoch Cameron (1847–1930). Photograph (*Wellcome Library, London*).

4.34 Andrew Duncan (1744–1828). Oil on canvas. Painting by Sir Henry Raeburn (*RCPEd*).

4.35 The poet Robert Fergusson (1750–1774). Oil on paper. Painting by Alexander Runciman *c*1772 (*Scottish National Portrait Gallery*).

4.36 The Crichton Institute. Engraving (*Wellcome Library, London*).

4.37 Alexander Morison (1779–1866). Painting by Richard Dadd (*National Portrait Gallery of Scotland*).

4.38 Sir Alexander Morison (1779–1866). Painting (*RCPE*).

4.39 Dorothea Lynde Dix (1802–1887). Photograph (*Library of Congress, USA*).

4.40 Craiglockhart War Hospital for Officers. Photograph (*Edinburgh Napier University*).

4.41 Sir Henry Littlejohn (1826–1914). Portrait by Sir George Reid (*Scottish National Portrait Gallery*).

4.42 Children in a city street in 1910. Photograph (*Mitchell Library, Glasgow*).

4.43 James Burn Russell (1837–1904). Photograph (*Wellcome Library, London*).

4.44 Sophia Jex Blake (1840–1912). Drawing (*Edinburgh University Library*).

4.45 Bruntsfield Hospital, Edinburgh. Photograph (*Lothian Health Service Archive*).

4.46 Sir German Sims Woodhead (1855–1921). Photograph (*Wellcome Library, London*).

4.47 The Research Laboratory at the Royal College Physicians of Edinburgh. Drawing (*RCPEd*).

4.48 Sir Patrick Manson (1844–1922). Photograph (*Wellcome Library, London*).

4.49 Diarmid Noel Paton (1859–1928). Photograph (*RCPSG*).

4.50 David Livingstone (1813–1873). Photograph (*Library of Congress, USA*).

4.51 Anderson's University in Glasgow. Drawing (*Glasgow Caledonian University*).

4.52 David Livingstone attacked by a lion. Drawing (*Wellcome Library, London*).

4.53 Livingstone at home with his daughter. Photograph (*corbisimages.com*).

4.54 Dr Elsie Inglis (1864–1917). Photograph (*Lothian Health Service Archive*).

4.55 Doctors of the Scottish Women's Hospitals in France (*Mitchell Library, Glasgow*).

4.56 The Scottish Women's Hospital at Royaumont. Painting by Norah Neilson Gray (*Imperial War Museum*).

4.57 A physical education class in Glasgow. Photograph (*Glasgow City Council Archives*).

4.58 A Milk Depot in Glasgow. Photograph (*Glasgow City Council Archives*).

4.59 David Lloyd George at Burns' Mausoleum, Dumfries, 1925 (© *Dumfries and Galloway Museums Service, licensor www.scran.ac.uk*).

4.60 Lachlan Grant. Photograph (*Scottish Life Archive, National Museum of Scotland*).

4.61 District Nurse, Ness, Isle of Lewis, 1930s (*Scottish Life Archive, National Museums of Scotland*).

4.62 Margaret Cairns, District Nurse, Fair Isle, Shetland, 1956 (*Scottish Life Archive, National Museums of Scotland*).

4.63 Aerial view of the Edinburgh Royal Infirmary. Photograph.

4.64 Rebecca Strong, matron, with nursing staff, Glasgow Royal Infirmary. Photograph (*copyright NHS Greater Glasgow and Clyde Archives, ref. HB14/8/53*).

4.65 Randolph Wemyss Memorial Hospital, Buckhaven. Photograph (*Fife Council Museums and Heritage Service*).

4.66 Bruntsfield Hospital. Photograph (*Lothian Health Service Archive*).

4.67 Gertrude Herzfeld (1890–1981). Oil on canvas. Painting by Sir William Hutchison (*RCSEd*).

4.68 X-ray Department at Glasgow Royal Infirmary. Photograph (*copyright NHS Greater Glasgow and Clyde Archives, ref HB14/24/6/1*).

4.69 The polygraph invented by Sir James Mackenzie. Drawing from *The Future of Medicine* by Sir James Mackenzie (*Wellcome Library, London*).

4.70 Sir David Wilkie (1882–1938). Photograph (*RCSEd*).

INDEX

———

General themes such as medical education and surgery are covered extensively in all chapters and so are not indexed, though there are entries for all individual colleges, surgeons etc. who are mentioned.

AUTHOR BIOGRAPHIES

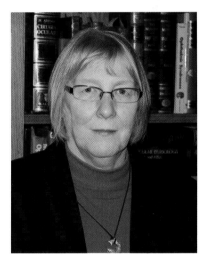 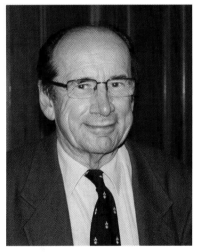 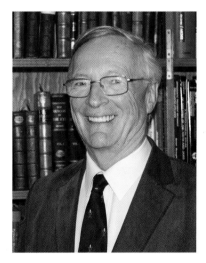

Helen Dingwall is an Honorary Lecturer (formerly Senior Lecturer) in the School of Arts and Humanities, University of Stirling. Her publications include *Late-Seventeenth Century Edinburgh: A Demographic Study* (1994), *Physicians, Surgeons and Apothecaries: Medical Practice in Seventeenth-Century Edinburgh* (1995), *A History of Scottish Medicine: Themes and Influences* (2003) and '*A Famous and Flourishing Society': The History of the Royal College of Surgeons of Edinburgh* (2005).

David Hamilton is an honorary senior lecturer at St Andrews University's Bute Medical School and he worked as a consultant surgeon in the Western Infirmary, Glasgow. He was the first Director of Glasgow University's Wellcome Unit for the History of Medicine and his books include *The Healers – A History of Scottish Medicine* (1981), *A History of Organ Transplantation* (2012) and *The Monkey Gland Affair* (1986).

Iain Macintyre, who worked as a general surgeon in Edinburgh, was Vice President of the Royal College of Surgeons of Edinburgh and a surgeon to the Queen in Scotland. His previous publications include *Surgeons Lives*, an anthology of biographies of Fellows of the Royal College of Surgeons of Edinburgh over 500 years. He is currently history editor of the *Journal of the Royal College of Physicians of Edinburgh*, and an Apothecaries' Lecturer in the History of Medicine at Edinburgh University.

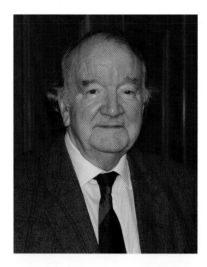

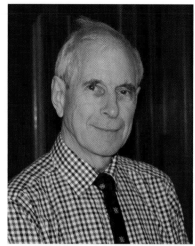

Morrice McCrae has been House Physician and House Surgeon at the Glasgow Royal Infirmary, Hall Fellow at Glasgow University and Consultant Physician at the Royal Hospital for Sick Children, Edinburgh. He is a Fellow of the Royal Colleges of Physicians of Edinburgh and of Glasgow, and College Historian of the Royal College of Physicians of Edinburgh. He is the author of *The National Health Service in Scotland: Origins and Ideals* (2003), *The New Club: A History* (2004), *Physicians and Society* (2008) and *Simpson: The Turbulent Life of a Medical Pioneer* (2010).

David Wright was a Consultant Anaesthetist, with an interest in Intensive Care, at the Western General Hospital in Edinburgh. He has been President of the Scottish Society of the History of Medicine and of the British Society for the History of Medicine. Between 2002 and 2008 he was the English Language Editor of *Vesalius*, the Journal of the International Society of the History of Medicine. He is an Apothecaries' Lecturer in the History of Medicine at Edinburgh University.